RECOGNITION AND SPECIFICITY IN PLANT HOST-PARASITE INTERACTIONS

RECOGNITION AND SPECIFICITY IN PLANT HOST-PARASITE INTERACTIONS

Edited by

J.M. DALY AND IKUZO URITANI

JAPAN SCIENTIFIC SOCIETIES PRESS, Tokyo
UNIVERSITY PARK PRESS, Baltimore

JSSP No. 01722-1104
Printed in Japan

Published jointly by
Japan Scientific Societies Press
Tokyo
and
University Park Press
Baltimore

Library of Congress Cataloging in Publication Data

Main entry under title:

Recognition and specificity in plant host-parasite interactions.

Bibliography: p.

1. Plant diseases—Congresses. 2. Host-parasite relationships—Congresses. 3. Host plants—Congresses. 4. Microorganisms, Phytopathogenic—Congresses.

I. Daly, Joseph Michael, 1922– II. Uritani, Ikuzō, 1919–
SB727. R42 581.2′3 79-10438
ISBN 0-8391-1440-0

PARTICIPANTS AND OBSERVERS

U. S. Participants

Aist, J. R.	Cornell University Ithaca, New York 14850
Bushnell, W. R.	USDA, University of Minnesota St. Paul, Minnesota 55101
Day, P. R.	Connecticut Agricultural Experiment Station P.O. Box 1106 New Haven, Connecticut 06504
Durbin, R. D.	USDA, University of Wisconsin Madison, Wisconsin 53706
Ellingboe, A. H.	Michigan State University East Lansing, Michigan 48823
Hanchey, P.	Colorado State University Fort Collins, Colorado 80521
Kuć, J.	University of Kentucky Lexington, Kentucky 40506
Nester, E. W.	University of Washington Seattle, Washington 98105
Paxton, J. P.	University of Illinois Urbana, Illinois 61801
Sequeira, L.	University of Wisconsin Madison, Wisconsin 53706
Siegel, A.	Wayne State University Detroit, Michigan 48202
VanEtten, H.	Cornell University Ithaca, New York 14850

U.S. Observers

Bell, A. A.	USDA, ARS, P.O. Box JF College Station, Texas 77840
Goodman, R. N.	University of Missouri Columbia, Missouri 65201
Gracen, V. E.	Cornell University Ithaca, New York 14850
Keen, N.	University of California Riverside, California 92502
Kosuge, T.	University of California Davis, California 95616
Murakishi, H.	Michigan State University East Lansing, Michigan 48823
Scheffer, R. P.	Michigan State University East Lansing, Michigan 48823
Wheeler, H.	University of Kentucky Lexington, Kentucky 40506
Wynn, W. K.	University of Georgia Athens, Georgia 30601
Yoder, O. C.	Cornell University Ithaca, New York 14850

Japan Participants

Asada, Y.	College of Agriculture Ehime University Matsuyama 790
Kojima, M.	Faculty of Agriculture Nagoya University Nagoya 464
Nishimura, S.	Faculty of Agriculture Tottori University Tottori 680
Oku, H.	College of Agriculture Okayama University Okayama 700
Ouchi, S.	College of Agriculture Okayama University Okayama 700

Sakai, R.	National Institute of Agricultural Sciences Kita-ku, Tokyo 114
Tani, T.	Faculty of Agriculture Kagawa University Miki-cho 761-07
Tomiyama, K.	Faculty of Agriculture Nagoya University Nagoya 464
Uritani, I.	Faculty of Agriculture Nagoya University Nagoya 464

Japan Observers

Doke, N.	Nagoya University Nagoya 464
Kono, Y.	Institute of Physical and Chemical Research Saitama 351
Takai, S.	Canadian Science Service Sault Sainte Marie Canada

PREFACE

Each year plant diseases cause a substantial, but largely unmeasurable, reduction in the harvest of man's only real renewable resource—the energy captured by green plants during the process of photosynthesis. Some of the loss in energy from plant diseases around the world can be estimated for many cultivated crops, but often overlooked are the losses of natural resources not so easily monitored, such as our forests and the managed or wild grazing lands that support animals, and upon which many cultures are dependent. In addition, we should not forget the aesthetic damage caused by disease to plant species that furnish beauty and relief from the vagaries of the elements. Disease is a normal, perhaps essential, component of all biological systems and mankind has been able and must continue, to accept some of the resultant loss. As with human disease, the ever present danger is the threat that a particular disease (or combination of diseases) will explode to epidemic proportions causing, at best, economic loss to individuals and communities or, at worst, famine and its fateful consequence to cultures and nations. The potato blight centuries ago in Europe or the corn rust in Africa of 25 years ago remain grim reminders of the potential that exists.

Plant pathology emerges as a scientific discipline in direct response to the human misery resulting from the potato famine. During the ensuing years, the scientific study of plant disease considerably reduced the economic hazards to world agriculture through the formation of control measures based on a sound understanding of the biology of plant disease. Cultural practices and sanitation, coupled with genetic manipulation of crops and the development of reliable organic fungicides, are possible only because of detailed knowledge of the life cycles of pathogens and the infectious processes within hosts. In a certain sense, however, current control practice is empirical and must be developed after, rather than before, the outbreak.

We can breed resistance into a crop or develop new fungicides but the disease already has been acknowledged as an economic problem. Although we recognize, and effectively use, genes for resistance after the fact of disease, we know little of what the gene does or how its product affects the pathogen. Owing to this ignorance, we do not know what effects such genes have on other processes within the plant in the absence of disease. Nor do we know what physiological limitations the continued incorporation of genes for resistance to pathogens will have for future crop productivity. This possibility is not an idle thought if one considers the diversity of insects and diseases even for a single crop.

In recent years, the concepts and techniques of modern, quantitative cell biology have led to a swell in the basic understanding of the physiology and biochemistry of plant host-pathogen interactions. It is possible to trace the onset of pathogenesis by the switch of normal plant metabolism to abnormal or little-used pathways and to obtain from the pathogen some of the chemical factors that induce the switch. Yet a fundamental problem remains. Despite our sophistication, the changes observed and induced appear to be general changes that a number of agents other than pathogens also may induce. In short, we lack the key to the remarkable specificity which is inherent in plant disease as it occurs in nature. In nature, plants are continually exposed, in soil or atmosphere, to a bewildering array of bacteria and fungi armed with diverse battery of devices for potential virulence. One species becomes an effective pathogen in corn but will not infect wheat, while another will destroy wheat or barley but finds corn incompatible. Even more remarkable is the varietal selectivity exhibited by many pathogens in a single crop species. It is now apparent that a necessary step for further progress in economic disease control is the identification of mechanisms whereby a host and pathogen "recognize" the potential for establishing a compatible (susceptible) or incompatible (resistant) relationship, and the devices whereby specificity for that relationship is established.

From June 27 to July 1, 1977, a cooperative U.S.-Japan Seminar convened at the Nebraska Center for Continuing Education, University of Nebraska, Lincoln, to review the topic "Recognition and Specificity in Host-Parasite Interactions." The formal papers and the subsequent discussions of them are the contents of this volume. This seminar was part of the U.S.-Japan Cooperative Science Program implemented by the National Science Foundation (USA) and the Japan Society for Promotion of Science who previously had supported cooperative conferences on related topics at

Gamogori, Japan in 1966 and the East-West Center at Hawaii in 1970. The proceedings of both conferences have appeared in book form.

The difficult job of developing the theme and soliciting speakers for an intellectually demanding topic was the cooperative task of two committees (J. M. Daly, Chairman, L. D. Dunkle, and J. VanEtten for the U.S.; I. Uritani, Chairman and K. Tomiyama for the Japanese). In addition to the speakers, a group of scientists of equal stature were invited to attend in order to share their expertise and critical analysis. For the U.S., the following participated: A. A. Bell, R. N. Goodman, V. E. Gracen, N. Keen, T. Kosuge, H. Murakishi, R. P. Scheffer, H. Wheeler, W. K. Wynn, and O. C. Yoder. The invited Japanese observers were: N. Doke, Y. Kono, and S. Takai. In addition, staff of the Departments of Plant Pathology and Agricultural Biochemistry were frequent visitors throughout the Conference.

The format agreed to by the U.S. and Japan organizing committees is illustrated with the table of Contents. The opening four papers developed the genetic constraints which any biochemical mechanisms to explain host-parasite interactions must follow. Two eminent geneticists first outlined the current status of the inheritance of disease reaction in plants, while the two subsequent papers in this group presented theoretical arguments and experimental work designed to translate such information into testable biochemical models. A set of three speakers then outlined some of the common features of cellular responses to infection from a cytochemical perspective. A third large group of presentations was concerned with the identity and mode of action of chemical components which determine specificity for either a pathogen or host, or both. It is now clear that some pathogens produce materials which contribute to the specific virulence of pathogens toward certain hosts and these received considerable attention. There is a small but increasing body of evidence, however, that there are constitutive components of the host which specifically serve as devices for recognition and this work was discussed next. Finally, the conference attempted to analyze the host response to infection for clues to recognition and specificity. It is generally assumed that resistance is the end result of an induced active host process which either kills or inhibits a potential pathogen. The final group of papers explored such topics as the role of phytoalexins, the acquisition of resistance, the role of nucleic acid, *etc.* in determining either recognition or specificity.

It is appropriate for the editors to say that many of the current concepts of plant host-parasite interactions were developed by the speakers and observers themselves. Thus, the papers in this volume deal directly with the authors' research activities; some of them are summarized here for the first time. We wish to call the attention of the readers to the discussions which occurred after each presentation. Publication limitations and the technical difficulties of recording and rephrasing each exchange require that the reader must be aware that much of the full flavor of free intellectual exchange has been lost. The exchange was open, often vigorous, and the most spontaneous that either editor has ever observed at an international meeting. Thanks largely to Dr. S. Ouchi's instantaneous and accurate help in translation of certain phrases, critical scientific points were raised and settled without interruption of the ready flow of stimulating comments. In preparing the summaries of those discussions, we were forced to eliminate much of this and the summaries thus may appear inbalanced. We have striven first to dispense with many comments on techniques and research protocol which were important for discussion. We have tried to retain the exchange which deal in a broad way as outlined by the title of this volume. Even some of these comments regrettably were lost due to the considerable technical difficulty of tape recording the fast intellectual exchanges of approximately 30 peers seated face to face in a conference setting, rather than a lecture room configuration.

The editors and the U.S. and Japan organizing committees must acknowledge the assistance of individuals and organizations making this volume possible. Drs. James Partridge, Gary Payne, and Wayne Pedersen were invaluable in handling the equipment for talks and discussions as well as overseeing the innumerable details required to make the conference successful. Dr. M. Kojima made a great effort to help us edit this book.

We should like to express our sincere gratitude to the National Science Foundation and the Japan Society for Promotion of Science for supporting the conference organization and the book publication. The encouragement of Chancellor Roy Young of the University as well as that of the Vice-Chancellor for Agriculture Martin Massengale was much appreciated. Nebraska Agricultural Experiment Station Directors Howard Ottoson and Robert Kleis provided needed advice and financial support as did the University of Nebraska Foundation. Our thanks to all.

November 1978

J. M. Daly
I. Uritani

CONTENTS

Participants and Observers v
Preface ix

GENETIC INFORMATION AND SPECIFICITY

Inheritance of Specificity: The Gene-for-gene Hypothesis
Albert H. ELLINGBOE 3
Modes of Gene Expression in Disease Reaction
P. R. DAY 19
Modes of Metabolic Determination of Specificity
Joseph KUĆ 33
The Induction of Resistance or Susceptibility
Seiji OUCHI, Chihaya HIBINO, Hachiro OKU, Michinori FUJIWARA, and Hideto NAKABAYASHI 49

CYTOLOGICAL EVENTS IN RECOGNITION AND SPECIFICITY

The Hypersensitive Response of Resistant Plants
Kohei TOMIYAMA, Noriyuki DOKE, Masayuki NOZUE, and Yukio ISHIGURI 69
Papillae and Penetration: Some Problems, Procedures and Perspectives
James R. AIST, Margaret A. WATERMAN, and Herbert W. ISRAEL .. 85
Induction of Lignification in Response to Fungal Infection
Yasuji ASADA, Tomizo OHGUCHI, and Isao MATSUMOTO 99

CONSTITUTIVE RECOGNITION OF SPECIFICITY

What Art Thou, O Specificity?
R. D. DURBIN and J. A. STEELE 115
The Role of Host-specific Toxins in Saprophytic Pathogens
Syoyo NISHIMURA, Keisuke KOHMOTO, and Hiroshi OTANI 133

Cerato-ulmin, a Semipathotoxin of *Ceratocystis ulmi*
Shozo TAKAI, W. C. RICHARDS, Yasuyuki HIRATSUKA, and K. J. STEVENSON 147
Elicitors of Incompatible Host Responses: The Role of Host Cell Membranes
Jack D. PAXTON 153
The Relation between Bacterial Toxic Action and Plant Growth Regulation
Ryutaro SAKAI, Koushi NISHIYAMA, Akitami ICHIHARA, Kunio SHIRAISHI, and Sadao SAKAMURA 165
Spore Agglutinating Factor and Germ Tube Growth Inhibiting Factor in Host Plant
Ikuzo URITANI and Mineo KOJIMA 181
The Role of Host Cell Membranes
Penelop HANCHEY and Harry WHEELER 193
The Nature of Basic Compatibility: Comparisons between Pistil-pollen and Host-parasite Interaction
W. R. BUSHNELL 211

INDUCTION OF HOST RESPONSES FOR INCOMPATIBILITY AND COMPATIBILITY

The Acquisition of Systemic Resistance by Prior Inoculation
Luis SEQUEIRA 231
Recognition and Specificity in Plant Virus Infection
Albert SIEGEL 253
RNA and Protein Synthesis and Enzyme Changes during Infection
Toshikazu TANI and Hiroyuki YAMAMOTO 273
Molecular Studies on Crown Gall Tumors
Eugene W. NESTER 289
Relationship between Tolerance to Isoflavonoid Phytoalexins and Pathogenicity
Hans D. VANETTEN 301
The Role of Phytoalexins in Host-parasite Specificity
Hachiro OKU, Tomonori SHIRAISHI, and Seiji OUCHI 317
Differential Growth Response of Various Fungal Strains to Divalent Cations and Phytoalexins
Mineo KOJIMA, Akira TAKEUCHI, and Ikuzo URITANI 335

SUBJECT INDEX 351
LIST OF MICROORGANISMS 355

GENETIC INFORMATION AND SPECIFICITY

Recognition and Specificity in Plant Host-Parasite Interactions, pp. 3–17, 1979

INHERITANCE OF SPECIFICITY: THE GENE-FOR-GENE HYPOTHESIS

ALBERT H. ELLINGBOE

Genetics Program and Department of Botany and Plant Pathology, Michigan State University, East Lansing, Michigan, U.S.A.

In this paper an attempt will be made to look at the genetics of interactions between host and parasite from the view of what the inheritance of variability, in both host and parasite, tells us about those interactions. Can we draw conclusions about how genes in host and parasite function to affect interactions between host and parasite? Is there a positive function in the parasite for virulence or avirulence? Is there a positive function in the host for resistance or susceptibility? These questions have to be stated in a manner which specifies their relationship to the genetic variability we are attempting to explain. We must distinguish between primary effects and secondary effects of the activity of genes which determine the specificity of interactions.

We must also distinguish between naturally-occurring variability and induced variability. Of the naturally-occurring variability we must distinguish between the most common patterns and the rarer patterns of interactions. We must look at the hard data and see which hypotheses are consistant with the facts.

I. DETECTION OF VARIABILITY

Most experiments have started with a demonstration of variability in both host and parasite. A collection of host lines is usually inoculated with a large number of strains of a parasite. One type of data collected is presented in Table I. Viewed from the standpoint of the host, a "—" means the host is resistant and a "+" means the host is susceptible. Viewed from the standpoint of the parasite, a "—" means the parasite is restricted in its development in the host and a "+" means the parasite can develop in the host. I have presented the data as an interaction because that is what it is. The "+" and "—" is a simplified version of a range in reactions.

The parasite strains are commonly classified as physiological races. They are usually morphologically indistinguishable. The host lines may or may not be morphologically distinguishable but are almost always of one species.

The reactions of the six host lines to the ten parasite strains show that no two host lines are genetically identical, and that no two parasite strains are genetically identical. Host line A does not help to distinguish the ten parasite strains.

TABLE I

The Reaction[a] of 6 Host Lines to 10 Strains of a Parasite

Parasite strains	Host lines					
	A	B	C	D	E	F
1	+	—	—	+	—	+
2	+	—	+	—	+	—
3	+	+	+	+	—	—
4	+	—	+	—	+	—
5	+	—	+	—	—	—
6	+	+	+	—	—	—
7	+	—	+	—	—	+
8	+	—	+	—	+	+
9	+	+	—	+	—	+
10	+	+	+	+	+	+

[a] —, incompatible host-parasite relationship; +, compatible host-parasite relationship.

II. BASIC GENETIC PATTERN

The procedure used by Flor (1947) (*1*) to begin an analysis of the inheritance of these differences was to select a host line on which all strains of the parasite could be maintained. In the example given, that would be host line A. Each of the other host lines was crossed to A. Parasite strain 5 can be used to distinguish between host lines A and B. If F2 plants of a cross between A and B were inoculated with strain 5, they may show that one gene can explain the difference between A and B when inoculated with strain 5. If one gene can explain the difference between A and B, a cross between strain 5 and strain 10 will also show one gene segregation. This one-for-one correspondence is found in essentially all genetic studies of naturally-occurring variability. The basic pattern which comes out of these studies is presented in Table II.

Had parasite strain 1 been used to inoculate the segregating F2 population of a cross between host lines A and B, we may have seen a two gene segregation ratio. Had parasite strain 1 been used to cross to strain 10, we would have seen a two gene segregation ratio. The basic pattern for two genes would have been as presented in Table III.

It has frequently been argued to me that the pattern presented in Table II is an artifact of the selection of particular parasite strains and host lines. For example, if from Table I we took host lines B and C and parasite strains 1 and 2 we would have three parasite/host genotypes which give an incompatible relationship and one which gives a compatible relationship. That is the reciprocal of the pattern given in Table II. Detailed genetic analyses of patterns which are reciprocal to the pattern in Table II have shown them to be due to more than one gene in host and/or parasite (Moseman, 1959)

TABLE II

The Basic Genetic Pattern of Interactions between Host and Parasite

Parasite genotype	Host genotype	
	Rx	*rx*
Px	−	+
px	+	+

−, incompatible host-parasite relationships; +, compatible host-parasite relationships.

TABLE III

The Basic Genetic Pattern of Interactions for Two Parasite/Host Gene Pairs (Two Loci in Each Organism and Two Alleles at Each Locus)

Parasite genotype	Host genotype			
	R1 *R2*	*R1* *r1*	*r1* *R2*	*r1* *r2*
P1 P2	−	−	−	+
P1 p2	−	−	+	+
p1 P2	−	+	−	+
p1 p2	+	+	+	+

−, incompatible parasite/host genotype; +, compatible parasite/host genotype.

(*3*). When the genes are separated so that we look at one gene at a time in host and parasite, the pattern presented in Table II emerges again.

III. INTERPRETATION OF BASIC PATTERN

Studies on the physiology and comparative biochemistry of host-parasite relations have commonly used either one strain of the parasite and two host lines, or two strains of the parasite and one line of the host. The first combination has been common for investigations of the "nature of resistance." Host lines may have been of different species or the other extreme of highly isogenic host lines. The second combination has been common for studies of "parasitism" and/or "pathogenesis." Let's suppose we were to study the biochemical differences between the reaction of host lines A and B (from Table I) to parasite strain 5. With only two host lines, any biochemical differences between the two host lines following inoculation will be absolutely associated with resistance or susceptibility. One can make an equally valid conclusion that resistance is a positive function or that susceptibility is a positive function. If we select one host line, B (from Table I), and parasite strains 5 and 10, all biochemical differences between plants inoculated with strain 5 or 10 will be absolutely associated with "parasitism" or "pathogenicity." One can make an equally valid conclusion that there is an active function for virulence or avirulence. If, on the other hand, we do these comparative studies with two host lines *and* two parasite strains as presented in Table II, the simplest interpretation is that specific interaction of these host and parasite genes is for an incompatible relationship. This interpretation means that we have to explain only one parasite/host genotype, namely *Px*/*Rx*. With the other three parasite/host genotypes, *i.e.*, *Px*/*rx*, *px*/*Rx*, and *px*/*rx*, there is no interaction of these genes. I interpret Table II to mean that the product of *Px* interacts with the product of its corresponding gene *Rx* to give an incompatible interaction between host and parasite. Viewed from the standpoint of the host, resistance is a positive function, *i.e.*, the production of the functional *Rx* gene product. Viewed from the standpoint of the parasite, avirulence is a positive function, *i.e.*, the production of the functional *Px* gene product.

There are two points we can now get out of Table III. One is that *P1* will interact with *R1*, but not *R2*, to give an incompatible relationship. This specificity is one of the bases of the gene-for-gene hypothesis presented by Flor (1955) (*2*). The second point to get from Table III is that if one parasite/host gene pair specifies incompatibility, that gene pair will be epistatic to all parasite/host gene pairs which would give a compatible relationship.

IV. ALLELIC HOST GENES

The argument for specific recognition for an incompatible relationship is also supported by the data with allelic genes in the host. It is common to find *R* genes in the host to be allelic. (Whether they are true alleles or closely linked genes is not known in most cases.) The evidence for true alleles at the *L* locus in flax is very good. The pattern with 6 of 14 alleles is presented in Table IV. A homozygous host line can have only one *L* allele. The corresponding *P* genes in the parasite are not allelic so each parasite has all six of the *P* loci. It is possible to have only six homozygous host lines. It is possible to have 2^6 or 64 homozygous parasite strains.

The first listed parasite strain in Table IV has one *P* gene and five *p* genes. It has an incompatible relationship with host line of genotype *Lo* but a compatible relationship with host lines with each of the other five *L* alleles. Is the relation an incompatible one on the basis of the *Po*/*Lo* interaction? What is the interaction between *p1* and *Lo*? What is the interaction between *p2*, *p6*, *p8*, or *p11* and *Lo*? What is the interaction between *Po* and *L1*? What is the interaction between *Po* and *L2*? Which genes are responsible for giving the first listed parasite strain the ability to give a compatible relationship with host lines with *L1*, *L2*, *L6*, *L8*, or *L11*? To explain these types of data on the basis of a positive function of these genes for compatibility requires

TABLE IV

The Interaction between Six *L* Alleles in *Linum usitatissimum* and the Corresponding Genes at Six Loci in *Melampora lini*[a]

Parasite genotype	Host genotype					
	L0	*L1*	*L2*	*L6*	*L8*	*L11*
Po p1 p2 p6 p8 p11	–	+	+	+	+	+
po P1 p2 p6 p8 p11	+	–	+	+	+	+
po p1 P2 p6 p8 p11	+	+	–	+	+	+
po p1 p2 P6 p8 p11	+	+	+	–	+	+
po p1 p2 p6 P8 p11	+	+	+	+	–	+
po p1 p2 p6 p8 P11	+	+	+	+	+	–
Po P1 p2 p6 p8 p11	–	–	+	+	+	+
Po p1 P2 p6 p8 p11	–	+	–	+	+	+
Po p1 p2 P6 p8 p11	–	+	+	–	+	+
Po p1 p2 p6 P8 p11	–	+	+	+	–	+
Po p1 p2 p6 p8 P11	–	+	+	+	+	–

[a] To simplify the diagram, the hosts lines and parasite strains are assumed to be homozygous and are written as though they were haploid. –, an incompatible host-parasite relationship; +, a compatible host-parasite relationship.

very complicated hypotheses. The explanation of these data on the basis of a positive function for incompatibility is quite simple. The first listed parasite strain in Table IV gives an incompatible relationship with the host line with *Lo* because of a *Po*/*Lo* interaction. The other host lines give a compatible relationship with strain one because they represent no interaction between the products of host and parasite genes. We must remember that these are the genes, and the patterns of interactions, which affect naturally-occurring host-parasite variability.

V. DOMINANCE

There has been much said in the literature about the dominance or recessiveness of genes affecting host-parasite relationships. One of the problems in evaluating dominance is presented in Table V. *R1a* is dominant to *R1b* with the first listed strain of the parasite. *R1b* is dominant to *R1a* with the second-listed strain of the parasite.

TABLE V

The Dominance Relationships between Two Alleles of an *R* Locus in a Host and Two Strains of a Parasite

Parasite genotypes	Host genotypes		
	R1a R1a	*R1a R1b*	*R1b R1b*
P1a p1b	−	−	+
p1a P1b	+	−	−

−, incompatible host-parasite relationship; +, compatible host-parasite relationship.

VI. TEMPERATURE SENSITIVITY

Temperature sensitivity is a very informative characteristic of some of the genes controlling naturally-occurring variability in host-parasite interactions. Temperature sensitivity is best illustrated with *Triticum aestivum* and *Puccinia graminis* f. sp. *tritici* and the *P6/Sr6* interaction as illustrated in Table VI. At 20°C the *P6/Sr6* genotype gives an incompatible relationship. At 25°C the *P6/Sr6* genotype gives a compatible relationship. Most temperature-sensitive mutations lead to a protein product which has biological activity at the normal temperature but which loses it biological activity at the elevated temperature. The observations that the *P6/Sr6* genotype specifies an incompatible relationship at the normal temperature 20°C, and a compatible relationship at the elevated temperature, 25°C, suggest that there is specific interaction between *P6* and *Sr6* at 20°C but no or reduced interaction at 25°C.

The genetic analysis of naturally-occurring variability in host-parasite interactions suggests that the specific recognition between products of corresponding host and parasite genes is for incompatible relationships. Compatible relationships result from the lack of interaction of certain alleles of these genes.

Based on the temperature-sensitive nature of some of these genes, I assume their important gene products are proteins. In Table II, the product of *Px* interacts with the product of *Rx*, possibly to form a dimer, and the result of that interaction is to set in motion the activity necessary for an incompatible relationship. The product of *Px* does not interact with the product of *rx* and, therefore, the requirements for an incompatible relationship are not met. The latter also holds for parasite/host genotypes *px/Rx*

TABLE VI

The Interaction between *Sr6* in *Triticum aestivum* and the Corresponding *P6* in *Puccinia graminis* f. sp. *tritici* at Two Temperatures

Parasite genotype	Host			
	20°C		25°C	
	Sr6	*sr6*	*Sr6*	*sr6*
P6	−	+	+	+
p6	+	+	+	+

−, incompatible host-parasite interaction; +, compatible host-parasite interaction.

and *px*/*rx*. If this hypothesis is correct, any mutation of *Px* which results in a loss of recognition of *Rx* should lead to a compatible relationship between host and parasite. Mutations to increased virulence *i.e.*, *Px* to *px**, should be easy to get, and they are. Mutations from *rx* to *Rx* are mutations to a specific specificity so they should be rare, and they are.

VII. UNIVERSALITY OF BASIC PATTERN

The analysis of the inheritance of variability in interactions between host and parasite given above seems to hold for most organisms. Over 90% of the variability reported in the literature is consistent with this pattern (Table II). As more detailed analyses are made with other hosts and parasites, the same basic pattern emerges. The same pattern seems to hold for fungi, bacteria, nematode, insect, and possibly viral, interactions with plants. The same pattern may also hold for interactions between animals and disease-causing non-antigenic entities.

VIII. EVOLUTION OF GENETIC INTERACTIONS

The interpretation of these data is that there is specific interaction of these genes for an incompatible relationship between host and parasite. These genes function to either prevent the establishment of compatible relationships or they function to destroy a compatible relationship once it is established. Failure of mutual recognition between corresponding genes leads to a compatible relationship. These corresponding genes, therefore, must be

TABLE VII

The Pattern of Interactions Expected of Corresponding Host and Parasite Genes whose Function was Necessary for Compatible Relationships

Parasite genotype	Host genotypes	
	Rx	*rx*
Px	+	–
px	–	–

–, incompatible host-parasite relationships; +, compatible host-parasite relationships.

superimposed on a basic compatibility between host and parasite. If the host and parasite had first evolved a basic compatibility, then it is easy to rationalize the existence of a system of corresponding genes whose function is to either prevent the establishment of compatible relationships or destroy compatible relationships once established.

In the evolution of host-parasite relationships I would expect there to be some genes in the parasite whose function was crucial to successful parasitism. There ought to be parasite genes whose function is crucial to the development of penetration structures, mobilization of nutrients in the host, alteration of host metabolism, *etc.* We can even surmise that genes in the parasite whose function is regulation might have corresponding genes in the host. If there is a correspondence of genes whose function is necessary for compatible relationships between host and parasite, they would be expected to follow a pattern presented in Table VII. The first thing to note is that the pattern given in Table VII is the reciprocal of the pattern given in Table II. Why don't we see variability of the pattern presented in Table VII? A mutation from *Px* to *px* may well be lethal to the parasite. A mutation from *Rx* to *rx* in the host may also be lethal to the parasite. Constitutive mutations at these loci may be lethal to the parasite. It may be possible to identify genes whose function is crucial to successful parasitism by inducing conditional mutations of these genes in a parasite. A temperature-sensitive mutation of a gene whose function is crucial to successful parasitism would be expected to develop and give a compatible relationship with its host at a normal temperature but would not be expected to develop at the elevated temperature. Its temperature sensitivity would be the reciprocal of the pattern presented in Table VI. We have been successful in inducing a large number of temperature-sensitive mutations in *Erysiphe graminis* f. sp. *tritici* and *Colletotrichum lindemuthianum* which can produce disease at 22°C but cannot produce disease at 25° and 28°C, respectively.

IX. A RECIPROCAL PATTERN?

The fungi which produce host specific toxins seem to follow the pattern given in Table VII. Strains of *Helminthosporium victoriae* which produce a toxin can develop in lines of *Avena sativum* which contain the *Vb* (=*Pc2*) gene. Strains which do not produce the toxin cannot develop in any host lines, with *Vb* or *vb*. Host lines with *vb* are resistant to all strains of *H. victoriae*. I would feel much more comfortable with this interpretation if the parasite lines which do not produce a toxin assayable on host lines with *Vb* would be capable of developing in host lines of other genotypes, such as lines with mutant *Vb** genes. In no parasite-host combination in which a host-specific toxin is demonstrated to be involved has there been a detailed genetic analysis. The data to date, however, are consistent with the pattern given in Table VII.

In another paper in this symposium there are data presented which suggest that DNA from *Agrobacterium tumifaciens* is transferred to the host in the transformation required in the crown gall disease. These data suggest a positive function for transformation of differentiated host tissue to neoplastic tissue. It will be interesting to see, in future research, if specificity of that DNA segment with host genotype can be demonstrated, and if that specificity follows the pattern given in Table II or Table VII.

X. DISCUSSION

In host-parasite interactions, we seem to be dealing with two types of gene interactions. More than 90% of the genetic variability studied to date is consistent with the pattern given in Table II. These genes are involved in a mutual recognition which determines the fate of the interactions. The mutual, specific recognition is for incompatible relations. What events transpire after that recognition are for incompatible relations. What events transpire after that recognition seem to be numerous and have varied effects. We know from comparative biochemical and physiological studies that there can be many differences in compatible and incompatible interactions. The decision for compatible or incompatible interactions, the result of *P*/*R* interactions, frequently seems to be made early in interactions. The result of that decision can be a cascade of changes. The problem in research, and in the discussions to follow, is to distinguish between the genes, and their products, which determine the specificity, and the secondary effects of that decision. *P/R* genes are like regulatory genes which can set into motion a large number of secondary changes, the manifestations of which can be numerous. The genes affecting interactions with the toxins, such as the hypothetical binding sites, are probably structural genes. Genes in host or parasite which are not part of a corresponding set are also probably structural genes.

Our problems in research and in discussion of research results with various approaches, are to formulate hypotheses which help to explain our results and are consistent with the results from many different approaches to the problems of specificity in interactions between host and parasite.

In this paper I have not tried to make a comprehensive analysis of the genetics of host-parasite interactions. I have tried to focus on the genetic aspects which deal with the fundamental arguments crucial to the simple question of whether specific interactions are for compatible or incompatible relationships between host and parasite.

For those of you who are not intimately familiar with the genetics of host-parasite interactions dealt with in the first part of this paper, I am including a list of 13 postulates of the gene-for-gene hypothesis. Also included are 3 postulates relating to the evolution of genetic variability. I hope these have the effect of simplifying the basic genetics.

XI. POSTULATES OF THE GENE-FOR-GENE THEORY OF HOST-PARASITE RELATIONSHIPS

1. There are allelic pairs of genes in the host (*RR,Rr,rr*) and in the parasite (*PP,Pp,pp*) that determine interactions between host and parasite.
2. The parasite/host genotype determines interactions between the host and parasite.
3. Gene *P1* in the parasite recognizes only *R1,* not *R2, R3, R4, etc.*, in the host.
4. Gene *R1* in the host recognizes only *P1,* not *P2, P3, P4, etc.*, in the parasite.
5. There may be multiple alleles at some *R* loci in the host.
6. *R* loci may be clustered in closely linked groups.
7. The corresponding *P* genes in the parasite are not necessarily allelic because the host *R* genes are allelic.

8. There may be a limited number of R loci in the host for reaction to a given parasite.
9. Specific recognition and interaction are necessary for an incompatible interaction between host and parasite.
10. Specific recognition is usually between dominant genes in host and parasite.
11. All non-recognized alleles behave as though they are a single recessive gene.
12. A parasite/host gene pair which specifies incompatibility is epistatic to all gene pairs specifying compatibility.
13. Modifier genes in the parasite affect the dominant P/R genes.

XII. DEFINITIONS

1. In this paper the term "compatible" refers to the type of response of the host and the parasite to invastion by the parasite. A "compatible" relation implies that the host and parasite, either upon contact or through adjustment and adaptation after contact, do not adversely alter the host, the parasite, or both. The term is intended to imply a harmonious relationship between host and parasite.
2. The base for compatibility comparisons is the parasite/host genotype P/r. Incompatibility is defined as a measurable difference from that observed in genotype P/r.

XIII. POSTULATES RELATING TO THE EVOLUTION OF GENETIC VARIABILITY IN HOST-PARASITE INTERACTIONS

1. The evolution of the gene-for-gene interactions can be rationalized if they are assumed to be superimposed on a basic compatibility between host and parasite. The first mutation was $r \rightarrow R$, the second $P \rightarrow p$. Mutation $P \rightarrow p$ led to loss of recognition of R in the host.
2. Different parasite/host gene pairs, P/R, for incompatibility affect unique systems of interaction between host and parasite if not a part of an allelic series in host or parasite.
3. Unnecessary p genes are commonly a handicap to the survival of the parasite. Therefore the P loci must have some other function to the parasite.

SUMMARY

Almost all naturally-occurring variability in host and parasite affecting interactions is controlled by genes which follow the pattern of gene-for-gene interactions. The simplest explanation of this pattern is that there is specific recognition between host and parasite genes for incompatibility. This conclusion is supported by detailed genetic analysis in both host and parasite of a single parasite/host gene pair, the epistasis of incompatibility, analysis of allelic host genes, dominance for incompatibility, and temperature sensitivity of interactions. The basic genetic pattern seems to be quite universal in interorganismic genetics.

Acknowledgment

I want to acknowledge my appreciation for the many valuable discussions with Profs. W. Q. Loegering and R. W. Lewis. The research supported in part by Grants GB-42124 and PCM 77-05343 from the National Science Foundation.

REFERENCES

1. Flor, H. H. 1947. Inheritance of reaction to rust in flax. *J. Agric. Res.* **74**: 241–262.
2. Flor, H. H. 1955. Host-parasite interaction in flax rust-its genetics and other implications. *Phytopathology* **45**: 680–685.
3. Moseman, J. G. 1959. Host-pathogen interaction of the genes for resistance in *Hordeum vulgare* and for pathogenicity in *Erysiphe graminis* f. sp. *hordei*. *Phytopathology* **49**: 469–472.

Discussion of Paper by Dr. Ellingboe

Ellingboe responded to several questions on the pattern of interactions between host and parasite as shown by the quadratic check. In summarizing he emphasized the characteristic pattern of the expected 3 and 1 ratios even when test crosses of the parasite, instead of host, are compared. This fact tends to eliminate bias due to the selection of individual strains in establishing a quadratic check for a single host. His interpretation is that avirulence in the pathogen is the result of a positive function while virulence is the lack of that function. A considerable dialogue among all participants arose by Wheeler's comments that the pattern in a quadratic check occurs because of the underlying assumptions and prescribed rules for describing inheritance. His feeling is that at present it is not possible to choose between positive or negative functions and called attention to Favret's proposed test of this hypothesis by physically deleting the proposed gene for avirulence. Ellingboe then pointed out that Favret did not consider other sorts of evidence such as the data for 4 possible parasite/host genotypes, or the patterns with multiple alleles, temperature sensitive genes, mutations, *etc.* Ellingboe also amplified the utility of the quadratic check by pointing out it appears to apply to small differences in disease reaction that generally have been assumed not to involve specific genes for resistance, such as lesion numbers, generation times, *etc.* It was apparent from the discussion that such theoretical considerations must be pursued more extensively. Siegel asked Ellingboe if he would comment on the possible nature of gene products causing compatibility or incompatibility. Ellingboe stated that no gene products for resistance or susceptibility are known. His working concept is that a product of a parasite avirulence gene may interact with the product of resistance gene of the host to form a complex regulating the activity of other genes. In the absence of the complex, normal successful parasitism occurs which must assume a basic compatibility between host and parasite. He recognized the theoretically valid argument favoring a positive gene product for successful establishment of the parasite but he emphasized the naturally-occurring variability and all possible genotype combinations point to the positive function of incompatibility genes as a fine control. For example, *Puccinia graminis* f.sp. *tritici* is a parasite in wheat but not corn indicating genes for compatibility for wheat but the disease reaction of individual wheat varieties involves resistance genes.

Recognition and Specificity in Plant Host-Parasite Interactions, pp. 19–31, 1979

MODES OF GENE EXPRESSION IN DISEASE REACTION

P. R. DAY

Genetics Department, The Connecticut Agricultural Experiment Station, New Haven, Connecticut, U.S.A.

The outcome of interaction between host and parasite is determined by a number of factors. They include temperature, humidity, light, the age, nutrition, and stage of growth of the host, and the genotypes of the host and the parasite. In this paper I explore what we know of the modes and the nature of this gene expression in fungal parasites. I will then discuss this in the context of gene expression in genetically better known saprophytic fungi finishing with some speculations about the possible impact of still newer analytical methods.

There are two kinds of effects of gene expression in disease reaction. The first, specificity, determines that a given host plant is susceptible or resistant to different pathogen strains, and that a given pathogen strain is avirulent or virulent on different host cultivars. Host and parasite each can exhibit two phenotypes depending on the genotype of the other. The second kind of effect of gene expression is non-specific and is discussed later.

I. SPECIFIC INTERACTIONS

In spite of fairly intensive efforts during the last few years we know surprisingly little about the nature of the controls of specificity in interactions between host and parasite. It now seems clear that the elegance and simplicity of Flor's gene-for-gene hypothesis was in some respects misleading. It was reasonable to assume that effects manifestly controlled by single alleles in either host or parasite must intrinsically be more easily explained in biochemical terms than effects whose genetic controls are not known. However, the result was to focus attention on clear cut and therefore probably highly evolved specificity. Unfortunately these systems appear to have unexpectedly complex mechanisms. The major break throughs have come instead from work with bacterial and fungal pathogens that produce pathotoxins. The isolation and characterization of a pathotoxin and analysis of its effects on the host has until now been a more persuasive simplification (see Refs. *29* and *30*) but it is limited to host-parasite interactions where pathotoxins play a majorrole. Attempts to find pathogen products that determine the outco me of the host-parasite interaction among the many other systems have so far been unsuccessful.

Specificity and Induced Mutation

Mutations that confer virulence on plant pathogens can be induced by mutagen treatment and selected by inoculation to resistant host plants. Such mutants have been recovered in several systems (*9*) but have had surprisingly little effect in furthering our understanding. Extensive searches for new specificities of mating type alleles of higher basidiomycetes and of self-incompatibility alleles governing pollen-style interactions in higher plants have in every case only generated mutants that can be interpreted as having lost a function rather than acquired a new specificity. The same is true of mutants of flax rust dikaryons heterozygous for dominant avirulence where the simplest explanation is that virulence results from the deletion of a segment of chromosome carrying the dominant allele.

In some respects it is not surprising that the study of induced virulent mutants has advanced so little. Beyond confirming that new races of pathogens arise by mutation there seems to be very little else to be gained in terms of immediate practical benefits. Studies of induced resistance in the host on the other hand could lead to new and perhaps very useful resistant cultivars. However, in spite of numbers of induced mutants in such crops as barley, maize, wheat, rice, capsicum, mint, and apple resistant to such pathogens as mildew, leaf blight, rust, blast, and wilt there is little or nothing to show by way of an improved understanding of resistance mechanisms (*35*). Indeed we still do not even know whether any of these induced mutations to resistance are race specific. Nearly all of our knowledge of the mode of gene action in molecular biology come from the study of induced mutants of microorganisms with defects in metabolism. The following very brief account of some findings obtained with *Neurospora* and yeast indicate the kinds of complexities found in the genetic controls of relatively simple metabolic steps in fungi. A more detailed account can be found in Fincham and Day (*14*). Auxotrophic mutants were isolated by detecting their failure to grow at all, or their abnormal growth on chemically defined media. Many mutants could be restored to normal, or near normal, growth by the addition of metabolites to the medium. Nutritional tests showed that a single compound would often suffice. Sometimes several compounds were required, for example when the mutational block prevented formation of a common precursor. The identification of accumulated intermediates showed the position of the mutational block and revealed the responsible enzyme that was either absent or altered to a non-functional form in the mutant. This was a very powerful tool. Specific mutants could be looked for to test hypotheses. But there were sometimes unsuspected difficulties. For example in aromatic metabolism in *Neurospora crassa* there are three separate 3-deoxy-D-arabinoheptulosonate-7-phosphate (DAHP) synthases inhibited by tyrosine, phenylalanine, and tryptophane respectively. If one or two are inactive the remaining activities can function well enough to support growth. To produce mutants defective in any of the three DAHP synthases the other two had to be shut down or repressed by feedback inhibition (*16*). Only the triple mutant is an auxotroph on minimal medium.

Another source of difficulty was that occasionally the enzyme that appeared most logically to be responsible for the step was in fact not involved. For example in an ornithine requiring *Neurospora* mutant unable to carry out the synthesis of ornithine from glutamic-γ-semialdehyde the enzyme ornithine δ-transaminase was present (*7*). This enzyme catalyses formation of ornithine from glutamic-γ-semialdehyde *in vitro*. However *in vivo* the N-acetyl derivative of glutamic-γ-semialdehyde is the immediate precursor and the mutant was blocked in this step. The enzyme ornithine δ-transaminase evidently has only a catabolic role *in vivo*.

Examples of a single mutation abolishing several steps in the same metabolic pathway were another puzzle. This was mostly due to the aggregation of several polypeptide chains into a complex with several different activities. If their structures are interdependent it is not difficult to see how disruption of one can destroy the function of the others.

A reverse case of complexity follows from examples where two or more genes appear to be responsible for the same enzyme activity. For example in *Neurospora* mutations at *arg-2* and *arg-3* can eliminate arginine specific carbamoyl phosphate synthetase. A current hypothesis is that the enzyme contains two polypeptide chains determined by the two genes (*33*). There is still no satisfactory explanation of the ten unlinked genes in yeast any one of which can mutate to block inositol phosphate synthetase activity creating a requirement for inositol (*6*).

Defects in pathways may be repaired by shunts and bypasses, a fact that emphasizes the interconnections in metabolism. For example yeast mutants with requirements for serine or glycine were suppressed when grown on acetate instead of glucose as a C source. The induction of glyoxylate cycle enzymes as a result of transfer to acetate included glyoxylate transaminase which converts glyoxylate to serine (*31*).

Mutations affecting synthesis of macromolecules have been especially rewarding. Unlike the simple compounds required by auxotrophs macromolecules can rarely be supplied to remedy the defect and as a consequence these mutations are nearly always lethal. Their analysis was made possible by using conditional mutants. These are lethal in one environment but able to grow in another. The most useful conditional lethals are temperature sensitive. They include not only forms that are sensitive to relatively high temperatures but others sensitive to relatively low temperatures.

Temperature sensitivity is determined by conformational instability of the mutant protein. Since enzyme function is dependent on molecular conformation if the protein is only stable at relatively low temperatures then it will only function at those low temperatures. The best known temperature sensitive system in host-parasite interaction is the *Sr6* gene from Red Egyptian wheat for resistance to *Puccinia graminis tritici* (*21*). This has been the subject of intensive study here in Lincoln in Dr. Daly's Laboratory. However, the hypothetical conformationally unstable protein produced by *Sr6* has not, as far as I know, been identified and thus its function in metabolism is unknown.

Mutants defective in DNA replication, RNA synthesis, and the systems involved in protein synthesis have all been described in fungi (*14*). Of particular interest are mutants with altered tRNAs which cause mistranslation; so called super-suppressors. These can be selected where mistranslation will restore a function lost in a missense or chain-termination mutant.

The prospect of introducing a super-suppressor in a haploid plant pathogen with well defined specificity is intriguing but hardly likely to be carried out in the very near future. Let us examine some of the obstacles. The pathogen could not be obligate such as a rust or mildew because identification of the suppressor would at present probably require testing its effects on a variety of auxotrophic mutants that could only be grown on defined culture media. A convenient system for genetic recombination must be available to incorporate the suppressor in a variety of genetic backgrounds. This excludes imperfect fungi and forms where the recombination systems, sexual or otherwise, are too clumsy, take too long, or are not sufficiently characterized. For all but a very few plant pathogens such as the gram negative bacteria *Pseudomonas, Erwinia,* and *Agrobacterium tumefaciens,* the prospect of analyses at this level appears so daunting that entirely different methods such as those of the newly emerging recombinant DNA systems or the synthesis by end-to-end ligation of DNA fragments to create recombinant DNA molecules may in the long run be much more profitable. I will return to this topic later.

Recent work by Lawrence, Mayo, and Shepherd (unpublished) in Adelaide on flax rust revealed one or several dominant suppressor-genes in the rust (*Melampsora lini*) that interfere with certain interactions expected to be avirulent. Four reactions involving the flax resistance genes M^1, L^1, L^7, and L^{10}, and their corresponding rust avirulence genes, that normally give avirulent or resistant reactions (low infection types) were affected and gave high infection types instead. None of the four avirulence alleles in the rust (A_{M^1}, A_{L^1}, A_{L^7}, and $A_{L^{10}}$) are linked. The alleles for resistance at the *L* locus in flax include nine others not affected by identified suppressors. At the *M* locus there are six other alleles that are also not affected. Unfortunately there is no evidence to indicate the mode of action of these suppressors.

In bacteria and fungi much useful information has been derived from study of the pathways involving the major nutrients such as nitrogen, carbon, and phosphate sources. The methods used to isolate auxotrophic mutants can be employed here, for example by modifying minimal medium so as to require utilization of the metabolite under study. Non-utilization can also be detected very efficiently by using a toxic analogue of the substance. The only snag is that this tends to produce numbers of mutants that fail to take up the analogue rather than not metabolize it.

With respect to mutation to resistance to toxic substances plant pathogens are clearly no less versatile than saprophytes. There are now many examples of mutation to resistance to fungicides (*9*). However, I am not aware of examples of mutation to resistance to toxic metabolites such as phytoalexins formed in the host as the result of triggering a resistance mechanism. While pea pathogens degrade pisatin (*11*) and spores of *Stemphylium botryosum* degrade alfalfa phytoalexin (*17*) this sort of mutation is not obviously responsible for specificity at the level of physiologic races. It appears to be more a difference involving species or genera.

Our knowledge of the molecular biology of plant parasites is sparse and the variety of techniques we can employ with them limited compared with *E. coli*, yeast, and *Neurospora*. The information we have on our host plants is even more limited. The reasons are plain. Biomedical science is largely concerned with mammals and primates. Plant pathologists have to work with fifteen major and at least 135 minor crops to mention only economically important food crops (*8*). Fiber, drug, and ornamental crops perhaps double these numbers. Each one has its own problems although some are common to many. It is no wonder that in plant pathology no systems have emerged as pre-eminently suited for concentrated investigation.

Since the effects of induced mutation to disease resistance in plant hosts seem to be for the most part non-specific they are considered in the next section.

II. NON-SPECIFIC INTERACTIONS

The second general class of gene expression is non-specific. An example is the finding that induced purine auxotrophs of pathogenic fungi are generally non-pathogenic (*22*). No host cultivars are known on which these auxotrophs can produce disease. They show only one phenotype. In fact some may be restored by adding purines to the host tissue whereas others show no response. Several authors have looked for and described non-pathogenic mutants. There are probably many ways in which the growth of a facultative parasite on its host may be impaired without affecting its growth on a defined nutrient medium. The capacity to grow on a minimal medium was employed to eliminate auxotrophs of *Penicillium expansum* by MacNeill and Barron (*23*). Some 10^5 cultures growing on minimal medium after mutagen treatment were tested on apple fruits and 7 mutants with altered pathogenicity were recovered. Only 2 were avirulent but normal in culture.

Ellingboe and Gabriel (*13*) recently reported isolating temperature sensitive mutants of *Colletotrichum lindemuthianum* and *Phyllosticta maydis* which vary in their ability to either grow on supplemented culture medium, or to produce expanding lesions on plants, depending on the temperature. In this work simple auxotrophy was eliminated by showing that supplementation did not restore growth on culture medium at the non-permissive temperature. Both approaches of isolating non-pathogenic mutants, conditional or otherwise, could well lead to the identification of metabolic systems that play key roles in the host-parasite interaction. Clearly if differences between induced non-pathogenic mutants and wild type can be seen in culture identification of the pathways involved will be very much easier than if the host plant must always be employed.

Another approach is to select mutants that are impaired in metabolic pathways assumed to be of importance in pathogenicity. For example mutants of *Fusarium* and *Verticillium* defective in pectolytic enzymes were selected to see what roles these enzymes play in inducing wilting (*18, 24*). In both organisms induction of wilt by mutants defective in various pectinase activities was unimpaired suggesting either that these activities are relatively unimportant or that they were produced in some other way *in vivo*.

In general auxotrophic mutants of plant pathogens have proved to be of limited interest in spite of claims for differential host reaction (*15, 22*).

A cursory examination of examples of induced mutations for resistance has failed to reveal to me any that are race specific. This may be because the deployment of such resistant mutants in agriculture has so far been too limited to reveal virulent mutants. There remains however, the possibility that some, if not many, will prove to be non-specific perhaps because the burden imposed on a potentially virulent race would be too great. They may turn out to be what Van der Plank (*32*) called "strong" resistance genes.

The host genes involved in general or horizontal resistance by definition have been considered to be non-specific. Several workers have re-examined the evidence for specificity among these interactions. For example Caten (*4*), continuing the approach begun by his colleagues in Birmingham, has shown that among isolates of race 0 of *Phytophthora infestans* on R_0 varieties of potato there are strains that are differentially adapted to the varieties on which they are found growing in the field. Essentially similar findings were reported independently by Clifford and Clothier (*5*) and Parlevliet (*27, 28*) for isolates of *Puccinia hordei* on "partially resistant" barley cultivars in Europe. Horizontal resistance as defined by Van der Plank does not admit such differential interactions. Leonard (personal communication) has stressed the importance in epidemiology of recognizing that horizontal resistance can apparently be overcome by pathogen adaptation involving specificity due to minor genes with quantitative effects. He distinguished vertical virulence from horizontal virulence preferring the latter term to aggressiveness. Ellingboe (*12*) would have us go still farther and regards horizontal resistance as that which has not yet been shown to be vertical. The implication that all resistance can be overcome as a result of pathogen adaptation is probably too sweeping. After all most pathogens have a very limited host range and this is surely largely because the uncongenial hosts they may infect are beyond their adaptive capacity. The inability of potato blight to parasitise wheat or grass is a case in point.

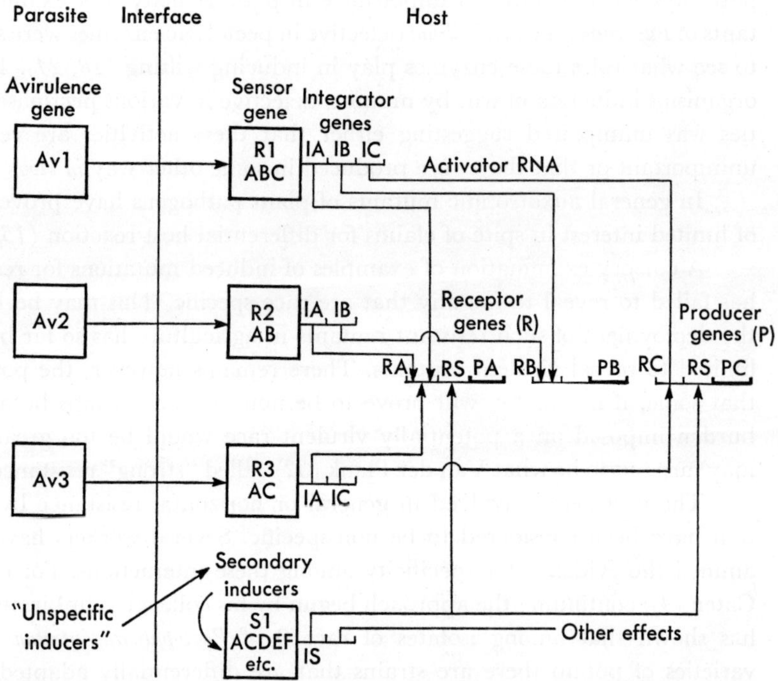

Fig. 1. A model for host-parasite interaction. The sensor genes *R1*, *R2*, and *R3* are resistance genes in the host that bind with the product of a specific avirulence gene from the parasite. The synthesis and diffusion of activator RNA to receptor genes results in the activation of their linked producer genes, producing the changes in metabolism associated with resistance. Sensor gene *S1* represents the class of sensor that responds to unspecific inducers. (After Britten and Davidson (*2*)). From Day (*9*).

Much of what we know of host-parasite interactions suggests that they are highly evolved. Since the products of resistance genes and of virulence or avirulence alleles have not been identified they seem unlikely to be involved in functions less complicated than regulation. Recent work on lectins as agents of cell recognition (*1, 25*) suggest that these compounds may be involved in triggering either of the chains of reactions that we call resistance or susceptibility.

Several years ago I proposed (*9*) the model shown in Fig. 1 based on a speculation of Britten and Davidson (*2*). It is not a good model because it has not led to any easy methods of testing its validity.

Several recent kinds of evidence are of interest. McIntyre and his colleagues (*26* and unpublished) reported that DNA extracts of several pathogens including fireblight and black shank when inoculated to host tissue (pear or tobacco) confer on it localized resistance to the pathogen. In Japan Yamamoto and Matsuo (*34*) reported similar protection of potatoes by treatment with DNA from blight resistant potato cultivars. Unfortunately the DNA extracts are relatively unspecific as inducers. For example DNA from susceptible potatoes was as effective as DNA from resistant cultivars or plants of other genera in inducing resistance. For fireblight, DNA from virulent and avirulent strains was equally effective. Evidently these materials are less subtle in their action than are the products of resistance genes.

A second piece of evidence is an account of the use of dichloro-dimethyl cyclopropane-carboxylic acid (see structural formula below) to potentiate the resistance mechanism of rice to blast disease (*Piricularia oryzae*) (*3*).

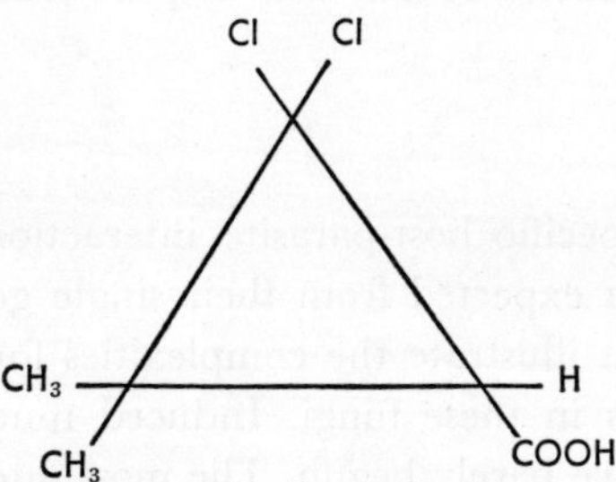

This compound is not toxic to *Piricularia* in complex media and its antifungal effects in plants treated with it (*19*) are probably not related to its fungicidal activity on defined media (Tamari's medium). Applications as soil drenches equivalent to 3 kg/ha (3 mg per 12.5 cm pot) resulted in protection of the plants (*20*) apparently by formation of the diterpene phytoalexins momilactone A and B. No phytoalexin was formed in treated plants unless or until they were inoculated with *Piricularia*. The phytoalexins were not formed in untreated plants in response to infection. However, they were formed in response to ultra violet (*U.V.*) irradiation of either leaves or coleoptiles and the compound (WL 28325) had no effect in this case. Treated and control plants were the same after *U.V.*

Evidently this compound increases the capacity of rice to synthesize phytoalexins in response to infection but does not itself stimulate their synthesis.

III. FUTURE PROSPECTS

For gram negative bacteria there are no technical obstacles to the isolation of functional regions of chromosomal or plasmid DNA and their study by using the plasmid or bacteriophage DNA-cloning vectors of *E. coli* K12. Studies of the plasmids of *Agrobacterium*, *Pseudomonas*, and *Erwinia* and their role in pathogenicity are now underway. Recent successes in experiments to introduce and clone specific fragments of DNA from yeast and *Neurospora* detected by their functional expression in *E. coli* suggest that these opportunities will also be available for pathogenic fungi and their plant hosts. For example if the structural gene for phenylalanine ammonia lyase were cloned and expressed in *E. coli* the prospects for studying its regulation and mutation might be greatly improved (see Ref. *10*). The technique holds great promise also for large scale production of the products of the genes that determine these interactions. It may also help in their identification.

SUMMARY

The mechanisms of specific host-parasite interaction appear to be more complex than was first expected from their single gene controls. Findings in *Neurospora* and yeast illustrate the complexities found in the controls of simple metabolic steps in these fungi. Induced mutation studies of host-parasite interaction have barely begun. The most interesting results to date reveal the effects of mutation on non-specific interactions. Further advances depend on concentration on one host-parasite system and the development of simple testable models.

REFERENCES

1. Albersheim, P. and A. J. Anderson-Prouty. 1975. Carbohydrates, proteins, cell surfaces, and the biochemistry of pathogenesis. *Annu. Rev. Plant Physiol.* **26**: 31–52.
2. Britten, R.J. and E.H. Davidson. 1969. Gene regulation for higher cells: A theory. *Science* **165**: 349–357.
3. Cartwright, D., P. Langcake, R. J. Pryce, D. P. Leworthy, and J. P. Ride. 1977. Chemical activation of host defence mechanisms as a basis for crop protection. *Nature* **267**: 511–513.
4. Caten, C.E. 1974. Intra-racial variation in *Phytophthora infestans* and adaptation to field resistance for potato blight. *Ann. Appl. Biol.* **77**: 259–270.
5. Clifford, B.C. and R. B. Clothier. 1974. Physiologic specialization of *Puccinia hordei* on barley hosts with non-hypersensitive resistance. *Trans. Br. Mycol. Soc.* **63**: 421–430.
6. Culbertson, M.R., T.F. Donahue, and S.A. Henry. 1976. Control of inositol biosynthesis in *Saccharomyces cerevisiae*: Inositol-phosphate sythetase mutants. *J. Bact.* **126**: 243–250.
7. Davis, R.H. and J. Mora. 1968. Mutants of *Neurospora crassa* deficient in orni thine-δ-transaminase. *J. Bact.* **96**: 383–388.
8. Day, P. R. 1973. Genetic variability of major crops. *Annu. Rev. Phytopathol.* **11**: 293–312.
9. Day, P. R. 1974. *Genetics of Host-parasite Interaction.* Freeman, San Francisco, p. 238.
10. Day, P. R. 1977. Plant genetics: Increasing crop yield. *Science* **197**: 1334–1339.
11. DeWit-Elshove, A. and A. Fuchs. 1971. The influence of the carbohydrate source on pisatin breakdown by fungi pathogenic to pea (*Pisum sativum*). *Physiol. Plant. Pathol.* **1**: 17–24.
12. Ellingboe, A. H. 1975. Horizontal resistance: An artifact of experimental procedure? *Aust. Plant Pathol. Soc. Newsl.* **4**: 44–46.
13. Ellingboe, A. H. and D. W. Gabriel. 1977. Induced conditional mutants for studying host/pathogen interactions. *In*: *International Symposium on the Use of Induced Mutations for Improving Disease Resistance in Crop Plants.* I.A.E.A., Vienna, (in press).
14. Fincham, J. R. S., P. R. Day, and A. Radford. 1978. *Fungal Genetics.* Blackwell, Oxford, 4th Ed. (in press).
15. Garber, E. D. 1960. The host as a growth medium. *Ann. N.Y. Acad. Sci.* **88**: 1187–1194.
16. Halsall, D. M. and C. H. Doy. 1969. Studies concerning the biochemical genetics and physiology of activity and allosteric inhibition mutants of *Neurospora crassa* 3-deoxy-D-arabino-heptulosonate-7-phosphate synthase. *Biochim. Biophys. Acta* **185**: 432–446.

17. Higgins, V. J. and R. L. Millar. 1969. Degradation of alfalfa phytoalexin by *Stemphyllium botryosum*. *Phytopathology* **59**: 1500–1506.

18. Howell, C. R. 1976. Use of enzyme-deficient mutants of *Verticillium dahliae* to assess the importance of pectolytic enzymes in symptom expression of *Verticillium* wilt of cotton. *Physiol. Plant Pathol.* **9**: 279–283.

19. Langcake, P. and S. G. A. Wickins. 1975. Studies on the mode of action of the dichlorocyclopropane fungicides: Effects of 2,2-dichloro-3,3-dimethyl cyclopropane carboxylic acid on the growth of *Piricularia oryzae. Cav. J. Gen. Microbiol.* **88**: 295–306.

20. Langcake, P. and S. G. A. Wickins. 1975. Studies on the action of the dichlorocyclopropanes on the host-parasite relationship in the rice blast disease. *Physiol. Plant Pathol.* **7**: 113–126.

21. Loegering, W. Q. and J. R. Geis. 1957. Independence in the action of three genes conditioning stem rust resistance in Red Egyptian wheat. *Phytopathology* **47**: 740–741.

22. Loprieno, N. 1964. I mutanti nutrizionali nello studio dei rapporti ospite-patogeno nelle fitopatie da microorganismi. *Agric. Ital.*, 1–15.

23. MacNeill, B. H. and G. L. Barron. 1966. Avirulence in prototrophs of *Pencillium expansum*. *Can. J. Bot.* **44**: 355–358.

24. Mann, B. 1962. Role of pectic enzymes in the Fusarium wilt syndrome of tomato. *Trans. Br. Mycol. Soc.* **45**: 169–178.

25. Marx, J. L. 1977. Looking at lectins: Do they function in recognition processes? *Science* **196**: 1429.

26. McIntyre, J. L., J. Kuć, and E. B. Williams. 1975. Protection of Bartlett pear against fire blight with deoxyribonucleic acid from virulent and avirulent *Erwinia amylovora*. *Physiol. Plant Pathol.* **7**: 153–170.

27. Parlevliet, J. E. 1976. Evaluation of the concept of horizontal resistance in the barley/*Puccinia hordei* host-pathogen relationship. *Phytopathology* **66**: 494–497.

28. Parlevliet, J. E. 1977. Evidence of differential interaction in the polygenic *Hordeum vulgare-Puccinia hordei* relation during epidemic development. *Phytopathology* **67**: 776–778.

29. Scheffer, R. P. 1976. Host-specific toxins in relation to pathogenesis and disease resistance. *In*: R. Heitefuss and P. H. Williams (eds.). *Encyclopedia of Plant Physiology*. vol. 4. Springer-Verlag, Berlin, 890 pp.

30. Strobel, G. A. 1977. Toxins of plant pathogenic bacteria and fungi. *In*: J. Friend and D. R. Threlfall (eds.). *Biochemical Aspects of Plant-Parasite Relationships*. Academic Press, New York, p. 354.

31. Ulane, R. and M. Ogur. 1972. Genetic and physiological control of serine and glycine biosynthesis in *Saccharomyces*. *J. Bact.* **109**: 34–43.

32. Van der Plank, J. E. 1968. *Disease Resistance in Plants*. Academic Press, New York, p. 206.

33. Williams, L. G. and R. H. Davis. 1970. Pyrimidine-specific carbamyl phosphate synthetase in *Neurospora crassa*. *J. Bact.* **103**: 335–341.
34. Yamamoto, M. and K. Matsuo. 1976. Involvement of DNA in resistance of potatoes to invasion by *Phytophthora infestans*. *Nature* **259**: 63–64.
35. 1974. *Induced Mutations for Disease Resistance in Crop Plants*. I.A.E.A., Vienna, p. 193.

Recognition and Specificity in Plant Host-Parasite Interactions, pp. 33-47, 1979

MODES OF METABOLIC DETERMINATION OF SPECIFICITY

JOSEPH KUĆ

Department of Plant Pathology, University of Kentucky, Kentucky, U.S.A.

Susceptibility and resistance are subjective evaluations of disease. A susceptible plant does, and a resistant plant does not, have its development affected severely enough to cause significant economic or aesthetic loss. Resistance and susceptibility, therefore, are not absolute. Environment, inoculum density, resistance to vectors are some factors which influence resistance or susceptibility. A small fleck on a tobacco leaf may be an example of susceptibility, whereas the same size fleck on wheat may be an example of high resistance. Investigators studying economic susceptibility may at times be studying metabolic resistance, and resistance or susceptibility may be poor criteria to determine specificity of recognition in plant-parasite interactions.

Does resistance depend upon the activation of a mechanism in the host which is unique for its role in defense against disease, and is this activation elicited by structural components or metabolites unique to the infectious agent? A metabolic process which is uniquely a defense reaction against disease has not been demonstrated in plants. Nevertheless, many cases of induced resistance in plants, when considered on the nonmolecular level, resemble immunization in animals. Cultivar nonpathogenic races of pathogens, attenuated pathogens, avirulent forms of pathogens, nonpathogens, metabolites of infectious agents, and the pathogen itself protect plants against disease, and in some cases the protection appears systemic (*5, 6, 9, 11, 13–15, 40, 42, 43, 45, 47, 48*). Induced resistance may or may not be dependent on the same mechanism as resistance initiated by a pathogen in a resistant host. Many reports are available on the effect of environmental factors on disease registance, *e.g.*, soil nutrients, soil pH, temperature, daylength, hormonal balance, frost injury, hail damage. Investigators, however, are often less intrigued by the reports of the effect of environmental conditions on resistance than they are of the effects of infections agents on resistance. The implication is often that resistance induced by an infectious agent is due to the activation of a unique defense mechanism comparable to the antibody-antigen reaction in animals. Evidence to support this contention is meager; nevertheless, plants have extremely effective mechanism, unique or not unique, which protect them from disease. A study of these mechanisms is complicated by the difficulty in differentiating metabolic processes which determine specificity in plant-parasite interaction from those that are the result of disease.

I. THE PLANT SURFACE

Cutin and suberin are structural components localized at plant surfaces. A major role assigned to these polymers is the protection of the plant from dehydration and infection (*16, 34, 46*). Components of the cuticle and suberin, however, may provide more than a physical barrier to pathogens. Some of the hydroxy and epoxy acid monomers of cutin and suberin are highly toxic to infectious agents. If the pathogen hydrolyzes these polymers to gain entry into the plant, the covalently bound toxicants are released and can provide protection for the plant. The covalent attachment of toxic materials to the polymers provides protection when needed, *i.e.*, in the presence of an infectious agent, but the insoluble storage form of the monomers is not toxic to the plant. The epoxy acids, which are components of cutin from many plants, are highly toxic to plants when administered as the free monomers (*35*). Aromatic compounds are also covalently attached to cutin and suberin. Recently, *p*-hydroxycinnamic acid and other phenolics were isolated from apple fruit cutin hydrolyzed with alkali (*34*). *Fusarium solani* f. *pisi* utilized cutin as a source of carbon and produced two extracellular enzymes, a cutinase and *p*-nitrophenyl esterase (*49*). The cutinase released many cutin monomers, whereas the *p*-nitrophenyl ester hydrolase may be specific for the hydrolysis of phenolic components. The fungus detoxicated liberated epoxy acids by producing an epoxide hydrase (*36*). Suberization has been recognized for centuries as a protective mechanism in Irish potato tubers, and seed pieces of tuber are commonly allowed to suberize before planting. Suberized potato slices, even of cultivars lacking major "*R*" genes for resistance, are resistant to *Phytophthora infestans* (*52*). Unlike cutin which generally contains lower quantities of covalently bound phenolics, as much as two-thirds of suberin may consist of phenolic compounds (*27*). Thus, infectious agents on or in suberized tissue would be potentially exposed not only to liberated hydroxy and epoxy acids but also liberated or bound phenolics and their oxidation products. The suberin of wound periderm in Irish potato tubers appears identical in its major components to the suberin in the peel of tubers (*34*), and suberin and the rate of suberization may represent both passive and active mechanisms for disease resistance in plants.

In addition to suberization, lignification also rapidly occurs around wounds in foliage and storage tissues, and the process is quite common in the plant kingdom (*17*). The lignins are not merely phenolic polymers resistant to degradation by microbial enzymes, but they also often contain phenolic acids esterified to either a lignin core or polysaccharide components (*20, 41*). The esterified acids are easily liberated by dilute alkali or microbial esterase. Lignin has been frequently suggested to function as a physical barrier to the development of pathogens or interfere with the action of extracellular microbial hydrolases by making pectic substances and other carbohydrates resistant to degradation. An additional mechanism for restricting development of infectious agents may be based upon oxidizable phenolics bound to lignins, polysaccharides or lipid components of cutin or suberin. Phenolics covalently bound to a core polymer might still be subject to oxidation by phenoloxidases and peroxidases, but they would not be subject to polymerization. The stabilized quinones could disrupt oxidationreduction potentials and participate in 1, 4 additions to components on the walls of infectious agents or detoxicate extracellular hydrolases or toxins produced by infectious agents. Phenolics might function, therefore, as rather non-specific binding and detoxication agents localized at plant surfaces and cell walls.

II. WOUND RESPONSE AS RELATED TO INFECTION

A defense mechanism does not become less interesting or effective because it is part of a generalized wound response or repair mechanism in plants, and the defense against disease in plants may be based in part on a response to injury. In animals, it is seldom that an infectious agent reaches the highly specific immune response. Similarly in plants, high specificity may only be applicable to less than 1% of the interactions where the infectious agent has coped with numerous non-specific mechanism for resistance. Many metabolic responses to infection, including the accumulation of phytoalexins, seem to be enhancements of the wound or repair response. Infected host-tissues, however, are also subjected to extracellular enzymes and metabolites produced by non viral infectious agents or to a reorientation of metabolism as directed by a virus. It is not surprising, therefore, that some qualitative as well as quantitative differences are often apparent between the metabolic responses to wounding and infection.

The interactions of potato tuber with *P. infestans* and sweet potato root with *Ceratocystis fimbriata* have received a great deal of attention. Both are characterized by profound shifts in metabolism and the accumulation of terpenoid and phenolic phytoalexins. A high concentration of the steroid glycoalkaloids α-solanine and α-chaconine is localized in the peel of potato tubers and to a depth of 1 or 2 mm below the cut surface of slices (*29, 31, 44*). The concentration which accumulates in the top mm of peeled tissue may reach or surpass that in the peel (*51, 52*). Steroid glycoalkaloid accumulation is suppressed and the accumulation of sesquiterpenoids is enhanced in slices inoculated with incompatible races of *P. infestans* or some nonpathogens of potato (*44*). Compatible races of *P. infestans* suppress accumulation of both groups of terpenoids (*12, 44, 57*). The level of the major furanoterpenoid, ipomeamarone, may reach 1–2% of the fresh weight of the upper mm of sweet potato slices infected with *C. fimbriata* (*54*). A considerable amount of carbon and energy are required to accomplish these biosyntheses. It is unlikely that fatty acids are the principal source of acetyl CoA and energy required for terpenoid synthesis in potato tubers. The tubers are low in storage lipids and, though acyl hydrolases and lipoxygenases are liberated and α- and β-oxidation are active in cut tissue (*18, 19, 26, 33*), overall fatty acid metabolism becomes rapidly directed toward the synthesis of suberin and various cytoplasmic and mitochondrial membranes (*33*).

The synthesis of suberin and new cells necessary for periderm formation requires an increased availability of fatty acids and the incorporation of acetate-1-^{14}C into lipids is enhanced several fold during the first 4 hr after cutting (*61*). The incorporation of acetate -1-^{14}C into total lipids, polar lipids, and neutral fats reaches a maximum within 10–12 hr and is subsequently appreciably slowed down. The rapid synthesis of fatty acids and their incorporation into new membranes may be a key factor of the repair mechanism to return the tissue to "normalcy." The contribution of lipids to respiration of potato slices appears significant only during the first 24 hr after cutting, and subsequently the source of carbon is predominantly carbohydrate, probably starch (*30*).

Starch degradation is evident 9–12 hr after slicing potato tubers, and after 48 hr most of the starch in the phellogen and phellem cells is degraded (*33*). Starch degradation is largely due to enhanced phosphorylase activity (*33*); therefore, glucose-1-P is likely to be the major carbon precursor entering the metabolic pool from which terpenoids are synthesized. One level of metabolic control of terpenoid accumulation is at the fundamental step which liberates glucose from starch. Pathways competing for acetyl CoA could be additional points of control. What is the signal which initiates the profound metabolic changes associated with the "wound response" and which have as one consequence the increased accumulation of terpenoids? Slicing a potato tuber does not introduce a polysaccharide elicitor from a fungus; nevertheless, the rapid accumulation of steroid glycoalkaloids is initiated. Slicing a potato tuber has been reported to immediately release CO_2 trapped in the tuber (*33*). The periderms of the potato tuber and sweet potato root may function as a barrier to diffusion of CO_2, and levels above 5% have been reported in potato tuber and sweet potato root (*21, 33, 60*). The release of CO_2 is temporary and within 1–2 hr is ended. At this time, respiratory activity of cut tuber discs is 5–10 times that of tissue within the intact tuber. The signal for terpenoid biosynthesis and accumulation may be the sudden release of CO_2 which removes a brake to metabolic activity and activates phosphorylase. Within 10–12 hr fatty acid synthesis markedly declines (*1*), and if the activity of glucose metabolism *via* the pentose pathway and glycolysis has not declined, acetyl CoA may accumulate and be shunted off to the synthesis of terpenoids. Indeed, the accumulation of steroid glycoalkaloids beneath a slice surface in potato tubers requires a lag period of 12–24 hr and does not reach a maximum until 96–144 hr after slicing (*51, 52*). The steroid glycoalkaloids may represent a trap for acetyl CoA until periderm and suberin formation are sufficient to once again brake metabolism. The steroid glycoalkaloids may, however, be more than a "metabolic safety valve." Their antibiotic activity (*2*) and localization at the wounded surface may make them an important part of the wound repair process.

Some enzymes of the acetate-mevalonate pathway increase in activity to accomodate the accumulation of furanoterpenoids in sweet potato roots as well as steroid glycoalkaloids and norsesqui and sesquiterpenoids in potato tubers (*55*). In addition, increased glucose oxidation *via* the pentose pathway and tricarboxylic acid cycle occurs shortly after slicing. Glucose-6-P dehydrogenase and gluconate-6-P dehydrogenase activities increase 100–500% within 2 days of slicing potato tubers or sweet potato root (*33*). The activations are not dependent upon a specific elicitor present or produced by infectious agents, and reagents as simple as mercuric chloride elicit the accumulation of considerable quantities of furanoterpenoids.

Neither furanoterpenoids nor the norsesqui and sesquiterpenoids of potato are stable end products of metabolism (*24, 29, 39*). They reach a peak in accumulation 96–120 hr after infection or treatment with elicitors and the levels decrease until they are barely detectable 7–10 days after treatment. Their accumulation, therefore, may be as much a result of decreased degradation as a result of increased synthesis. Thus, elicitors for the accumulation of these phytoalexins may be inhibitors of degradation or elicitors of increased synthesis.

Many of the metabolic alterations described for wounded potato tubers and sweet potato roots are also valid for other storage organs (*33*). Similar wound responses may occur in nonstorage tissues, and they must be evaluated when considering the "specific" elicitation of phytoalexin accumulation and the biosynthesis and degradation of phytoalexins.

III. COORDINATED DEFENSE

During the past twenty years considerable progress have been made in elucidating the modes of elicitation, structure, biosynthesis, and degradation of phytoalexins. The work has catalyzed research in the field of plant pathology and plant biochemistry and contributed significantly to our understanding of factors influencing the interaction of plants with infectious agents. To my knowledge, however, phytoalexins have not unequivocally explained a single case of varietal resistance or susceptibility. Much evidence supports their role in protecting nonhosts against infectious agents (*38*); however, they are not elicited by all nonpathogens of a plant. The presence of substantial quantities of pisatin in young expanding lesions containing the pisatin-sensitive root rot pathogen *Apanomyces euteiches* is not consistent with the suggested role of pisatin as a phytoalexin (*56*). Phytoalexins are not initial determinants of specificity (*40*), and various forms of stress elicit their accumulation (*38, 40, 53*). Nevertheless, phytoalexins have been isolated and characterized in many species of the leguminosae and other plant families (*11, 38*). They accumulate in or around infection sites to levels which inhibit the development of many infectious agents *in vitro*. Whether they accumulate quickly enough to be the first, only, or major factors restricting growth of infectious agents is under debate. The evidence supporting the role of phytoalexins is largely circumstantial; nevertheless, they cannot be ignored, and in my judgment, they have a role in disease resistance. Another class of compounds, the phytoagglutinins (plant lectins), may also contribute to determining specificity and may augment the action of phytoalexins. These compounds are proteins or glycoproteins that bind to specific carbohydrates.

Induced resistance has been observed with numerous bacterial and fungal diseases (*5, 11, 37, 38, 40, 47*). Since heat-killed cells often elicited protection, it seems quite likely that a chemical substance might be the active elicitor. Huang, Huang, and Goodman (*28*) and Goodman, Huang, Huang and Thaipanich (*22*) reported the rapid agglutination of avirulent, but not virulent, *E. amylovora* in apple shoots. Even more exciting was their observation that *Pseudomonas pisi* and *E. amylovora* elicited the accumulation of soluble agglutinins. Professor Sequeira's chapter deals in depth with his interesting work associating lectins with resistance of tobacco to *Ps. solanacearum*. The mechanism for the recognition of compatible or incompatible bacteria that is suggested by his work involves the interaction of three components: a) Bacterial lipopolysaccharide, which may represent the binding site for host lectin; b) bacterial extracellular polysaccharide, which interferes with binding; and, c) host cell wall lectin.

Investigators in the field may argue about which is the initial or most important mechanism for disease resistance (or susceptibility) in plants. Such arguments may be fruitless in that two or more distinct mechanisms may be operative and the presence of both mechanisms and their coordination may determine the specificity of the interaction. Interactions in which phytoalexins accumulate but the plant is judged susceptible may be due to a lack of or inadequacy in a second mechanism. The second mechanism may be the presence or induced production of agglutinins.

A thought-provoking paper by Uritani and his colleagues (*55*) presents data which support this view. They report that resistance of sweet potato root to nonpathogenic isolates of *C. fimbriata* is based on at least two mechanisms. In the initial stage of infection, agglutinating factors in host cells may agglutinate spores and germinating hyphae thereby localizing the fungus. In the second stage, both pathogenic and nonpathogenic strains of the fungus elicit the accumulation of furano-terpenoids in host tissue. The implication is that the speed of development of the pathogenic strain exceeds the accumulation of fungitoxic levels of furanoterpenoids due to a lack of agglutination, whereas spread of the nonpathogenic strain is limited by agglutination which allows furanoterpenoids to accumulate to fungitoxic levels in and around the site of interaction between host and fungus. This concept is consistent with our investigations of the systemically induced resistance of cucumber to *Colletotrichum lagenarium* by *C. lagenarium* (*7, 8, 32, 42, 45*). Infection of a cotyledon or first true leaf (leaf one) of cucumber with *C. lagenarium* systemically protects cucumber plants against disease caused by subsequent challenge with the pathogen. Protection is evident as a reduction in the number and size of lesions and lasts for 4–5 weeks. A second or booster inoculation, 3 weeks after the first inoculation, extends the time of protection into the fruiting period. A single lesion produces significant protection.

Watermelon and muskmelon are similarly protected. Cucumber plants are also systemically protected against the disease by prior infection with *Ps. lachrymans* or tobacco necrosis virus (TNV). Since protection is elicited by infection with a virus, metabolites synthesized by infectious agents or polysaccharide cell wall components of fungi are not the only factors capable of eliciting protection. Protection was not elicited against TNV either by TNV or by *C. lagenarium*, but *Ps. lachrymans* and *C. lagenarium* were mutually protective.

Cucumber and watermelon are also protected in the field. In one trial with cucumbers, the total area occupied by lesions on protected plants was less than 2% of the lesion area of unprotected plants. Similarly, 47 of 69 unprotected challenged watermelons died, whereas 1 of 66 protected challenged plants died.

There is no evidence that the systemic accumulation of classical phytoalexins is alone responsible for the protection. A chloroform-soluble inhibitor of the growth of *C. lagenarium* has been obtained from tissue surrounding lesions on protected and unprotected plants. The inhibitor may be important in restricting lesion development and account for the normally restricted lesions characteristic of cucurbit anthracnose. Spore germination and appresoria formation are not inhibited on protected plants, but development from the appresoria appears reduced in protected plants. Penetration from appresoria was 20 to 40% and from less than 1 to 5% in unprotected and protected plants, respectively. The presence of a preformed agglutinin appears associated with resistance of cucumber to scab (*25*). Studies also indicate an agglutinating factor accumulates in unchallenged plants systemically protected by *C. lagenarium.* It is possible that at least three mechanisms contribute to acquired resistance of cucurbits to *C. lagenarium.* One mechanism restricts penetration into the host, a second agglutinates developing hyphae in penetrated tissue to minimize spread, and the third is the production of phytoalexins around the site of infection. The agglutinins may restrict spread of bacteria and fungi by agglutinating the infectious agent or by reacting with their extracellular hydrolytic enzymes or toxins. The systemic protection of cucurbits resembles the systemic elicitation of protease inhibitors in wounded plants (*23, 59*) though injury does not itself elicit protection. Injury of leaves of plants representing several plant families or the introduction of extracts from injured tissues into plants elicits the systemic accumulation of protease inhibitors. Protein in responding tissues markedly changes and as much as 12% of the protein in affected tissues is protease inhibitor with a high content of disulfide cross linkages.

The elicitor of protease inhibitor accumulation is still uncharacterized but the implications of this "long distance" communication are profound in relation to disease resistance and practical control of disease. Several possible ingredients of a defense system become apparent: 1) A rapid "long distance" system of communication; 2) presence and/or elicitation of protein or glycoprotein enzyme inhibitors and agglutinins; 3) presence and/or elicitation of phytoalexins. In a coordinated defense against disease, any one or two mechanisms for resistance may be active, but if a third is inactive it may become the limiting factor for resistance and the plant is susceptible. Plants with mechanisms for resistance, therefore, can in fact be susceptible. Induced resistance may be based on the marked activation of a mechanism which is not limiting to defense to a level that overcomes the limitation of a deficient factor, *e.g.*, phytoalexins accumulate rapidly enough and with sufficient magnitude to eliminate the need of an agglutinin. In other situations, induced resistance may enhance a limiting factor in the coordinated mechanism. The key to disease resistance in plants may be the functioning of multiple mechanisms for resistance and the key concept in understanding their interaction is one of "coordinated defense." Of course, the infectious agent also influences the effectiveness or coordination of host defense. The active contribution of the infectious agent makes the interaction complex but at the same time increases many-fold the possibilities for specificity.

IV. ELICITORS

The work with elicitors has emphasized only a single possible aspect of defense—the accumulation of phytoalexins. The importance of elicitors studied to date, therefore, is dependent on the importance of phytoalexins in resistance. Cruickshank (*10*) reported monilicolin A, a peptide produced by *Monilinia fructicola*, elicited phaseollin accumulation in green bean at 2.5×10^{-9} M, but it did not elicit the accumulation of phytoalexins in pea or broad bean. Elicitors of phytoalexins accumulation have also been isolated from culture filtrates and mycelia of *C. lindemuthianum* (*3*) and *P. megosperma* var. *sojae* (*4*). These probably have a basic carbohydrate core of β 1→3 and β 1→6 glucopyranose units, but other sugars or polyols may be important for elicitation. There is no evidence to indicate that elicitors determine varietal resistance or the resistance of nonhosts. It is intriguing to speculate that since some of the elicitors are extracellularly produced or located on or in cell walls, and, since some are extremely active elicitors of phytoalexin accumulation, that they are important in activating defense mechanisms in a host. The list of phytoalexin elicitors, however, includes hundreds of chemical compounds as well as various form of injury. Recently, Robinson and Wood (*50*) reported that sucrose, galactose, glucose, and raffinose increased the accumulation of pisatin in pea leaf discs. It is not evident that the elicitors of phytoalexin accumulation characterized to date determine specificity. A recent article (*58*) supports this point of view: "Phytoalexin production is regarded as considerably more remote, and certainly without direct relation to specificity. In fact there is evidence that it represents only part of a major stimulation of secondary metabolic activity that follows a hypersensitive response, a part that has been recognized because its products are fungitoxic. . . ."

SUMMARY

Coordinated defense may be a key to resistance. It may encompass explanations for the presence of mechanisms for resistance in susceptible plants, genetic control of resistance, and complexity of the resistance phenomenon. Though many factors may contribute to coordinated defense, three seem highly intriguing and there is some evidence to support each: a) Rapid systemic communication of signals in higher plants; 2) presence and production of phytoagglutinins; 3) presence or production of phytoalexins.

Acknowledgments

Journal paper No. 77-11-161 of the Kentucky Agricultural Experiment Station, Lexington, Kentucky 40506, U.S.A. The author's work reported in this paper was supported in part by a grant from the Herman Frasch Foundation and Grant 316-15-51 of the Cooperative State Research Service of the United States Department of Agriculture.

REFERENCES

1. Abdelkader, A., P. Mazliak, and A. Catesson. 1969. Biogenese des lipides mitochondriaux aux cours de la "survie" (ageing) de disques de parenchyme de tubercule de pomme de terre. *Phytochemistry* **8**: 1121–1133.
2. Allen, E. and J. Kuć. 1968. α-Solanine and α-chaconine as fungi-toxic compounds in extracts of Irish potato tubers. *Phytopathology* **58**: 776–781.
3. Anderson-Prouty, A. and P. Albersheim. 1975. Isolation of a pathogen-synthesized fraction rich in glucan that elicits a defense response in the pathogen's host. *Plant Physiol.* **56**: 286–291.
4. Ayers, A., B. Valent, J. Ebel, and P. Albersheim. 1976. Composition and structure of wall-released elicitor fractions. *Plant Physiol.* **57**: 766–774.
5. Bell, A. and J. Presley. 1969. Heat-inhibited or heat-killed conidia of *Verticillium albo-atrum* induce disease resistance and phytoalexin accumulation in cotton. *Phytopathology* **59**: 1147–1151.
6. Braun, J. and A. Helton. 1971. Induced resistance to *Cytospora* in *Prunus persica*. *Phytopathology* **61**: 685–687.
7. Caruso, J. and J. Kuć. 1977. Field protection of cucumber against *Colletotrichum lagenarium* by *Colletotrichum lagenarium*. *Phytopathology* **67**: 1290–1292.
8. Caruso, J. and J. Kuć. 1977. Protection of watermelon and muskmelon against *Colletotrichum lagenarium* by *Colletotrichum lagenarium*. *Phytopathology* **67**: 1285–1289.
9. Cruickshank, I. and M. Mandryk. 1960. The effect of stem infestation of tobacco with *Peronospora tabacina* on foliage infection to blue mould. *J. Aust. Inst. Agric. Sci.* **26**: 369–372.
10. Cruickshank, I. and D. Perrin. 1968. The isolation and partial characterization of monilicolin A, a polypeptide with phaseollin-inducing activity from *Monilinia fructicola*. *Life Sci.* **7**: 449–458.
11. Deverall, B. 1977. *Defense Mechanisms in Plants*. Cambridge Univ. Press, London, p. 110.

12. Doke, N. 1975. Prevention of the hypersensitive reaction of potato cells to infection with an incompatible race of *Phytophthora infestans* by constituents of zoospores. *Physiol. Plant Pathol.* **7**: 1–7.
13. Elliston, J., J. Kuć, and E. B. Williams. 1971. Induced resistance to bean anthracnose at a distance from the site of the inducing interaction. *Phytopathology* **61**: 1110–1112.
14. Elliston, J., J. Kuć, and E. B. Williams. 1976a. Protection of *Phaseolus vulgaris* against anthracnose by *Colletotrichum* species nonpathogenic to bean. *Phytopathol. Z.* **86**: 117–126.
15. Elliston, J. E., J. Kuć, and E. B. Williams. 1976b. A comparative study of the development of compatible, incompatible, and induced incompatible interactions between *Colletotrichum* spp. and *Phaseolus vulgaris. Phytopathol. Z.* **87**: 289–303.
16. Ende, G. and H. Linskens. 1974. Cutinolytic enzymes in relation to pathogenesis. *Annu. Rev. Phytopathol.* **12**: 247–258.
17. Friend, J. 1976. Lignification in infected tissue. *In*: J. Friend and D. Threlfall (eds.). *Biochemical Aspects of Plant-Parasite Relationships*. Academic Press, London, New York, pp. 291–303.
18. Galliard, T. 1973. Lipids of potato tubers. *J. Sci. Food Agric.* **24**: 617–622.
19. Galliard, T. 1975. Degradation of plant lipids by hydrolytic and oxidative enzymes. *In*: T. Galliard and E. Mercer (eds.). *Recent Advances Chemistry and Biochemistry of Lipids*. Academic Press, New York, pp. 319–357.
20. Gee, M., I. Nelson, and J. Kuć. 1968. Abnormal lignins produced by the brown midrib mutants of Maize II. Comparative studies on normal and brown midrib-1-dimethylformamide lignins. *Arch. Biochem. Biophys.* **123**: 403–408.
21. Gerhardt, F. 1942. Simulaneous measurement of the carbon dioxide and organic volatiles of the internal atmosphere of fruits and vegetables. *Agric. Res.* **64**: 207–219.
22. Goodman, R., P. Huang, J. Huang, and V. Thaipanich. 1976. Induced resistance to bacterial infection. *In*: K. Tomiyama, J. M. Daly, I. Uritani, H. Oku, and S. Ouchi (eds.). *Biochemistry and Cytology of Plant-Parasite Interaction*. Kodansha Ltd., Tokyo and Elsevier, New York, pp. 35–42.
23. Gustafson, G. and C. Ryan. 1976. Specificity of protein turnover in tomato leaves. Accumulation of proteinase inhibitors induced with the wound hormone PIIF. *J. Biol. Chem.* **251**: 7004–7010.
24. Haard, N. and P. Weiss. 1976. Influence of exogenous ethylene on ipomeamarone accumulation in black rot infected sweet potato roots. *Phytochemistry* **15**: 261–262.
25. Hammerschmidt, R. and J. Kuć. 1977. Agglutinins as factors in the resistance of cucumber to scab. *Proc. Am. Phytopathol. Soc.* **4**: 159.
26. Hasson, E. and G. Laties. 1976. Separation and characterization of potato lipid acylhydrolases. *Plant Physiol.* **57**: 142–147.

27. Holloway, P. 1972a. Composition of suberin from the corks of *Quercus suber, Betula pendula,* and some *Ribes* species. *Chem. Phys. Lipids* **9**: 158–170, 171–179.

28. Huang, P., J. Huang, and R. Goodman. 1975. Resistance mechanisms of apple shoots to an avirulent strain of *Erwinia amylovora. Physiol. Plant Pathol.* **6**: 283–287.

29. Ishizaka, N. and K. Tomiyama. 1972. Effect of wounding or infection by *Phytophthora infestans* on the contents of terpenoids in potato tubers. *Plant Cell Physiol.* **13**: 1053–1063.

30. Jacobson, B., B. Smith, S. Epstein, and G. Laties. 1970. The prevalence of carbon-13 in respiratory carbon dioxide as an indicator of the type of endogenous substrate. *J. Gen. Physiol.* **55**: 1–17.

31. Jadhav, S. and F. Solunkhe. 1975. Formation and control of chlorophyll and glycoalkaloid in tubers of *Solanum tuberosum* L. and evaluation of glycoalkaloid toxicity. *Adv. Food Res.* **21**: 307–354.

32. Jenns, A. and J. Kuć. 1977. Localized infection with tobacco necrosis virus protects cucumber against *Colletotrichum lagenarium. Physiol. Plant Pathol.* **11**: 207–212.

33. Kahl, G. 1974. Metabolism in plant storage tissue slices. *Bot. Rev.* **40**: 263–314.

34. Kolatlukudy, P. 1975. Biochemistry of cutin, suberin, and waxes, the lipid barriers on plants. *In*: T. Galliard and E. Mercer (eds.). *Recent Advances in the Chemistry and Biochemistry of Plant Lipids.* Academic Press, New York, pp. 203–246.

35. Kolatlukudy, P., T. Walton, and R. Kushawaha. 1973. Biosynthesis of the C_{18} family of cutin acids: ω-Hydroxyoleic acid, ω-hydroxy-9,10-epoxystearic acid, 9,10,18-trihydroxystearic acid, and their Δ^{12} unsaturated analogs. *Biochemistry* **12**: 4488–4497.

36. Kolatlukudy, P. and L. Brown. 1975. Fate of naturally occurring epoxy acids: A soluble epoxide hydrase which catalyzes *cis* hydration, from *Fusarium solani pisi. Arch. Biochem. Biophys.* **166**: 599–607.

37. Kuć, J. 1968. Biochemical control of disease resistance in plants. *World Rev. Pest Control* **7**: 42–55.

38. Kuć, J. 1972. Phytoalexins. *Annu. Rev. Phytopathol.* **10**: 207–232.

39. Kuć, J. 1975. Teratogenic constituents of potatoes. *Rec. Adv. Phytochem.* **9**: 139–150.

40. Kuć, J. 1975. Phytoalexins and the specificity of plant-parasite interaction. *In*: R. K. S. Wood and A. Graniti (eds.). *Specificity in Plant Disease.* Plenum Press, New York, pp. 253–271.

41. Kuć, J. and O. Nelson. 1964. The abnormal lignins produced by the brown-midrib mutants of maize. *Arch. Biochem. Biophys.* **105**: 103–113.

42. Kuć, J., G. Shockley, and K. Kearney. 1975. Protection of cucumber against *Collectotrichum lagenarium* by *Collectotrichum lagenarium. Physiol. Plant Pathol.* **7**: 195–199.

43. Kuć, J., W. W. Currier, J. Elliston, and J. McIntyre. 1976. Determinants of plant

disease resistance and susceptibility: A perspective based on three plant-parasite interactions. *In*: K. Tomiyama, J. Daly, I. Uritani, H. Oku, and S. Ouchi (eds.). *Biochemistry and Cytology of Plant-Parasite Interaction.* Kodansha Ltd., Tokyo and Elsevier, New York, pp. 168–180.

44. Kuć, J., W. Currier, and M. Shih. 1976. Terpenoid phytoalexins. *In*: J. Friend and D. R. Threlfall (eds.). *Biochemical Aspects of Plant-Parasite Relationships.* Academic Press, London, pp. 225–257.
45. Kuć, J. and S. Richmond. 1977. Aspects of the protection of cucumber against *Colletotrichum lagenarium* by *Colletotrichum lagenarium. Phytopathology* **67**: 533–536.
46. Martin, J. 1964. Role of cuticle in the defense against plant disease. *Annu. Rev. Phytopathol.* **2**: 81–100.
47. Matta, A. 1971. Microbial penetration and immunization of uncongenial host plants. *Annu. Rev. Phytopathol.* **9**: 387–410.
48. McIntyre, J., J. Kuć, and E. B. Williams. 1975. Protection of Bartlett pear against fireblight by deoxyribonucleic acid from virulent and avirulent *Erwinia amylovora. Physiol. Plant Pathol.* **7**: 153–170.
49. Purdy, R. and P. Kolatlukudy. 1975. Hydrolysis of plant cuticle by plant pathogens. Properties of cutinase I, cutinase II, and a nonspecific esterase isolated from *Fusarium solani pisi. Biochemistry* **14**: 2832–2840.
50. Robinson, T. and R. K. S. Wood. 1976. Factors affecting accumulation of pisatin by pea leaves. *Physiol. Plant Pathol.* **9**: 285–297.
51. Shih, M. and J. Kuć. 1973. Incorporation of ^{14}C from acetate and mevalonate into rishitin and steroid glycoalkaloids by potato slices inoculated with *Phytophthora infestans. Phytopathology* **63**: 826–829.
52. Shih, M., J. Kuć, and E. Williams. 1973. Suppression ot steroid glycoalkaloid accumulation as related to rishitin accumulation in potato tubers. *Phytopathology* **63**: 821–826.
53. Stoessl, A., J. Stothers, and E. Wood. 1976. Sesquiterpenoid stress compounds of the *Solanaceae. Phytochemistry* **15**: 855–872.
54. Uritani, I. 1963. The biochemical basis of disease resistance induced by infection. *Conn. Agric. Expt. Sta. Bull.* **663**: 4–19.
55. Uritani, I., K. Oba, M. Kojima, W. Kim, I. Oguni, and H. Suzuki. 1976. Primary and secondary defense actions of sweet potato in response to infection by *Ceratocystis fimbriata. In*: K. Tomiyama, J. Daly, I. Uritani, H. Oku, and S. Ouchi (eds.). *Biochemistry and Cytology of Plant-Parasite Interaction.* Kodansha Ltd., Tokyo and Elsevier, New York, pp. 239–252.
56. Van Etten, H. and S. G. Pueppke. 1976. The relation between pisatin and the development of *Apanomyces euteiches* in diseased *Pisum sativum. Phytopathology* **66**: 1174–1185.
57. Varns, J. and J. Kuć. 1972. Suppression of the resistance response as an active mechanism for susceptibility in the potato—*Phytophthora infestans* interaction.

In: R. K. S. Wood, A. Ballio, and A. Graniti (eds.). *Phytotoxins in Plant Diseases.* Academic Press, London and New York, pp. 465–468.

58. Ward, E. and A. Stoessl. 1976. On the question of "elicitors" or "inducers" in incompatible interactions between plants and fungal pathogens. *Phytopathology* **66**: 940–941.
59. Walker-Simmons, M. and C. Ryan. 1977. Wound induced accumulation of trypsin inhibitor activities in plant leaves. *Plant Physiol.* **59**: 437–439.
60. Whiteman, T. and H. Schomes. 1945. Respiration and internal gas content of injured sweet-potato roots. *Plant Physiol.* **20**: 171–182.
61. Willemot, C. and P. Stumpf. 1967. Fat metabolism in higher plants. *Plant Physiol.* **42**: 391–397.

Recognition and Specificity in Plant Host-Parasite Interactions, pp. 49-65, 1979

THE INDUCTION OF RESISTANCE OR SUSCEPTIBILITY

SEIJI OUCHI, CHIHAYA HIBINO,*1 HACHIRO OKU, MICHINORI FUJIWARA, AND HIDETO NAKABAYASHI *2

College of Agriculture, Okayama University, Okayama, Japan

After one-to-one relationship between genes in the plant and the pathogen was established by Flor (*14*), genetic approaches to the host-parasite interaction became a new avenue of research in plant pathology (*10–12, 15–18, 25, 27, 39*), although Flor's gene-for-gene concept may not unitarily account for all the patterns of interactions occurring in versatile plant-parasite combinations. Powdery mildews of barley and wheat, however, are in the list of diseases to which the concept can be applied (*10–12, 15*). Genetic analysis of these powdery mildews clearly demonstrated that a particular race elicites a genetically defined response in a given host cultivar, either susceptibility or resistance depending on their genetic constituents, and thus provides useful information in the establishment of the biochemical basis of specificity (*11, 12, 44*).

Even though molecular mechanisms of genic regulation in higher organisms are still at the stage of speculation, it seems necessary for plant pathologists to integrate biochemical data accumulated in the past in terms of gene function. Day (*10*) reviewed biochemical studies on plant-parasite

*1 Chuno Senior High School, Mugi-cho, Gifu 501–35, Japan.
*2 Shimonoseki West Senior High School, Toyoura-cho, Yamaguchi 759–63, Japan.

interactions from this aspect and put forth a model of genic regulation, and Albersheim (*2*) proposed a hypothesis on molecular basis of varietal specificity in gene-for-gene systems.

Induced resistance or susceptibility associated with obligate parasitism has been the subject of many studies (*18, 20, 21, 35, 36, 45, 49*). However, molecular mechanism of cross protection in obligate parasitism has not yet been elucidated clearly, although phytoalexin activity is likely involved in this phenomenon (*23, 30, 31*), and practically nothing is known about the mechanism of induced susceptibility. Induced susceptibility, accessibility in our terminology, especially when it was triggered by biotrophs, is thought to provide useful information for analysing the function of genes in plant-parasite interaction, and, at a practical level, may help the exploitation of molecular mechanisms of mutual recognition between hosts and parasites. Thus we discuss in this paper some biological phenomena associated with interactions between powdery mildew fungi and their host plants with an emphasis on induced resistance or susceptibility.

I. INDUCTION

Preliminary infection often predisposes the plant to other etiological agents (*48, 50*), and much information has become available on induced susceptibility against powdery mildews (*28, 35, 36, 46, 49*). Moseman, Scharen, and Greeley (*28*) demonstrated that wheat powdery mildew propagated on barley leaves which had been inoculated with compatible race of barley powdery mildew. Tsuchiya and Hirata (*46*) showed that among 51 powdery mildew fungi collected from different species of plants 45 were capable of growing on barley leaves that had been infected by *Erysiphe graminis hordei*. Our results presented in this treatise extend these previous information on induced susceptibility and elucidate with genetically defined materials that induction of resistance or susceptibility (accessibility) depends largely on genetic constituents of the host and parasite involved in the primary interaction.

Three cultivars of barley (*Hordeum vulgare*), H.E.S. 4(compatible with race Hh4), Russian 74(compatible with race Hr74), and cultivar Kobinkatagi(compatible with race 1) were mainly used. A near-isogenic line derived from Kobinkatagi X *Hordeum spontaneum nigrum*(immune to any race found in Japan) was also used in some experiments. As pathogens, *E. graminis hordei* races 1, Hh4, Hr74, *E. graminis tritici* race t_2, and *Sphaerotheca fuliginea* from melon were used. All these races were propagated on their respective compatible host plants and partially synchronized before use by a modified procedure of Nair and Ellingboe (*29*).

Leaves of H.E.S. 4 were first inoculated with conidia of race Hh4(compatible) or Hr74(incompatible) and incubated at 20°C for 48 hr. The primary inoculum on the leaves was removed by rubbing with a wet cotton ball, and the leaves were then challenge-inoculated with either race. The percentage of conidia with elongated secondary hyphae and the length of hyphae were measured 48 hr after the challenge inoculation. The results (*35*) showed that the leaves inoculated with an incompatible race became resistant, inaccessible in our term, to a primarily compatible race, giving rise to a lower infection frequency and shorter hyphal length, while those that had been induced with a compatible race became more susceptible than non-induced ones to the originally incompatible race, as was reflected on higher infection frequency and longer hyphal length. Essentially similar results were obtained when Russian 74 was used as a test plant (*35*). Induced susceptibility(accessibility) was more clearly demonstrated when the leaves that had been inoculated with a compatible race were challenged by race t_2 of the wheat fungus (*35*). A fact worth noting here is that the leaves that had been induced with incompatible race(Hr74) supported a significant growth of race t_2 while they inhibited establishment and hyphal growth of a compatible race of barley fungus. The most explicit demonstration of induced accessibility was made by inoculating *Sph. fuliginea*, the melon fungus, on leaves that had been induced with compatible or incompatible race of barley fungus. Barley leaves supported the growth of the nonpathogenic melon fungus provided they had been preliminarily inoculated with compatible race, as had been expected (Fig. 1). The leaves that had been inoculated with incompatible race (Hr74) or wheat fungus also permitted the melon fungus to grow in contrast with the expectation that these leaves should have been induced to become inaccessible (*36*). At first glance, these were puzzling and seemed to contradict with the concept of induced accessibility, but were accounted for by setting forth the following two assumptions; (1) regardless of their compatibility, conidia that succeeded in breaking the primary barrier (recognition) and established a pseudosymbiotic relation with cell it invaded might actively and continously suppress operation of cellular defense mechanisms; (2) the area that this suppression is effective might be extremely limited. The validity of these assumptions will be elaborated in detail in the following sections.

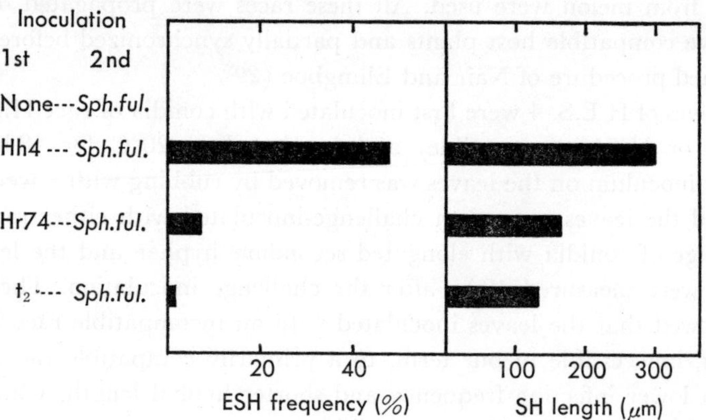

Fig. 1. Infection by *Sph. fuliginea* (*Sph. ful.*) of barley leaves that had been condi tioned by compatible or incompatible race of *E. graminis hordei*. Barley leaves (H.E.S.4) were first inoculated with compatible (Hh4) or incompatible (Hr74) of *E. graminis hordei* or race t_2 of *E. graminis tritici* and 48 hr later were reinoculated with conidia of *Sph. fuliginea*. Affinity indices were determined 48 hr after challenge inoculation (*36*).

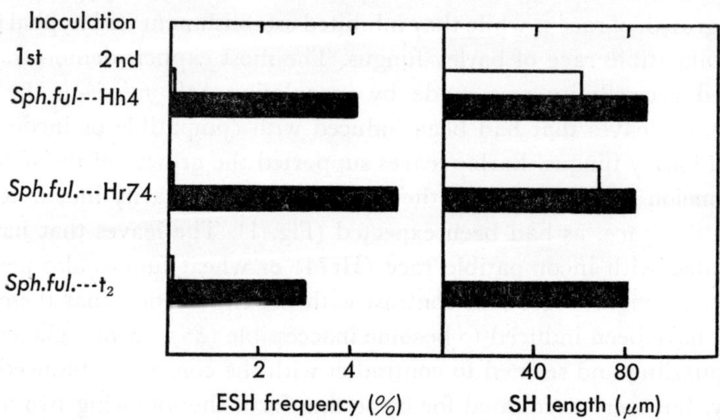

Fig. 2. Infection by *E. graminis hordei* and *E. graminis tritici* of melon leaves that had been primarily infected by *Sph. fuliginea*. Melon leaves (Earl's Favorite) were inoculated with conidia of *Sph. fuliginea* and were then challenged by conidia of races (Hh4, Hr74) of *E. graminis hordei* or race t_2 of *E. graminis tritici*. The infection frequency and hyphal growth of barley and wheat fungi on non-induced (open bars) and induced (closed bars) leaves were determined 48 hr after challenge inoculation (*36*).

Counterpart experiments with melon leaves elucidated that melon leaves became accessible to otherwise nonpathogenic barley and wheat powdery mildews provided they had been preliminarily infected by melon powdery mildew (Fig. 2) (*36*).

II. TIME REQUIRED FOR ESTABLISHING CELLULAR CONDITIONING

Time required for plant cells to establish an irreversible conditioning toward either rejection or permission was demonstrated by a double inoculation procedure. Barley leaves, H.E.S. 4, were inoculated either with wheat race t_2 to induce inaccessibility or with compatible race Hh4 to induce accessibility and challenged with Hh4 or melon fungus respectively with a 3-hr interval to estimate affinity indices of the challenger. Infection frequency of compatible race decreased to a statistically significant level when inoculated 6 hr after the inducer race t_2, indicating that rejection reaction had been established within 6 hr of incompatible interaction (*34*). The melon fungus, however, became capable of growing on barley leaves when it was inoculated 15–18 hr after the compatible race (*36*). This is consistent with the observation reported by Tsuchiya and Hirata (*46*). The results thus indicated that cellular conditioning toward accessibility, probably suppression of genes for resistance, requires longer period of time than that toward inaccessibility.

III. LOCALIZATION OF INDUCED RESISTANCE AND SUSCEPTIBILITY

The observation that the barley leaves that had been inoculated with wheat fungus became accessible to melon fungus which is otherwise incapable of growing on barley leaves led us to postulate that some conidia of wheat fungus which established a pseudosymbiotic association with barley cells eventually rendered the cellular state accessible to melon fungus. This assumption, however, must be followed by another assumption that the induced area might be quite restricted, to account for infection frequency of different challengers, as stated previously. The validity of these assumptions were tested by inoculating barley leaves. H.E.S. 4, with compatible Hh4 and subsequently challenging with melon fungus (*34*). The results (Fig. 3) showed that the nonpathogen colonized the cells harboring the compatible haustorium with a very high frequency, but was incapable of colonizing the

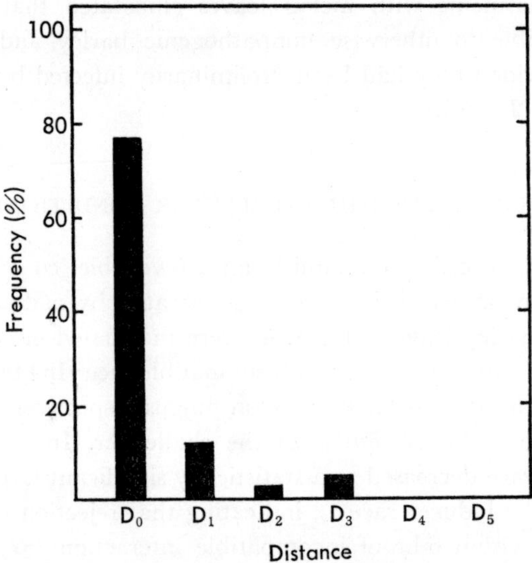

Fig. 3. Effect of preinoculation with *E. graminis hordei* (compatible race Hh4) on infection by *Sph. fuliginea* in barley leaves (H.E.S.4). Induction period was 48 hr. D_0 represents cell that harbored the haustorium of compatible race (Hh4), D_1 cells transversely adjacent to it, D_2 the one next to it, and so forth (*34*).

cells located 4 cell rows apart from the haustorium-harboring cell. Similar experiments for testing localization of induced resistance showed that the inaccessibility induced in barley leaves by race t_2 was also localized at the site where the nonpathogen had been inoculated as inducer (Fig. 4) (*34*). Thus both the induced resistance and induced susceptibility are localized in the area where the primary interaction was effectively completed. Érsek demonstrated that defense reaction induced in wheat leaves by the barley powdery mildew was localized (*13*). Localization of induced resistance (*4, 9, 23*) and susceptibility (*49*) has been reported in some other obligate parasitic diseases. Abnormal sensitivity to compatible race was also induced in cells located closely to the necrosis caused by an incompatible race in bean anthracnose (*43*). However, resistance information in cucumber anthracnose appears to become systemic (*22*).

IV. IRREVERSIBILITY OF INDUCED SUSCEPTIBILITY AND RESISTANCE

The fact that cells induced to become accessible or inaccessible lost their

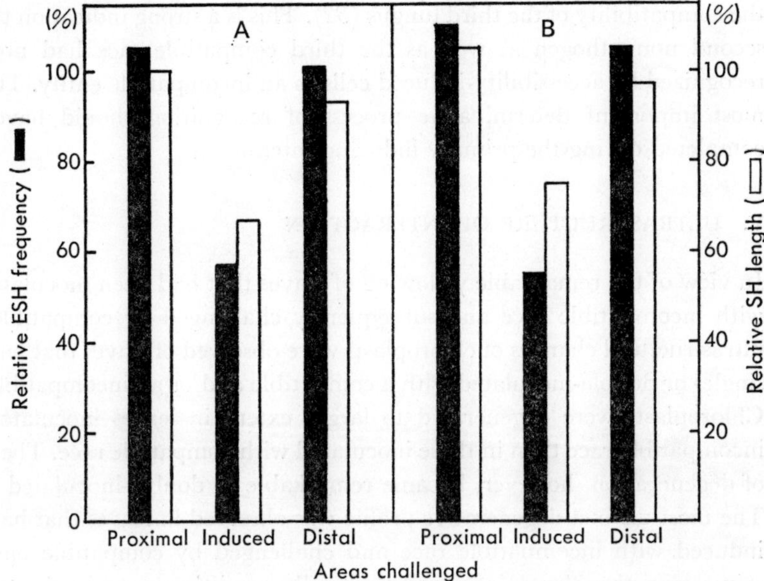

Fig. 4. Effect of induced resistance on establishment of infection by a compatible race on barley leaves. Leaves (H.E.S.4 or Kobinkatagi) were first inoculated with race t_2 of *E. graminis tritici*, then were challenged with compatible race Hh4. Indices of respective non-induced control were represented as 100. Tested with Kobinkatagi-race t_2-race 1 (compatible) (A), and H.E.S. 4-race t_2-Hh4 compatible) (B). Proximal and distal areas were separated respectively 5 mm from the induced middle part of leaves (10 mm long) (*34*).

inherent ability to recognize the challenger suggest that genic regulation of these cells related to recognition might have become irreversibly unfunctional. This irreversibility of the primary cellular conditioning was assured by the use of yellowing response of leaves that had been cross-inoculated and by a triple inoculation procedure (*34*). The leaves that had been induced to become inaccessible and was challenged by compatible race exhibited much more extensive yellowing than those challenged by incompatible race, suggesting that the cells that had been conditioned to be inaccessible now recognized the compatible race as incompatible. Unequivocal demonstration of irreversibility was further achieved by a triple inoculation. The results showed that the leaves with induced accessibility allowed the third fungus to grow to the same extent regardless of the second fungus and the hyphal length of the second fungus was essentially the same irrespective of the compatibility of the third fungus (*32*). This is a strong indication that the second nonpathogen as well as the third compatible race had not been recognized by accessibility-induced cells as an incompatible entity. Thus the most important determinative process of recognition should have been completed during the primary inducing interaction.

V. ULTRASTRUCTURE OF INTERACTION

In view of the remarkable yellowing of leaves that had been inoculated first with incompatible race and subsequently challenged by compatible race, ultrastructural changes of chloroplasts were observed of leaves that had been single- or double-inoculated with a compatible and/or an incompatible race. Chloroplasts were degenerated to larger extent in leaves inoculated with incompatible race than in those inoculated with compatible race. The extent of degeneration, however, became remarkable in double-inoculated leaves. The most distinct degenerative profile was observed in leaves that had been induced with incompatible race and challenged by compatible one, substantiating the above inference that cells conditioned to be inaccessible recognize a primarily compatible race as incompatible.

VI. HEAT-INDUCED SUSCEPTIBILITY

Since Salmon found that barley leaves touched with a hot knife became susceptible to powdery mildew (*41*), heat predisposition has been studied in numerous host-parasite combinations (*42, 48, 50*). It has been well established that heat treatment of plants causes remarkable changes in their response to pathogenic as well as nonpathogenic microorganisms, as could be exemplified in the modification of phenotypic expression of resistance genes (*24, 26*), and more specifically of the pattern of phytoalexin production (*3, 6, 7, 19, 30, 40*). In spite of this abundant information on heat predisposition, surprisingly little is known about the mechanism of the heat effect on the primary plant-pathogen interaction (*40*). Some characteristics of heat-induced susceptibility were studied with barley powdery mildew (*33, 37, 38*). Heat treatment above 45°C rendered leaves of an immune isogenic line susceptible to race 1 of *E. graminis hordei*. Treatment at 53°C induced susceptibility, but longer exposure at this temperature caused a decrease of once-induced susceptibility at an exponetial rate (*38*). Treatment at 55°C-10 sec rendered the leaves susceptible to race 1 to the extent that abundant sporulation, though one-tenth those formed on compatible host, was ensured for an incompatible race. The rate of recovery from heat shock was also exponential (*37*). These results suggest that some particular steps of recognition or subsequent conditioning might be especially heat sensitive. Noteworthy was the finding that an incomatible race was capable of inducing accessibility in heated leaves (*33*). Infection frequency of race 1 inoculated as challenger on immune leaves which had been heated and inoculated with the same race was significantly higher than that on leaves which had not received previous inoculation, indicating that the fungus succeeded in establishing a pseudosymbiotic association with cells it invaded prior to their recovery from heat shock was capable of inducing accessibility (*33*). However, the ability of the invaded fungus to induce accessibility was gradually overcome as recognition ability of cells recovered from heat shock (*33*). These results also suggest that accessibility induction is an active process.

In regard to heat predisposition, one should not overlook the fact that heat dosage that are therapeutic for one pathogen induced, in some cases, susceptibility to another pathogen (*49*), and also the observation that infection frequency of wheat powdery mildew fungus on heat-treated barley leaves was much lower compared with that of barley fungus on leaves treated similarly. These facts suggest that heat predisposition is not simply due to general metabolic suppression of host cell. It is possible that molecules involved in the primary recognition are rendered unfunctional by heat treatment.

Cytological studies of the initial phase of interaction is required for understanding the mechanism of heat predisposition, and in fact some has already been done (*1*).

VII. EFFECT OF INHIBITORS ON INTERACTION

If the recognition and/or subsequent cellular conditioning were processes which involve transcription and translation, the infection should be affected by inhibitors of these processes. Thus the effects of inhibitors of nucleic acid and protein syntheses, actinomycin D, cycloheximide, and blasticidin S, on the infection establishment by a compatible or incompatible race were studied with barley powdery mildew. The results indicated that there was always an inhibitor sensitive step for the fungus to establish in the early phase of interaction, 3 to 18 hr after inoculation. The inhibition of accessibility induction was confirmed by a double inoculation procedure. These results seem to substantiate the idea that accessibility induction is indeed an active and inducible process.

VIII. CONCLUDING REMARK

Plants inoculated with an avirulent race or nonpathogen often respond with resistance to a virulent pathogen inoculated as challenger. This phenomenon has been called "induced resistance" or "cross-protection" and has been the subject of many types of research (*4, 8, 9, 20, 23, 30, 31, 40, 45*). Information accumulated during the past two decades or so shows that versatile biochemical changes occur in plant cells invaded by etiological agents and that these changes differ qualitatively and quantitatively from compatible to incompatible interactions. In some cases phytoalexins are suggested to be involved in resistance, but in others are not (*21, 47*). It became also clear that these changes are inducible processes, hence it is most likely that these processes involve a derepressive operations of genes for resistance.

In contrast with the tremendous amount of information on induced resistance, little is known about induced susceptibility. As often stated, however, disease is an exception rather than rule. Among vast sum of microorganisms, only limited number of species cause a disease in a given plant or animal. Therefore the pathogens should have elaborate means to suppress general defense mechanisms which plants acquired during their evolutionary process. One of the most basic attributes of different types of cellular organisms is their ability to recognize foreign entity and operate regulatory systems to adapt the new environment. There is no reason to preclude this very intrinsic ability from possibilities that it plays a role in host parasite interactions. In fact recent trends in research of host-parasite specificity indicates that recognition of pathogen by host cell is the primary determinative process of specificity. The pathogens must suppress this ability as well as the subsequent physiological conditioning toward unfavorable environment for them to survive. This very primitive assumption finally leads to the concept of induced susceptibility. The results presented in this paper clearly showed that cells invaded by a compatible race were eventually rendered susceptible to incompatible race and some nonpathogens and suggested that this induction of accessibility is indeed an active process.

Genetic implication of these results led us to postulate that host genes such as those determining response to a particular race may probably function in the recognition process, hence should be called "recognition genes" instead of "resistance genes." As most living beings were accomodated with physical and chemical mechanisms to protect themselves, plants should have acquired devices to defend themselves from pathogens during their evolutional process. They may share a common genic constituents for resistance, especially when they were phylogenically close each other, as could be illustrated by the synthesis of common phytoalexin in different species of plants. By nature, the function of recognition genes must be qualitative rather than quantitative, and may probably be constitutive in some interactions and inducible in others. As Day illustrated in his model of genic regulation of host-parasite interaction (*10*), genes controlling biochemical processes associated with virtual resistance may be directly or indirectly controlled by recognition(sensor) genes, and are most likely inducible. Then the induction of accessibility should involve suppression of these recognition and/or resistance genes. Induced accessibility is then a type of gene complementation for some nonpathogens to establish infection. This type of coexistence, however, may probably be restricted to certain types of biotroph such as powdery mildews. Even in powdery mildews, there were exceptions. Leaves of *Pisum sativum* have never become accessible to *E. graminis hordei* and *tritici* by preliminary inoculation with virulent race of *E. pisi* (unpublished data). Barley leaves which had been inoculated with compatible race of *E. graminis hordei* did not permit the establishment of some nonpathogenic powdery mildews (*46*). These exceptions suggest that one cannot generalize the invariable presence of accessibility induction in various host-parasite interactions, but at the same time these indicate that accessibility is not due to mere depression of metabolic activity of host cells. Since induced accessibility is effective not only for the incompatible race but also to nonpathogens, it is hardly interpreted on the basis of gene-for-gene concept. One might argue that it is only a secondary effect. The exceptions stated above, however, do not lead to such a simple conclusion. There seem to be different levels, qualitative or quantitative, of recognitions among versatile host-parasite interactions. Biochemical approaches to the process of accessibility induction should unify these biological observations and provide useful information for understanding the primary recognition at molecular level.

SUMMARY

Preliminary inoculation with an incompatible race of *Erysiphe graminis hordei* or nonpathogenic *E. graminis tritici* rendered barley leaves inaccessible to compatible challenger race, while earlier interaction with a compatible race made leaves accessible to incompatible or nonpathogenic powdery mildews. Melon leaves inoculated with *Sphaerotheca fuliginea* became accessible to barley and wheat powdery mildews, permitting them to produce conidia on leaves of this non-host plant. By double- or triple-inoculation procedure it was elucidated that inaccessibility was established within 6 hr of incompatible interaction and accessibility was established during 15–18 hr of compatible interaction, and that both the induced accessibility and inaccessibility were localized and seemed to be irreversible. The results of heat-shock treatment prior to inoculation and application of inhibitors of protein and nucleic acid synthesis at the initial phase of interaction suggested that induced accessibility is most likely an active process.

Acknowledgments

We wish to express our gratitude to Prof. U. Hiura, Okayama University, for his continuous advice and kind supply of genetically defined cultivars and races used in this series of experiments. We also thank Mr. T. Shiraishi for his tireless help. This work was supported by grant from the Ministry of Education, Science, and Culture, Japan(Nos. 156033 and 13006).

REFERENCES

1. Aist, J. and H. W. Israel. 1977. Effects of heat shock inhibition of papilla formation on compatible host penetration by obligate parasites. *Physiol. Plant Pathol.* **10**: 13–20.
2. Albersheim, P. and A. J. Anderson-Prouty. 1975. Carbohydrates, proteins, cell surface, and the biochemistry of pathogenesis. *Annu. Rev. Plant Physiol.* **26**: 31–52.
3. Bell, A. A. and J. T. Presley. 1969. Temperature effects upon resistance and phytoalexin synthesis in cotton inoculated with *Verticilium albo-atrum. Phytopathology* **59**: 1141–1146.
4. Ben Arie, R. and S. Guelfat-Reich. 1969. Post harvest heat treatment to control storage rots of spadona pears. *Plant Dis. Reptr.* **53**: 363–367.
5. Burrows, V. D. 1970. Absence of lateral transfer within the oat leaf of substances responsible for crown rust resistance. *Can. J. Bot.* **48**: 198–199.

6. Chamberlain, D. W. and J. W. Gerdeman. 1966. Heat-induced susceptibility of soybeans to *Phytophthora megaspermae* var. *sojae, Phytophthora cactorum* and *Helminthosporium sativum*. *Phytopathology* **56**: 70–73.
7. Chamberlain, D. W. 1972. Heat-induced susceptibility to nonpathogens and cross-protection against *Phytophthora megaspermae* var. *sojae* in soybean. *Phytopathology* **62**: 645–646.
8. Chester, K. S. 1933. The problem of acquired physiological immunity in plants. *Quart. Rev. Biol.* **8**: 129–154.
9. Cheung, D. S. M. and B. J. Barber. 1972. Activation of resistance of wheat to stem rust. *Trans. Br. Mycol. Soc.* **58**: 333–336.
10. Day, P. R. 1974. *Genetic of Host Parasite Interaction*. Freeman and Co., San Francisco.
11. Ellingboe, A. H. 1972. Genetics and physiology of primary infection by *Erysiphe graminis*. *Phytopathology* **62**: 401–406.
12. Ellingboe, A. H. 1976. Genetics of host-parasite interactions. *In*: R. Heitefuss and P. H. Williams (eds.). *Encyclopedia of Plant Physiology*. vol. 4. Springer-Verlag, Heidelberg, pp. 761–778.
13. Érsek, T. 1973. Defense reaction induced by a primary inoculation with barley lowdery mildew on wheat seedlings. *Acta Phytopathol. Acad. Sci. Hung.* **8**: 261–263.
14. Flor, H. H. 1955. Host-parasite interaction in flax rust—its genetics and other implications. *Phytopathology* **45**: 680–685.
15. Flor, H. H. 1971. Current status of the gene-for-gene concept. *Annu. Rev. Phytopathol.* **9**: 275–296.
16. Hiura, U. 1960. Studies on disease resistance in barley. IV. Genetics of the resistance to powdery mildew. *Ber. Ohara Inst. Landw. Biol.* **11**: 235–300.
17. Hiura, U. 1964. Genetics of host-parasite interaction in barley mildew. *Ber. Ohara Inst. Landw. Biol.* **12**: 121–129.
18. Hooker, A. L. 1967. The genetics and expression of resistance in plants to rusts of the genus *Puccinia*. *Annu. Rev. Phytopathol.* **5**: 163–182.
19. Jerome, S. M. R. and K. O. Müller. 1958. Studies on phytoalexins. II. Influence of temperature on resistance of *Phaseolus vulgaris* toward *Sclerotinia fructicola* with reference to phytoalexin output. *Aust. J. Biol. Sci.* **11**: 301–314.
20. Johnston, C. O. and D. Huffman. 1958. Evidence of local antagonism between two cereal rust fungi. *Phytopathology* **48**: 69–70.
21. Kuć, J. 1972. Phytoalexins. *Annu. Rev. Phytopathol.* **10**: 207–232.
22. Kuć, J., G. Shockley, and K. Kearney. 1975. Protection of cucumber against *Colletotrichum lagenarium* by *Colletotrichum lagenarium*. *Physiol. Plant Pathol.* **7**: 195–199.
23. Littlefield, L. J. 1969. Flax rust resistance induced by prior inoculation with an avirulent race of *Melampsora lini*. *Phytopathology* **59**: 1323–1328.
24. Luig, N. H. and S. Rajaran. 1972. The effect of temperature and genetic back-

ground on host gene expression and interaction to *Puccinia graminis tritici*. *Phytopathology* **62**: 1171–1174.

25. McKeen, W. E. and D. K. Bhattacharya. 1970. Limitation of infection by *Erysiphe graminis* f. sp. *hordei* culture CR3 by the Algerian gene Mla in barley. *Can. J. Bot.* **48**: 1109–1113.
26. Mohamed, H. A. 1960. Predisposition of wheat seedlings to stem rust infection and development. *Phytopathology* **50**: 339–340.
27. Moseman, J. G. 1966. Genetics of powdery mildew. *Annu. Rev. Phytopathol.* **4**: 269–290.
28. Moseman, J. G., A. L. Scharen, and L. W. Greeley. 1965. Propagation of *Erysiphe graminis* f. sp. *hordei* on wheat. *Phytopathology* **55**: 92–96.
29. Nair, S. K. R. and A. H. Ellingboe. 1965. Germination of conidia of *Erysiphe graminis* f. sp. *tritici*. *Phytopathology* **55**: 365–368.
30. Oku, H., S. Ouchi, T. Shiraishi, T. Baba, and H. Miyagawa. 1975. Phytoalexin production in barley powdery mildew as affected by thermal and biological predispositions. *Proc. Japan Acad.* **51**: 198–201.
31. Oku, H., S. Ouchi, T. Shiraishi, Y. Komoto, and K. Oki. 1975. Phytoalexin activity in barley powdery mildew. *Ann. Phytopathol. Soc. Japan* **41**: 185–191.
32. Ouchi, S., C. Hibino, and H. Oku, 1976. Effect of preliminary inoculation on the infection establishment by a subsequent fungus as demonstrated in powdery mildew of barley by a triple inoculation. *Physiol. Plant. Pathol.* **9**: 25–32.
33. Ouchi, S., H. Nakabayashi, and H. Oku. 1977. Ability of an incompatible race of *Erysiphe graminis hrodei* to induce an accessibility to the same race in heat-predisposed barley leaves. *Ann. Phytopathol. Soc. Japan* **43**: 62–64.
34. Ouchi, S., H. Oku, and C. Hibino. 1976. Localization of induced resistance and susceptibility in barley leaves inoculated with powdery mildew. *Phytopathology* **66**: 901–905.
35. Ouchi, S., H. Oku, C. Hibino, and I. Akiyama. 1974. Induction of accessibility and resistance in leaves of barley by some races of *Erysiphe graminis*. *Phytopathol. Z.* **79**: 24–34.
36. Ouchi, S., H. Oku, C. Hibino, and I. Akiyama. 1974. Induction of accessibility to nonpathogen by a preliminary inoculation with a pathogen. *Phytopathol. Z.* **79**: 142–154.
37. Ouchi, S., H. Oku, H. Nakabayashi, and K. Oka. 1975. Some characteristics of the heat-induced susceptibility demonstrated in powdery mildew of barley. *Ann. Phytopathol. Soc. Japan* **41**: 453–460.
38. Ouchi, S. H. Oku, H. Nakabayashi, and K. Oka. 1976. Biphasic heat-induced susceptibility demonstrated in powdery mildew of barley. *Ann. Phytopathol. Soc. Japan* **42**: 131–137.
39. Powers, H. R., Jr. and W. J. Sando. 1960. Genetic control of the host-parasite relationship in wheat powdery mildew. *Phytopathology* **50**: 454–457.

40. Rahe, J. E. and J. Kuć. 1970. Metabolic nature of the infection limiting effect of heat on bean anthracnose. *Phytopathology* **60**: 1005–1009.
41. Salmon, E. S. 1905. Further cultural experiments with biologic forms of the Erysiphaceae. *Ann. Bot.* **19**: 125–148.
42. Schoeneweiss, D. F. 1975. Predisposition, stress, and plant disease. *Annu. Rev. Phytopathol.* **13**: 193–211.
43. Skipp, R. A. and B. J. Deverall. 1973. Studies on cross-protection in the anthracnose disease of bean. *Physiol. Plant Pathol.* **3**: 299–313.
44. Slesinski, R. S. and A. H. Ellingboe. 1970. Gene-for-gene interactions during primary infection of wheat by *Erysiphe graminis* f. sp. *tritici*. *Phytopathology* **60**: 1068–1070.
45. Tani, T., S. Ouchi, T. Onoe, and N. Naito. 1975. Irreversible recognition demonstrated in the hypersensitive response of oat leaves against crown rust fungus. *Phytopathology* **65**: 1190–1193.
46. Tsuchiya, K. and K. Hirata. 1973. Growth of various powdery mildew fungi on the barley leaves infected preliminarily with the barley powdery mildew fungus. *Ann. Phytopathol. Soc. Japan* **39**: 396–403.
47. Van Etten, H. D. and S. G. Pueppke. 1976. Isoflavonoid phytoalexins. *In*: J. Friend and D. R. Threlfall (eds.). *Biochemical Aspects of Plant Parasite Relationships.* Academic Press, New York, pp. 239–289.
48. Yarwood, C. E. 1959. Predisposition. *In*: J. G. Horsfall and A. E. Dimond (eds.). *Plant Pathology*. vol. 1. Academic Press, New York, pp. 521–562.
49. Yarwood, C. E. 1965. Predisposition to mildew by rust infection, hest, abrasion, and pressure. *Phytopathology* **55**: 1372.
50. Yarwood, C. E. 1976. Modification of the host response—Predisposition. *In*: R. Heitefuss and P. H. Williams (eds.). *Encyclopedia of Plant Physiology*. vol. 4. Springer-Verlag, Heidelberg, pp. 703–718.

Discussion of Paper by Drs. Ouchi et al.

YODER opened the session by asking if accessibility induced in barley by mildew resulted in increased compatibility to fungi other than *Erysiphe*. DALY asked the same question for induced resistance. OUCHI replied these possibilities had not been studied. SCHEFFER then asked a series of questions in order to establish if there were exceptions to observations that compatible strains induced accessibility and incompatible strains induced resistance. He pointed out that there are instances recorded with *Helminthosporium* where incompatible strains do not induce resistance to compatible strains. OUCHI indicated that exceptions had not been observed in the combinations so far tested. In response to questions by URTITANI and KEEN, OUCHI reported that simultaneous inoculation with compatible and incompatible strains always resulted in a compatible reaction (in fact this is the control for each experiment) but noted they were not able to establish if the incompatible pathogen developed as well, if at all. ELLINGBOE compared such results with studies of rust fungi where two sets of results can be obtained: the lowest infection type produces a higher infection type; in other instances the infection is the same. DALY observed that this system is not quite the same. The ectophytic mildew system permits a true mixed infection of individual cells whereas rust pustules arise from separate penetrations and which then appear to develop discretcly. KUĆ opened a very general discussion by remarking on the similarity of the mildew system to the potato-*Phytophthora* system which he and TOMIYAMA have investigated independently. In KUĆ's view, one interpretation is that once a hypersensitive response is elicited it can be reversed by a compatible strain but prior inoculation of a compatible strain suppresses the ability of an incompatible strain to cause the hypersensitive response. He wondered if the key was collapse of cells in resistance. OUCHI agreed that might be true in the potato system but he does not see any collapsed cells with incompatibility. DALY questioned whether suppression of an active resistance was an appropriate picture and asked if there was any direct evidence for the induction of incompatible response to any degree or any time in cases of challenges with incompatible strains against compatible reactions. OUCHI agreed with DALY's statement that existing data with obligate parasites at least do not permit a choice of whether the differences in fungal development observed in compatible and incompatible reactions are the result of active repression of the fungus in cases of incompatibility or stimulated development with compatibility. On the other hand, ELLINGBOE believed that in systems he worked with there was no indication that compatible host cells responded in any way to the presence of the parasite. TOMIYAMA expressed reservations about the indiscriminate use, at this time of development of the science, of the concepts of resistance and susceptibility in order to explain experimental results. His feeling is that the phenomena are much too complex and thus we should focus, for now, on specific phenomena, such as rapid cell death, to ascertain the factors causing it and its relationship to final disease reaction. In this way, step by step, newer and better understanding of resistance and susceptibility will accrue. GRACEN closed the session by agreeing with TOMIYAMA and commented that students of plant breeding quickly learn that resistance is relative. Further, that although we emphasize specific host and parasite genes for disease reaction, very little attention is paid to the interaction of these genes with other components of the host or parasite genome. He believes the interaction among host or parasite genes are important and as complex as those between host and parasite genes.

CYTOLOGICAL EVENTS IN RECOGNITION AND SPECIFICITY

Recognition and Specificity in Plant Host-Parasite Interactions, pp. 69–84, 1979

THE HYPERSENSITIVE RESPONSE OF RESISTANT PLANTS

KOHEI TOMIYAMA, NORIYUKI DOKE, MASAYUKI NOZUE, AND YUKIO ISHIGURI

Plant Pathology Laboratory, Faculty of Agriculture, Nagoya University, Nagoya, Japan

In 1902, H. M. Ward noted that the hypersensitivity of resistant host plants to parasites plays an important role in resistance of bromes to brown rust. It has been said that it was the first recognition of "hypersensitivity" in plants (*19*). He recognized that there was no difference between the behavior of the resistant and susceptible hosts until direct physiological contact with parasite is established, and then the tissue of an uncongenial host infected by the pathogen turned brown and died. At the same time the pathogen ceased to grow. Since that time, a great deal of experimental evidence has accumulated, suggesting that, in many diseases, hypersensitive response of host which can be recognized by browning of infected tissue accompanies the resistance phenomena of plants.

In 1959, Müller (*19*) extensively reviewed research on hypersensitivity in disease resistance of plants. He gave as one of several definitions of hypersensitivity the following "hypersensitive reaction encompasses all morphological and histological changes that, when produced by an infectious agent, elicit the premature dying off(necrosis) of the infected tissue as well as inactivation and localization of the infectious agent." In this excellent review, he put emphasis on the importance of phytoalexin production as a part of the hypersensitivity reaction. However, at that time, little data were

TABLE I

Relation between the Time from Inoculation to Death of 50% of Potato-cells Infected by *Phytophthora infestans* and Degree of Disease Resistance

Cultivars.	Tissues infected	Rresistance genes and races	Time from cutting[a] to inoculation (hr)	Time from inoculation to 50% cell death (hr)	Degree of resistance	Reference
Hokkai No. 10	Cut surface of leaf petiole	$R_1 \times$ race 0	Short time	10	mR[b]	*(30)*
Kennebec	Cut surface of leaf petiole	$R_1 \times$ race 0	Short time	12	mR	*(30)*
Rishiri	Cut surface of tuber	$R_1 \times$ race 0	Short time	12	mR	*(26)*
Rishiri	Cut surface of tuber	$R_1 \times$ race 0	20	3	hR	*(26)*
Eniwa	Cut surface of tuber	$R_1 \times$ race 0	Short time	20	wR	*(26)*
Eniwa	Cut surface of tuber	$R_1 \times$ race 0	20	3	mR	*(26)*
Hokkai No. 17	Cut surface of leaf petiole	$R_4 \times$ race 0	Short time	18	wR	*(30)*
Shimakei 278	Cut surface of leaf petiole	$R_4 \times$ race 0	Short time	19	wR	*(30)*
41089–8	Cut surface of leaf petiole	$R_1R_4 \times$ race 0	Short time	12	mR	*(30)*
41089–8	Intact surface of very young leaf midrib	$R_1R_4 \times$ race 0	Intact	4	hR	*(28)*
Hokkai No. 9	Intact surface of very young leaf midrib	$R_1 \times$ race 1	Intact	10	mR	*(28)*
Hokkai No. 10	Intact surface of very young leaf midrib	$R_1 \times$ race 0	Intact	3	hR	*(28)*
Hokkai No. 10	Intact surface of very young leaf midrib	$R_1 \times$ race 1	Intact	10	mR	*(28)*
Hokkai No. 10	Cut surface of leaf petiole	$R_1 \times$ race 1	Short time	About 3 days	S	*(30)*
Rishiri	Cut surface of leaf petiole	$R_1 \times$ race 1	Short time	2 days	S	*(28)*

[a] Tubers or leaf petioles were cut and cut surfaces were washed with water and then inoculated. [b] hR, Highly resistant (only one or a few cells invaded, no sporulation); mR, medium resistant (a few to several cells invaded, no sporulation); wR, weakly resistent (more than several cells invaded, spars sporulation); S, susceptible (abundant spores).

available for discussing direct causative relations between hypersensitive cell death and disease resistance, and for describing the physiological mechanism of the hypersensitive cell death.

As far as the physiology of hypersensitive cell death is concerned, the situation at present is not so much different from that at the time of Müller's review. Investigation on the meaning and physiological mechanism of hypersensitive cell death has been rather neglected, although researches on hypersensitivity in a broad sense or elicitors and blockers of tissue necrosis have been made by many authors (*2, 10, 15, 16, 35*). In some diseases doubt as to whether the hypersensitive cell death was a cause or a result of disease resistance was presented (*9, 26*). In the case of potato late blight there is a close correlation between the length of time from penetration to hypersensitive cell death and degree of disease resistance regardless of genetic background of host and parasite (Table I). Evidences was reported that cell death triggered accumulation of the phytoalexin, rishitin, and also that inhibition of intracellular hyphal growth paralleled accumulation of rishitin (*25, 31*). These results strongly suggest that hypersensitive cell death serves as a trigger for initiation of an inhibition process of disease development, at least in the case of potato late blight.

It may be reasonable to suppose that, in some diseases, timing of hypersensitive cell death may play a key role as a limiting factor for initiation of a successful defense reaction, and in some diseases, some other factors may play a more important role than hypersensitive cell death. Detailed studies of the process of cell death for each individual disease is necessary in order to draw general conclusions as to the meaning of hypersensitive cell death.

It is without question, however, that hypersensitive cell death constitutes an essential part in the series of physiological phenomena involving hypersensitivity. Knowing the mechanism of hypersensitive cell death is important for an understanding of how host plants respond to parasites.

Under appropriate conditions, a cell of the potato cultivar, Rishiri, having the R_1-gene die very rapidly upon infection by an incompatible race of *Phytophthora infestans*. In most rapid cell death, it dies within 30 min after penetration. In this paper we discuss the mechanism of hypersensitive cell death, and physiological phenomena closely related to hypersensitive cell death, based on our recent experimental results. In all experiments, potato cultivar "Rishiri"(R_1) and race 0(incompatible to Rishiri) and race 1 (compatible) of *P. infestans* were used.

I. *DE NOVO* PROTEIN SYNTHESIS AND HYPERSENSITIVE CELL DEATH

To determine how *de novo* protein synthesis relates to hypersensitive cell death, the following experiments were carried out.

More than several hours (usually about 20 hr) (aged disc) or soon (fresh disc) after preparation of tissue discs from tubers of potato cultivar Rishiri (R_1-gene), the discs were inoculated with *P. infestans*. Microscopic sections were made, at intervals, from the infected surface of the discs, and observed under a light microscope.

When an aged disc of potato tuber is inoculated with the incompatible race 0, the infected cells die very rapidly. On the contrary, in the case of fresh discs the hypersensitive death occurs very late (*29, 30*). These phenomena indicated that the cells at the surface of fresh disc lack the ability to respond hypersensitively to infection by the incompatible race, but they acquire this ability by 20 hr after the preparation of discs.

Fresh discs were treated with 10 ppm of blasticidin S(BcS) for 3 hr beginning 3 hr after preparation of the discs, and then inoculated with the incompatible race 1, 7 and 14 hr after the treatment, and then observed under a microscope. The results showed that the cells did not acquire the potential to react hypersensitively to infection by the incompatible race (Fig. 1). In this case, the infected cells survived for almost the same period as the cells infected by the compatible race 1. With the aged discs, whose hypersensitivity potential had been allowed to develop, on the contrary, treatment with BcS had no effect on the potential. Under these experimental conditions, it was demonstrated, using [^{3}H]leucine, that protein synthesis was definitely reduced (*4, 21*). These results indicated that *de novo* protein synthesis was necessary for cells of fresh discs to acquire the potential, but was not necessary in order for the infected cells to react hypersensitively after the hypersensitivity potential had been developed.

Development of the potential to react hypersensitively was found not only in the case of cut tuber tissue, but also in cut leaf-petiole tissue (*29*).

It has been reported that metabolic activity of storage-tissue discs is very low soon after preparation of the discs, and then it is activated in several hours (*13, 14*). In the case of potato-tuber discs, respiration of fresh discs are known to be malonate resistant and it was demonstrated that TCA cycle was not operating. The TCA cycle becomes operative during aging process, accompanied with rise in respiration and other metabolic activities. The

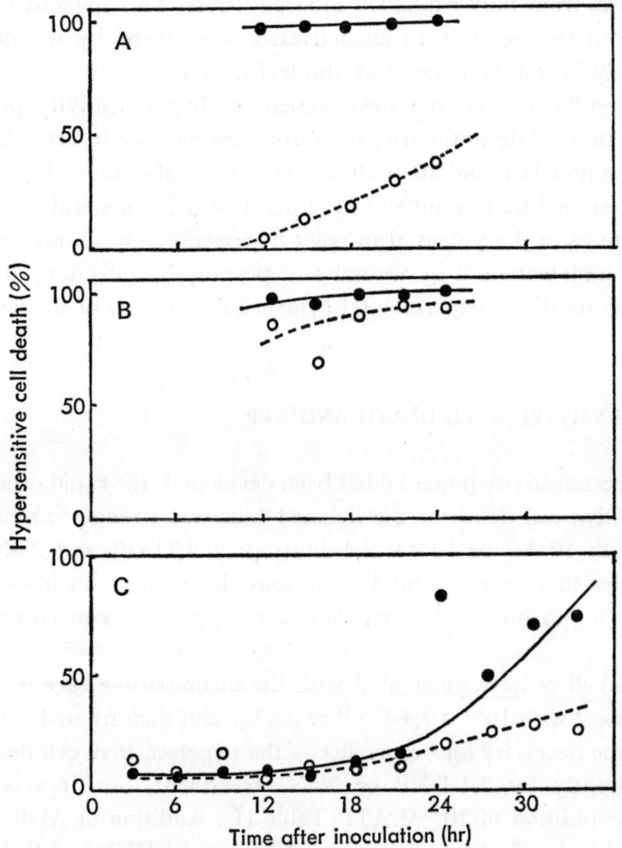

Fig. 1. Time from inoculation to hypersensitive death of the surface cells of potato-tuber discs treated with BcS (10 ppm, for 3 hr) 3 or 20 hr after preparations of discs and then inoculated with race 0 (incompatible) or race 1 (compatible) of *P. infestans*. A, Treated with BcS 3 hr after preparation of discs, and inoculated with race 0 13 hr after preparation (○), or inoculated without BcS treatment (control) (●); B, treated with BcS 20 hr, inoculated with race 0 24 hr (○), or control (●); C, treated with BcS 3 hr, and then inoculated with race 1 (○), non-treated with BcS and inoculated with race 1 (●) (*21*).

activation of metabolic activity is prevented only when a metabolic inhibitor, such as actinomycin D or puromycin, is applied within the first 6 to 8 hr after cutting.

Manicol (*17*) showed that a wound respiration phase, followed by induced respiration lasting several days, also was found only in peripheral regions of discs from fully expanded tobacco leaves. This suggests that the transition from resting state to an activated one caused by wounding is found not only in storage tissues but also leaf tissues.

These results suggest that development of hypersensitivity potential after cutting may relate to the transition from resting state to activated one. This phenomenon is found in both storage and leaf-petiole tissue. It is, therefore, presumed that an intact cell of plant tissue, in general, may be in a resting state as to the potential to react hypersensitively to infection and activated to high potential by wound and possibly by infection, although there is so far no direct experimental evidence in the case of induction by infection.

II. HYPERSENSITIVE CELL DEATH AND ATP

After the hypersensitivity potential has been developed, the rapid occurrence of hypersensitive cell death of the infected cells was strongly inhibited by treatment with 10^{-3} M or 10^{-4} M 2,4-dinitrophenol(DNP) and NaN_3 (*22, 28–30*). Under these experimental conditions, little effect on intracellular hyphal growth was observed when they were applied at concentration of 10^{-4} M (*22*).

The aged discs were inoculated with the incompatible race 0 after or before treatment with 10^{-4} M 2,4-DNP or NaN_3, and then treated with ATP (*22*). The time necessary for occurrence of the hypersensitive cell death was prolonged greatly by 2,4-DNP or NaN_3 treatment, but it was again shortened by addition of 10^{-4} M ATP(Table II). Addition of ADP, on the contrary, had little effect on this process. NaN_3 or 2,4-DNP had little effect no the time during which the cells of aged discs infected by the compatible

TABLE II

Effect of ATP and 2,4-DNP [on the Hypersensitive Death of Cells of Potato-tuber Discs Infected by the Incompatible Race

	Water		ATP[a]	
	Water	2,4-DNP[b]	Water	2,4-DNP[b]
% of dead cells	72.3±9.9[c]	28.0±7.4	72.2±15.2	60.3±12.7

[a] Addition of 0.1 mM ATP for 45 min 5 hr after inoculation. [b] Treated with 0.1 mM 2,4-dinitrophenol(DNP) before inoculation. [c] Observed 8 hr after inoculation.

race 1 survived. These results indicated that ATP directly related to the process of hypersensitive cell death in aged discs, and also suggest that the hypersensitive cell death is not simply the collapse of an infected cell, but an energyrequiring vital response to infection.

In fresh discs, in which the hypersensitivity potential has not yet been developed, ATP had only a little effect on the occurrence of hypersensitive cell death. This suggested that other important factors than ATP may play their role in the insensitivity of the fresh discs.

III. HYPERSENSITIVE CELL DEATH AND SH-REAGENTS

Preinfectional treatments of aged discs of potato tubers with low molecular weight SH-reagents *viz* 2,4-DNP, 2,4-dinitrofluorobenzene, N-ethylmaleimide, *p*-chloromercuribenzoic acid, and high molecular weight SH-reagent, dextran (MW 7×10^4) bound *p*-chloromercuribenzoic acid (PMDT) inhibited rapid occurrence of the hypersensitive death of cells of aged discs infected by incompatible race 0 (*8*). As PMDT is known not easily to penetrate into a human blood cell (*23*), it is supposed, in the case of tuber discs also, PMDT may act mainly on cell membrane of the aged discs.

These results suggest that modification of cell membrane with SH-reagents may inhibit recognition of incompatible parasites by the host cell.

IV. ALTERATION OF CELL MEMBRANE ACTIVITY BY INFECTION

Electric potential differences between surfaces of aged potato-tuber discs infected by incompatible race 0 and compatible race 1 or between each of them and noninfected one were determined during the initial period of infection (*18*). Electric potential difference began to increase almost simultaneously with host-wall penetration by both the incompatible and compatible races. The increase was larger in the former than in the latter soon after penetration. These results suggest that the cell membrane of the host cell undergoes severer alteration by infection with the incompatible race than with the compatible race very soon after penetration.

V. HYPERSENSITIVE CELL DEATH AND PHYTOALEXIN

To accumulate rishitin in an enough amounts to be chemically detectable in tuber discs infected by the incompatible race takes about 8 to 9 hr after about 20% of the infected cells have died, regardless of length of time from inoculation to hypersensitive cell death (*25*). Most of rishitin was found to accumulate in brown infected lesion (*24, 33*). However, it was demonstrated by using ^{14}C-acetate that rishitin was synthesized in the healthy cells of about 10 cell-layers neighboring the infected brown lesion (*20*). These results seemed to suggest that synthesis of rishitin was triggered by hypersensitive death of the infected cells, and synthesized in healthy cells neighboring the infected brown lesion. However, it was demonstrated in a recent experiment that it was not correct.

Experiments using ^{14}C-acetate showed that synthesis of rishitin was initiated about 3 hr after preparation of discs, even if the discs was not inoculated. When the discs were inoculated with the incompatible race soon after cutting, the rate of radioactivity in the rishitin fraction per total radioactivity absorbed was already greater as compared with that in noninfected discs before the hypersensitive cell death occurred (*1*) (Fig. 2).

Using ^{14}C-labeled rishitin it was demonstrated that rishitin was metabolized to other compounds in cut and noninfected healthy tuber tissue (*11*). The ability to metabolize rishitin could not be found in the fresh discs

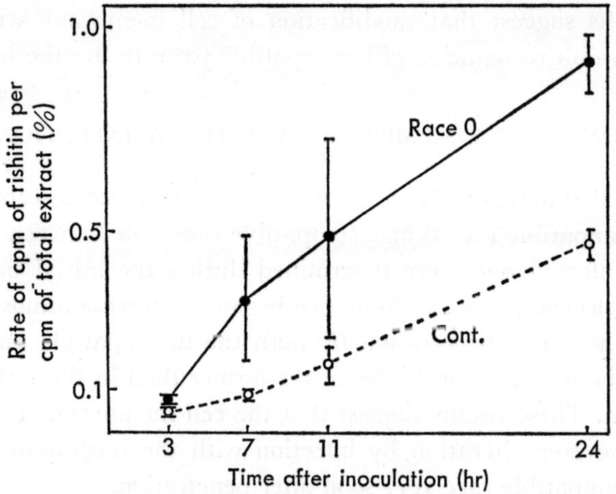

Fig. 2. Incorporation rate of radioactivity of acetate-2-^{14}C into rishitin in the potato tuber discs (cultivar Rishiri) infected by incompatible race 0 of *P. infestans* and non-infected discs. Inoculation was made soon after preparation of the discs. The radioactivity incorporation rate was expressed as the rate of cpm of rishitin fraction to cpm of total extract (extracted with chloroform: methanol, 2:1 v/v). Time indicated hours after cutting and inoculation.

within a few hours after preparation of the discs but then the discs became able to metabolize rishitin (*12*). It is, therefore, assumed that wound or infection induces rishitin synthesis, but rishitin is transformed to other compounds in healthy tissue without being accumulated, unless it it transported to dead lesion of the infection. In the dead lesion, rishitin may accumulate without transformation. These results presented evidence supporting the presumption that rishitin may be an intermediate and not an end product of metabolism (*16*).

VI. POSSIBLE SUBSTANCES OF *P. INFESTANS* CAUSING OR BLOCKING HYPERSENSITIVE CELL DEATH

It was previously reported (*31*) that hyphal homogenates of *P. infestans* had a toxic effect on potato-tuber discs. Both cultural filtrate of *P. infestans* and the precipitate obtained by treating the filtrate with ethanol (final 70%) had toxic effects on potato-tuber discs. However, there was no relation between the toxicity and host-parasite specificity.

In previous paper (*32, 34*), it was reported that treatment of protoplasts with the supernatant fraction obtained by centrifugation at $105{,}000 \times g$ of hyphal homogenate of the incompatible race 0 gave the most injurious effect on the protoplasts isolated from potato cultivar Rishiri(R_1) as compared with the case of compatible combinations: that is, race 1 × Rishiri, race 0 × Irish cobbler, race 1 × Irish cobbler. Leakage of preabsorbed ^{32}P from the protoplasts treated with the supernatant of hyphal homogenate obtained by centrifugation at $105{,}000 \times g$ also was greatest in the incompatible combination as compared with the compatible combinations. The ethanol(80%) insoluble fraction of the supernatant also had an injurious effect on the protoplasts (*32*).

Treatment of the tuber discs with sediment obtained by centrifugation of zoosporial homogenate (race 0 or race 1) at $110{,}000 \times g$ or $20{,}000 \times g$ caused leakage of electrolyte from the tissue, and also necrosis. This inducer of necrosis could be bound with proteinous substance having MW 40,000–45,000 contained in microsomal fraction, when the former was mixed with the latter, resulting in loss of its biological activity (*3, 5–7*).

Encystment and germination of zoospores were synchronized by shaking the zoospore suspension in the presence of $CaCl_2$ (8×10^{-4} M) at 18°C. High molecular weight substances were released during germination. These substances seemed partly to be released by rupture of the zoospores, but most of them seemed to be released from living germinating encysted zoospores. Pretreatment of the discs with these substances prolonged the time for occurrence of hypersensitive death of the cells which were caused by infection by the incompatible race.

SUMMARY

1) Fresh cut surface cells of potato-tuber and leaf petiole had little potential to react hypersensitively to infection by the incompatible race of *P. infestans*. During aging process, they acquire the hypersensitivity potential. This process need *de novo* protein synthesis.
2) When the hypersensitivity potential has been developed, *de novo* protein synthesis is not necessary for the occurrence of hypersensitive cell death upon infection. However, respiratory enzyme inhibitors (2,4-DNP or NaN_3) inhibit the occurrence of hypersensitive cell death. This inhibition could be restored with ATP, but not with ADP. ATP appears to be related to the process of hypersensitive cell death. These results suggest that the hypersensitive cell death is not simply collapse of an infected cell, but an energy-requiring vital response to infection.
3) High molecular weight SH-reagent (dextran bound *p*-chloromercuribenzoic acid) inhibited hypersensitive cell death, suggesting modification of cell membranes with SH-reagent inhibit the occurrence of hypersensitive cell death. This suggests that the cell membrane may be a recognition site of the incompatibility.
4) Systems synthesizing and metabolizing rishitin could be induced in healthy potato-tuber tissue by just cutting(wound). Synthesized rishitin may be metabolized soon in healthy wound tissue, resulting in accumulation of only a trace amount of rishitin, but may be accumulated in the brown dead lesion caused by infection.
5) These results seem to allow us to present a hypothesis that incompatibility established at cell membrane may cause a kind of irritated condition in a host cell which may result in commencement of phytoalexin synthesis on the one hand and hypersensitive cell death on the other hand. Accumulation of phytoalexin, however, cannot be the cause of hypersensitive cell death in the case of potato late blight.
6) By using potato-tuber tissue and protoplasts, elicitor of necrosis was found in hyphal and zoosporial homogenate of *P. infestans*. Ethanol(70–80%) precipitate of the homogenate also elicited necrosis. Blocker of the occur-

rence of necrosis was found in the germination fluid of the zoospores of *P. infestans*. Further investigation is necessary to know whether these substances really elicite or suppress the hypersensitive response of potato to *P. infestans*.

REFERENCES

1. Amami, S., K. Tomiyama, and N. Doke. 1976. On the phytoalexin production in potato late blight. *Ann. Phytopathol. Soc. Japan* **42**: 84; Amami, S. Master thesis, Nagoya University.
2. Daly, J. M. 1976. Induced susceptibility or induced resistance as the basis of host-parasite specificity. *In*: K. Tomiyama, J. M. Daly, I. Uritani, H. Oku, and S. Ouchi (eds.). *Biochemistry and Cytology of Plant-Parasite Interaction*. Kodansha Ltd., Tokyo and Elsevier, New York, pp. 144–156.
3. Doke, N. 1975. Prevention of the hypersensitive reaction of potato cells to infection with an incompatible race of *Phytophthora infestans* by constituents of the zoospores. *Physiol. Plant Pathol.* **7**: 1–7.
4. Doke, N. and K. Tomiyama. 1975. Effect of blasticidin S on hypersensitive death of potato leaf petiole cells caused by infection with an incompatible race of *Phytophthora infestans*. *Physiol. Plant Pathol.* **6**: 169–175.
5. Doke, N., K. Tomiyama, N. Nishimura, and H. S. Lee. 1975. *In vitro* interaction between components of *Phytophthora infestans* zoospores and components of potato tissue. *Ann. Phytopathol. Soc. Japan* **41**: 425–433.
6. Doke, N. and K. Tomiyama. 1976. Effect of zoosporial homogenate of *Phytophthora infestans* on cell membrane of potato tuber. *Ann. Phytopathol. Soc. Japan* **42**: 84.
7. Doke, N., K. Tomiyama, H. S. Lee, N. Nishimura, and N. Matsumoto. 1976. Mechanism of hypersensitive cell death in host-parasite interaction. K. Tomiyama, J. M. Daly, I. Uritani, H. Oku, and S. Ouchi (eds.). *Biochemistry and Cytology of Plant-Parasite Interaction*. Kodansha Ltd., Tokyo and Elsevier, New York, p. 157.
8. Doke, N. and K. Tomiyama. 1977. Effect of sulfhydryl-binding compounds on hypersensitive death of potato tuber cells following infection with an incompatible race of *Phytophthora infestans*. *Physiol. Plant Pathol.* **12**: 133–137.
9. Elnagly, M. A. and R. Heitefuss. 1976. Permeability changes and production of antifungal compounds in *Phaseolus vulgaris* infected with *Uromyces Phaseoli*. 2. Role of phytoalexins. *Physiol. Plant Pathol.* **8**: 269–277.
10. Goodman, R. N. 1976. Induced resistance to bacterial infection. *In*: K. Tomiyama, J. M. Daly, I. Uritani, H. Oku, and S. Ouchi (eds.). *Biochemistry and Cytology of Plant-Parasite Interaction*. Kodansha Ltd., Tokyo and Elsevier, New York, pp. 35–42.

11. Horikawa, T., K. Tomiyama, and N. Doke. 1976. Accumulation and transformation of rishitin and lubimin in potato tuber tissue infected by an incompatible race of *Phytophthora infestans*. *Phytopathology* **66**: 1186–1191.

12. Ishiguri, Y., K. Tomiyama, N. Doke, A. Murai, N. Katsui, F. Yagihashi, and T. Masamune. 1977. Induction of rishitin-metabolizing activity in potato tuber tissue by cutting and identification of its metabolites. *Phytopathology* **68**: 720–725.

13. Kahl, G. 1974. Metabolism in plant storage tissue slices. *Bot. Rev.* **40**: 263–314.

14. Kahl, G. and B. Wielgat. 1976. Regulation of transcriptional activity in wound potato tuber tissue. *Physiol. Veg.* **14**: 725–738.

15. Kuć, J. 1972. Phytoalexins. *Annu. Rev. Phytopathol.* **10**: 207–232.

16. Kuć, J. 1976. Phytoalexins. *In*: R. Heitefuss and P. H. Williams (eds.). *Encyclopedia of Plant Physiology*. vol. 4. Springer-Verlag, Berlin, pp. 632–652.

17. Manicol, P. K. 1976. Rapid metabolic changes in the wounding response of leaf discs following excision. *Plant Physiol.* **57**: 80–84.

18. Matsumoto, N., K. Tomiyama, and N. Doke. 1976. Alteration of membrane permeability of potato-tuber tissue infected by incompatible and compatible races of *Phytophthora infestans* during the initial phase of infection. *Ann. Phytopathol. Soc. Japan* **42**: 279–286.

19. Müller, K. O. 1959. Hypersensitivity. *In*: J. C. Horsfall and A. E. Dimond (eds.). *Plant Pathology*. vol. 1. Academic Press, New York, pp. 469–519.

20. Nakajima, T., K. Tomiyama, and M. Kinukawa. 1975. Distribution of rishitin and lubimin in potato-tuber tissue infected by an incompatible race of *Phytophthora infestans* and the site where rishitin is synthesized. *Ann. Phytopathol. Soc. Japan* **41**: 49–55.

21. Nozue, M., K. Tomiyama, and N. Doke. 1977. Effect of blasticidin S on development of potential of potato tuber cells to react hypersensitively to infection by *Phytophthora infestans*. *Physiol. Plant Pathol.* **10**: 181–189.

22. Nozue, M., K. Tomiyama, and N. Doke. 1977. Effect of adenosine 5′-triphosphate on hypersensitive death of potato tuber cells infected by *Phytophthora infestans*. *Phytopathology* **68**: 873–876.

23. Ohta, H., J. Matsumoto., K. Nagano., M. Fujita, and M. Nakano. 1971. The inhibition of Na, K-activated adenosintriphatase by a large molecule derivative of p-chloromercuribenzoic acid at the outer surface of human red cell. *Biochem. Biophys. Res. Commun.* **42**: 1127–1133.

24. Sato, N. and K. Tomiyama. 1969. Localized accumulation of rishitin in the potato-tuber tissue infected by an incompatible race of *Phytophthora infestans*. *Ann. Phytopathol. Soc. Japan* **35**: 202–217.

25. Sato, N., K. Kitazawa, and K. Tomiyama. 1971. The role of rishitin in localizing the invading hyphae of *Phytophthora infestans* in infection sites at the cut surfaces of potato tubers. *Physiol. Plant Pathol.* **1**: 289–295.

26. Tani, T., H. Yamamoto., T. Onoe, and N. Naito. 1975. Initiation of resistance and host collapse in the hypersensitive reaction of oat leaves against puccinia coronata avenae. *Physiol. Plant Pathol.* **7**: 231–242.
27. Tomiyama, K. 1956. Cytological studies on resistance of potato plants to *Phytophthora infestans.* (3). The time required for the browning of midrib cell of potato plants infected by *P. infestans. Ann. Phytopathol. Soc. Japan* **20**: 165–169.
28. Tomiyama, K. 1957. Cell physiological studies on the resistance of potato plants to *Phytophthora infestans.* (5). Effect of 2,4-DNP upon the hypersensitive reaction of potato plant cell to infection by *P. infestans. Ann. Phytopathol. Soc. Japan* **22**: 75–78.
29. Tomiyama, K. 1960. Some factors affecting the death of hypersensitive potato plant cells infected by *Phytophthora infestans. Phytopathol. Z.* **39**: 134–148.
30. Tomiyama, K. 1967. Further observation on the time requirement for hypersensitive cell death of potatoes infected by *Phytophthora infestans* and its relation to metabolic activity. *Phytopathol. Z.* **58**: 367–378.
31. Tomiyama, K. 1971. Cytological and biochemical studies of the hypersensitive reaction of potato cells to *Phytophthora infestans. In*: S. Akai and S. Ouchi (eds.). *Morphological and Biochemical Events in Plant-Parasite Interaction.* Phytopathol. Soc. Japan, Tokyo, pp. 387–401.
32. Tomiyama, K., H. S. Lee, and N. Doke. 1974. Effect of hyphal homogenate of *Phytophthora infestans* on the potato-tuber protoplasts. *Ann. Phytopathol. Soc. Japan* **40**: 70–72.
33. Tomiyama, K. and M. Fukaya. 1975. Accumulation of rishitin in dead potato-tuber tissue following treatment with $HgCl_2$. *Ann. Phytopathol. Soc. Japan* **41**: 418–420.
34. Tomiyama, K., N. Doke, and H. S. Lee. 1976. Mechanism of hypersensitive cell death in host-parasite interaction. *In*: K. Tomiyama, J. M. Daly, I. Uritani, H. Oku, and S. Ouchi (eds.). *Biochemistry and Cytology of Plant-Parasite Interaction.* Kodansha Ltd., Tokyo and Elsevier, New York, pp. 136–142.
35. Wacek, T. J. and L. Sequeira. 1973. The peptidoglycan of *Pseudomonas Solanacearum*: chemical composition and biological activity in relation to the hypersensitive reaction in tobacco. *Physiol. Plant Pathol.* **3**: 363–369.

Discussion of Paper by Drs. Tomiyama et al.

DALY asked if a single hypha initiating hypersensitive cell death could cause more than one cell to die. TOMIYAMA answered that it could: initial penetration from a zoospore is always directly into a cell; then the infected cell is killed. Sometime the hypha cease to grow after only a cell is killed. Sometime it invades a few or several cells and the infected cells are killed, and then the hypha cease to grow. The hypha generally, when the infected cells are not killed, enters into intercelluar space and grows intracellularly after it invaded one or a few cells and can kill a limited number of adjacent cells. DURBIN asked how an incompatible reaction with *P. infestans* on leaves, the natural situation, would compare with infection studied in cut tubers. In leaves there can be no aging process for induction of the hypersensitivity potential. TOMIYAMA replied although the situation in leaves is much more complex than in cut tubers, but the same phenomena are observed with leaf petioles. If the leaf petioles are cut and the fresh cut surfaces are inoculated with the incompatible race, the hypersensitive cell death occurs very late. However, when the cut surface tissue are aged, they respond very rapidly. It seems a reasonable presumption that, in the intact cells of all parts of potato plants, infection itself induces the hypersensitivity potential. KUĆ commented that he has found that elicitor from the fungus applied to a-potato slice causes the rishitin level to increase and then decrease, showing that it is degraded even in the first millimeter of tissue. Since TOMIYAMA's results with rishitin synthesis and breakdown are similar, KUĆ pointed out that perhaps the concept of an elicitor is not correct. If the rishitin that is measured is the difference between that which is synthesized and that which is degraded, it is impossible to tell whether the elicitors are inducing synthesis or whether synthesis is always taking place and they are instead interfering with degradation. DALY added that this makes it important to know the turnover rate in terms of concentrations in healthy tissue. KEEN asked if it were conceivable to think that plants would be continuously synthesizing phytoalexins. KUĆ answered that he thought it was a reasonable assumption and many phytoalexins may be transitory intermediates which do not accumulate in sufficient amounts to detect.

GOODMAN asked if the results with dextran-bound PMDT indicated that sites of the trigger for the hypersensitive reaction are SH-groups located on membrane surfaces. He had been able to induce the hypersensitive reaction in tobacco with low levels of SH-compounds. TOMIYAMA answered that SH-reagents such as PMDT might interact with the cell membrane but that he had no evidence of how they specifically inhibit hypersensitivity.

DAY noted that all experiments were done by using compatible and incompatible reactions in tubers with the R_1-gene. What would happen in a cultivar with no R_1-gene? Is there any way of triggering a hypersensitive response in such a cultivar by chemical treatments that would help explain the signal in an incompatible reaction? TOMIYAMA replied that blasticidin S has the same effect on both the incompatible and compatible host cells, *i.e.*, it prolongs survival of infected cells, on both compatible and incompatible reaction with R_1-genes as well as with cultivars containing no R_1-gene. He feels that the difference between compatibility and incompatibility in potato late blight is quantitative, not qualitative, as far as the physiology of host response is concerned. So far, there is no evidence that some chemical treatment can induce (rather, should be called "accelerate") the hypersensitive type of reaction in the case of compatible potato-*P. infestans* combination.

OKU asked how rishitin synthesis is affected by the inhibitors blasticidin S and DNP. TOMIYAMA stated that blasticidin S inhibits rishitin synthesis at early (3–5 hr) but not at later stages; however he had not checked DNP. TOMIYAMA added that he does not understand the relationships between hypersensitivity and phytoalexin production as shown by the inhibitor studies; however both phenomena are apparently the result of early host-pathogen interactions and are good criteria to use in the complex study of resistance.

TANI asked if increased growth of the incompatible fungus occurs in tissue in which the hypersensitivity potential is blocked by blasticidin S. TOMIYAMA said that the incompatible fungus grows well and even produces spores on the infected tissue when fresh discs are treated with blasticidin S. Thus the incompatible response is changed to a compatible one along with the blocking of the potential.

URITANI inquired if rapid cell death is a basic factor in the overall resistant reaction. TOMIYAMA replied that he believes the hypersensitive cell death is one of the most important factors in the disease resistance especially in the case of potato late blight, and also stated that the very rapid hypersensitive reaction he has been studying is a special case that allows him to approach a very complicated phenomenon. However, hypersensitive death in potato late blight normally occurs much more slowly, often 24 hr after penetration, and is comparable to incompatible reactions to other diseases such as powdery mildew.

Recognition and Specificity in Plant Host-Parasite Interactions, pp. 85-97, 1979

PAPILLAE AND PENETRATION: SOME PROBLEMS, PROCEDURES AND PERSPECTIVES

JAMES R. AIST, MARGARET A. WATERMAN, AND HERBERT W. ISRAEL

Department of Plant Pathology, Cornell University, Ithaca, New York, U.S.A.

All living tissues respond characteristically to wounding. Plant tissues may respond morphologically by producing new cells and modifying existing cells at the periphery of the injured region, thereby containing the damage (*16*). The accompanying metabolic changes include increased respiration and altered phenolic and protein metabolism (*9, 12*). It is largely because these and other wound healing responses closely resemble plant disease resistance reactions that wound healing is considered to be a major disease resistance mechanism (*12, 16, 17*).

An individual plant cell may respond rapidly to either localized wounding or fungal attack by accumulating a mass of seething cytoplasm (cytoplasmic aggregate) at the site of perturbation and depositing a localized, amorphous, heterogeneous mass of materials paramurally—between its plasmalemma and cell wall (*1*). Such paramural depositions are termed, collectively, wall appositions (*6*). They may be further classified according to how they are incited (*1*): those incited by fungi are termed papillae (*11*), whereas those incited by abiotic wounding are termed wound plugs (*1*). These terms usually denote structural, paramural entities, but it is important to remember that the deposition process would also alter portions of the cell wall and plasmalemma bounding the appositions (*2*). Because of chemical, structural, optical, and developmental similarities between papillae and wound plugs (*1, 2*), both structures may be considered to result from the same basic plant cell response to perturbation.

Various aspects of wall appositions were discussed in detail in a recent review (*1*). In the present paper, we discuss our views concerning a popular notion about wall apposition function, outline recent pertinent experimental work and suggest important areas for further investigation.

I. SOME FIRST STEPS IN IMPLICATING WALL APPOSITIONS IN DISEASE RESISTANCE

Before 1976, the evidence that wall appositions play a role in disease resistance consisted of several correlations between apposition incidence, shape or size and penetration failures (*1*). We will briefly review next the more important observations from some of those studies.

With certain hosts, Kusano (*10*) found a correlation between the size or shape of wall appositions and the number of protoplasts of the fungal parasite *Olpidium viceae* in the host cell: thick or bulb-shaped appositions were correlated with reduced numbers of parasites in the cell. Furthermore, in the case of bulb-shaped appositions, the parasite had apparently migrated through the penetration tube, only to be surrounded by an apposition at the end of the tube. Kusano concluded that, although there was no consistent correlation between apposition formation and overall disease resistance, certain kinds of appositions did reduce the number of infections.

Differential susceptibility of different cell types of the fungus *Allomyces* to infection by *O. allomycis* has been attributed to a corresponding difference in the production of wall appositions (*8*). In the rarely infected resting sporangia and hyphal cells of the host, growth of the appositions kept pace with that of the parasite penetration tubes until the tubes ceased to grow. No infection whatsoever was seen in several resting sporangia and hyphae which were attacked by over 30,000 encysted *Olpidium* zoospores. Rather, all of the parasites' penetration tubes were sealed off from the host protoplasts, and the cysts were unable to empty their contents. In contrast, appositions occurred only occasionally in thin-walled sporangia, which were heavily infected.

One of the best associations between wall appositions and resistance was described by Heath (*7*), who investigated early host and non-host reactions to the cowpea rust fungus, *Uromyces phaseoli* var. *vignae*. Susceptible hosts never formed appositions when penetrated, small appositions were infrequently seen in intermediate reactions, and in two immune cowpea varieties conspicuous appositions were formed in all invaded cells. In the non-host, *Phaseolus vulgaris*, wall appositions were formed at all points where hyphae touched host cells and were most evident bordering haustorial mother cells. It was assumed that appositions prevented formation of haustoria by 90% of the penetrating hyphae. In instances where haustoria did form, apposition growth was slight or unnoticed and the haustoria appeared to be similar to those in susceptible cowpea cultivars.

Finally, Vance and Sherwood (*13*), in a new approach to the problem,

TABLE I

Effects of Selected Treatments on Host-parasite Interactions[a]

	Treatment	Encounter sites (No.)	% With papillae	PE	% With papillae, and penetration failed
Experiment I	None	50	100	98	2
Olpidium-	NaH_2PO_4[c]	50	90	52	38
Brassica system[b]	Heat shock $+NaH_2PO_4$[d]	25	8	44	4
	Heat shock only	25	20	100	0
Experiment II		69	72	54	28
Erysiphe-	$Ca(H_2PO_4)_2$[f]	33	91	6	85
Hordeum system[e]	Heat shock $+Ca(H_2PO_4)_2$	59	2	8	2
	Heat shock only	50	2	54	2
Experiment III	None	32	69	47	34
Erysiphe-	Cinnamate[g]	35	66	0	66
Hordeum system	Heat shock +cinnamate	26	0	4	0
	Heat shock only	27	0	33	0

[a] All parts of each experiment were repeated at least twice except where noted. Since repeated experiments gave similar results, the data were pooled. [b] Data were taken 4–5 hr after inoculation. [c] Inoculated roots were immersed in 0.001 M NaH_2PO_4, pH 6.0, from 1.75 to 4.0 hr after inoculation. [d] Heat shock preceded inoculation. This part of the experiment was done once. [e] Data were taken 18–20 hr after inoculation. Heat shock preceded inoculation. [f] Coleoptiles were incubated over a solution containing 0.01 M $Ca(H_2PO_4)_2$, adjusted to pH 6.0 with $Ca(OH_2)$, from 10 to 18 hr after inoculation. [g] Coleoptiles were incubated over 0.0012 M sodium cinnamate, pH 6.0, from 10 to 18 hr after inoculation.

reduced protein synthesis, size of wall appositions and resistance to various non-pathogens of reed canary grass by pretreating leaf disks with cycloheximide. Appositions induced by the on-pathogen *Helminthosporium avenae* on untreated disks were 5–9 μm in diameter and 5–12 μm long, whereas those induced on treated disks, as illustrated in their Fig. 1, C and D, measured 8–12 μm in diameter by 2–3 μm long. They viewed formation of wall appositions as ". . . a dynamic response mechanism of the plant for containing the fungus at the penetration site."

In most of the above studies, it was *assumed* that if penetration failures occur in association with wall appositions, then the appositions *caused* the attempted penetrations to fail. What was missing in all studies was a compelling argument or demonstration that factors apart from the appositions did not cause the penetration failures (*1, 16*). The appositions could have been wound-healing depositions having nothing to do with resistance (*1*). Ideally, experiments adequate to rule out effects of possible resistance factors other than wall appositions should have been done. Until adequate experimentation has been done, it is appropriate to postpone the conclusion that wall appositions prevent fungal ingress. The need for caution in this regard is further emphasized in the next section where examples are given of appositions which were associated with, but did not cause, penetration failures.

II. RECENT INVESTIGATIONS OF THE ROLE OF WALL APPOSITIONS IN RESISTANCE

Convinced that the postulated role of wall appositions in resistance needed stronger evidence, we began a long-range project in 1973 to reinvestigate the matter in a more definitive manner. First, we sought optically suitable host cells that were known to produce appositions at sites of penetration failures. To guard against the possibility that host factors other than appositions (*e.g.*, phytoalexins) would cause penetration failures which might be mistakenly attributed to the appositions, we chose two compatible parasite-host combinations, *O. brassicae* on *Brassica oleracea* L. *gongyloides* (kohlrabi) and *Erysiphe graminis hordei* on *Hordeum vulgare* (barley). The choice of compatible hosts enabled us to answer two important questions: (i) do wall appositions cause penetration failures on unaltered host cells, and, if not, (ii) do they have a potential to cause penetration failures? Our investigative approach was two-fold. First, we examined the time courses of unaltered interactions in search of correlations which might suggest that wall appositions prevent penetrations. Second, we altered the timing, location and/or extent of apposition formation and looked for corresponding effects on penetration.

In these studies, penetration efficiency (PE) was defined as the number of successful penetrations per 100 test appressoria (*Erysiphe*) or zoospore cysts (*Olpidium*). Successful penetrations were recorded for *Erysiphe* when mature haustorial central bodies (4) were formed, and for *Olipidium* when zoospore cysts were totally emptied of the parasite protoplasts (*3*).

III. TIME COURSE STUDIES

Reports from other laboratories generally outlined the developmental time courses of *Erysiphe* and *Olpidium*. We further refined these for our particular cultures of the parasites. *Erysiphe graminis hordei* begins penetration from mature appressoria about 10.5 hr after inoculation, and by 18 hr all possible penetrations from primary hooks (*4*) have occurred. This latter point was twice confirmed in replicated experiments in which six randomly selected sites of penetration failure on each of two coleoptiles were thoroughly examined 18 hr after inoculation. Following an additional 24 hr incubation, the same sites were found to have neither haustoria nor additional wall apposition material. Thus, our attention in the *Erysiphe-Hordeum* system was focused on the period 10–18 hr after inoculation. For the *Olpidium-Brassica* system the corresponding time period occurred 1.75–4.0 hr after inoculation.

With both parasite-host systems, we then examined the time courses of events associated with penetration at 150 encounter sites (sites of actual or potential penetration) (*3,4*). Events at each site were observed by interference-contrast microscopy and recorded every 5 min (*Olpidium-Brassica* system) or 10 min (*Erysiphe-Hordeum* system). Part of the data was divided into groups, one containing encounter sites at which an apposition preceded host wall traversal and another containing those at which the reverse occurred. The rationale was this: if appositions prevent penetration, then those which precede penetration might be more effective than those which succeed penetration, resulting in a difference in fungal development between the two groups. Accordingly, we found that PE of both parasites was greatly reduced when appositions preceded penetration attempts. Although these results further implicated appositions as effective deterrents to invasion, encounter sites characterized by penetration failure in the absence of appositions made us suspect that the apposition-associated penetration failures were due to innate developmental deficiencies of some of the parasite propagules. Because such failures would occur even if wall appositions did not form, it seemed useful to prevent appositions from forming during penetration and to see whether the fungus would then be better able to penetrate.

IV. EXPERIMENTAL MANIPULATION OF WALL APPOSITIONS

The overall rationale of these experiments was this: if wall appositions are effective barriers to fungal attack, then inhibition or enhancement of their formation should result in a corresponding effect on penetration efficiency. However, for the results to be conclusive, other factors which could bring about the same results had to be ruled out. Because wall appositions are highly localized, they can be separated from other possible resistance mechanisms. One way we separated them was by creating appositions *before* inoculation and then determining the relative ability of subsequent inoculum to penetrate both the appositions and apposition-free sites on the *same* cell or tissue. Any host feature which conferred resistance only at the appositional site was probably a product of the deposition process (see Introduction). Another approach was to force host cells to restrict formation of appositions to one location during penetration; certain resistance mechanisms unrelated to appositions would then have spatial distributions different from the appositions. Direct interferring effects of experimental treatments on the fungi were routinely avoided by treating the host plants before inoculation, whereas taking comparative data on fungal units which were treated similarly ruled out *both* direct and indirect effects.

In the first experiment, tissues of both hosts were heat-shocked before inoculation to prevent them from producing wall appositions during penetration (*5*). Kohlrabi roots were exposed to 41°C for 20 min and barley coleoptiles to 50°C for 45 sec. Although the heat-shock strongly inhibited host cyclosis and apposition formation during penetration, the affected host cells recovered cyclosis soon thereafter and supported normal parasite development. With the *Olpidium-Brassica* system, PE and the number of unsuccessful cysts with penetration tubes were similar at 500 encounter sites on both shocked and unshocked host cells. With the *Erysiphe-Hordeum* system, PE was similar at 150 encounter sites on both shocked and unshocked host cells, and 11 penetration pegs failed to produce haustoria in shocked cells. These results showed that something other than wall appositions caused several penetration failures which, in unshocked cells, are fortuitously associated with appositions.

With the second method, wall appositions were mechanically induced by bending kohlrabi root hairs before they were inoculated with zoospores of *O. brassicae* (*2*). Pairs of cysts were selected before visible interactions began: one cyst of each pair was located over a mechanically induced apposition and the other was not. Both members of each pair were located on the same root hair. The outcome at each encounter site was recorded after the cysts had been given an extra hour to penetrate. Only 4 of 41 zoospore cysts located over mechanically induced appositions completed penetration, whereas 34 of 41 cysts located >10 μm from appositions on the same set of host cells penetrated. Thus, even compatible root hairs had the potential to prevent penetrations by forming wall appositions. This potential may not have been realized in the unaltered *Olpidium-Brassica* encounters discussed above because the appositions were not developed fast enough or because a feature conferring resistance to the mechanically induced appositions was absent from those induced by the fungus. A companion experiment compared interactions of cysts 2–4 μm from mechanically induced appositions to those of cysts >10 μm from appositions, and showed that the induced resistance was confined to the region of, or near, the appositions.

In a third experiment (*14, 15*), barley coleoptiles were inoculated with conidia of *E. graminis* hordei 8 hr before some of them were centrifuged for 12–14 hr at $4{,}750 \times g$. Centrifugation caused the host cytoplasm, and thus apposition formation, to be localized within each cell. Unusually large wall appositions were deposited at encounter sites over cytoplasm-rich (centrifugal) zones of the inoculated host cells, where PE was 22%. In contrast, no appositions were deposited at encounter sites over cytoplasm-poor (centripetal) zones of the host cells, where PE was 64%. Fungal development on cytoplasm-poor zones and uncentrifuged coleoptiles was similar, and only appressoria which induced wall appositions failed to penetrate into cytoplasm-rich zones of centrifuged coleoptiles. Data were presented to rule out effects other than those of a host cytoplasmic response. The results suggested that an enhanced host response, perhaps wall apposition formation, prevented penetration into the cytoplasm-rich zones of normally compatible host cells. Furthermore, since similar percentages of penetration pegs failed to produce haustoria in both the presence (uncentrifuged coleoptiles) and absence (cytoplasm-poor zones) of wall appositions, this study corroborated the conclusion, from the earlier heat-shock study, that wall appositions did not cause penetration failures in untreated coleoptiles.

V. IF NOT WALL APPOSITIONS, THEN WHAT?

Innate developmental deficiencies of propagules of our parasites could account for the apposition-associated failures we observed in untreated compatible host cells. However, similar deficiencies could not explain the failure of many fungi to penetrate incompatible hosts, since a high developmental potential of the fungi on compatible hosts can be demonstrated. Whether or not penetration attempts into incompatible hosts are stopped by wall appositions can only be determined by experimentation. In the meantime, we have done several experiments which provide examples of known factors other than wall appositions that can cause penetration attempts to fail at encounter sites where appositions occur.

We found that a number of chemical and physical treatments, when applied in an appropriate manner to inoculated kohlrabi roots and barley coleoptiles, greatly reduced PE with little or no reduction in wall apposition induction. This effect caused an increase in the percentage of encounter sites with both an apposition and a failure, *i.e.*, many cysts and appressoria which would have penetrated successfully on untreated host cells failed to penetrate, in the presence of wall appositions, on treated host cells. These additional penetration failures, however, were not caused by the appositions, since a comparable percentage of additional failures occurred on treated host cells which had first been heat-shocked to prevent apposition formation during penetration. The effectiveness of the treatments in preventing penetrations into shocked cells suggests further that the treatments may have had a direct inhibitory effect on the fungi.

Table I gives the results obtained with a few of the chemical treatments. Because some of the active chemicals are not normally considered toxic to fungi, especially at the concentrations employed, these results imply that besides commonly recognized inhibitors, a number of unsuspected and undetected inhibitory substances could be present at encounter sites on untreated plant cells and could act independently of wall appositions to prevent penetrations. Such substances could be part of a natural resistance mechanism, or they could be introduced or induced by way of the experimental procedures used. Regardless of the origin of the substances, their presence would lead to a false indication that wall appositions prevented penetrations. Thus, application of experimental procedures that isolate the effects of wall appositions from effects of other inhibitory factors is a necessary step in the demonstration of a role of wall appositions in disease resistance.

VI. PERSPECTIVES FOR FUTURE RESEARCH

Although there are long-standing correlations between wall appositions and penetration failures, only recently were successful attempts made to experimentally test the hypotheses that the appositions either do or could confer resistance. Such testing should now be extended from our parasite-host combinations to many others, especially where natural resistance is expressed, to determine whether or not wall appositions are the basis of resistance there. Experimentation of this nature opens the door to meaningful investigations of *how* wall appositions may prevent penetrations.

In specific cases where wall appositions have been shown to be capable of preventing fungal ingress, it may be worthwhile to explore the possibility of developing plant varieties with enhanced apposition forming ability and, thus, of enhanced disease resistance. Superficially, this may seem an attractive direction for future work, since the ubiquity of wall apposition induction may make it possible to deal simultaneously with several pathogens. However, known examples of wall appositions which are not effective against penetration or which are initiated too late to deter the fungus suggest the need to first obtain more information on the induction mechanisms and composition of wall appositions that have been shown to be effective.

SUMMARY

In time course studies, wall appositions seemed to prevent some penetrations when initiated before wall traversal, but a cause-and-effect relationship was not established. Heat shock experiments showed that wall appositions did not affect the PE on unshocked host cells; something other than wall appositions caused the penetration attempts to fail. Wall appositions which were mechanically induced to form in kohlrabi root hairs before inoculation with zoospores of *O. brassicae* were effective in preventing penetrations. Thus, even compatible root hairs had the potential to prevent penetrations by forming wall appositions.

Barley coleoptiles were inoculated with conidia of *E. graminis hordei* 8 hr before they were centrifuged for 12–14 hr at $4{,}750 \times g$. The results suggested that an enhanced host response, such as wall apposition formation, prevented penetration into the cytoplasm-rich zones of normally compatible host cells, and that papillae in uncentrifuged coleoptiles did not prevent penetrations. In other experiments, known factors apart from wall appositions caused penetration attempts to fail where appositions occurred.

Our studies point out the need for experimental testing of structure-function postulates and for information on the induction and composition of effective papillae.

Acknowledgment

These studies were supported by CSRS Special Grant No. 316-15-53 and NSF Grant No. PCM76-17209. S. Bucci, J. Piraino, and M. Strang provided technical assistance.

REFERENCES

1. Aist, J. R. 1976. Papillae and related wound plugs of plant cells. *Annu. Rev. Phytopathol.* **14**: 145–163.
2. Aist, J.R. 1977. Mechanically induced wall appositions of plant cells can prevent penetration by a parasitic fungus. *Science* **197**: 568–571.
3. Aist, J. R. and H. W. Israel. 1977. Timing and significance of papilla formation during host penetration by *Olpidium. Phytopathology,* **67**: 187–194.
4. Aist J. R. and H. W. Israel. 1977. Papilla formation: Timing and significance during penetration of barley coleoptiles by *Erysiphe graminis hordei. Phytopathology* **67**: 455–461.
5. Aist J. R. and H. W. Israel. 1977. Effects of heat-shock inhibition of papilla formation on compatible host penetration by two obligate parasites. *Physiol. Plant Pathol.* **10**: 13–20.
6. Bracker, C. E. and L. J. Littlefield. 1973. Structural concepts of host-pathogen interfaces. *In*: R. J. W. Byrde and C. V. Cutting (eds.). *Fungal Pathogenicity and the Plant's Response.* Academic Press, London, p. 499.
7. Heath, M. C. 1972. Ultrastructure of host and nonhost reactions to cowpea rust. *Phytopathology* **62**: 27–38.
8. Karling, J. S. 1948. An *Olpidium* parasite of *Allomyces. Am. J. Bot.* **35**: 503–510.
9. Kuć, J. A. 1976. Phytoalexins. *In*: R. Heitefuss and P. H. Williams (eds.). *Encyclopedia of Plant Physiology.* vol. 4. Springer-Verlag, Heidelberg, 890 pp.
10. Kusano, S. 1936. On the parasitism of *Olpidium. Japan. J. Bot.* **8**: 155–187.
11. Smith, G. 1900. The haustoria of the Erysipheae. *Bot. Gaz.* **29**: 153–184.
12. Uritani, I. 1976. Protein metabolism. *In*: R. Heitefuss and P. H. Williams (eds.). *Encyclopedia of Plant Physiology.* vol. 4. Springer-Verlag, Heidelberg, 890 pp.

13. Vance, C. P. and R. T. Sherwood. 1976. Cycloheximide treatments implicate papilla formation in resistance of reed canarygrass to fungi. *Phytopathology* **66**: 498–502.

14. Waterman, M. A., J. R. Aist, and H. W. Israel. 1977. A new technique for manipulating host-parasite interactions by low speed centrifugation. *Can. J. Bot.* **56**: 542–545

15. Waterman, M. A., J. R. Aist, and H. W. Israel. 1977. Centrifugation studies clarify the role of papilla formation in compatible barley powdery mildew interactions. *Phytopathology* **68**: 797–802

16. Wood, R. K. S. 1967. *Physiological Plant Pathology*. Blackwell Scientific Publ., Oxford, p. 570.

17. Yarwood, C. E. 1973. Some principles of plant pathology. II. *Phytopathology* **63**: 1324–1325.

Discussion of Paper by Drs. Aist et al.

PAXTON asked if there is any evidence that papillae in unsuccessful attempts at invasion are different, either in size or chemical composition, from papillae where successful penetration has occurred. AIST noted that no differences were observed by light microscopy except in the overall morphology and the structure against which they are deposited. DAY remarked that in spite of the fact that inoculation requires only 5 min, it is possible for one zoospore to encyst at the beginning of this period and another one 5 min later on the same root hair. Since the percentage of penetration failures is slightly higher where two cysts are observed on the same root hair, could the first penetration induce a reaction not associated with papilla development that might make a second penetration unsuccessful? AIST stated that he thought this could certainly occur although he had never observed anything which would indicate this in his experiments.

SIEGEL wondered if it would be possible to compare compatible and incompatible hosts having single gene differences in order to determine the numbers of successful and unsuccessful penetrations in relation to papilla formation. AIST remarked that this kind of study is being done by BUSHNELL. The problem is that the resistance may not be papilla-related. BUSHNELL commented that he did not find a relation between specific genes and papilla response in powdery mildew of barley when coleptile tissues were used. He has been finding some differences in leaves that correlate with this specific response.

URITANI asked if appositions contain membranes and organelles. AIST replied that membranes and vesicles are entrapped as enclaves of cytoplasm which are sequestered off as papillae grow; these later degenerate to become dark regions and result in the heterogeneous appearance of papillae. GOODMAN asked about the way in which membranes arrive in the area between the plasmalemma and the cell wall. AIST thought of two possibilities. Simple plasmalemmasomes may be formed which could fuse, cut off vesicles, and end up being pushed out and embedded in the apposition material.

There is more convincing structural evidence for a mechanism involving finger-like projections formed by papillae in areas where differential rates of deposition occur. These fingers invaginate the plasmalemma, grow around, coalesce, and enclose a portion of the cytoplasm.

BUSHNELL questioned the use of highly susceptible host material, particularly in the heat shock experiment in which papillae could have prevented penetration of only 14 out of 500 cysts. Would there be an advantage in using a compatible tissue in which there is no papilla response after heat shock and would there be larger differences with such a system? AIST agreed that the system he had chosen is not ideal for the heat shock type of experiments. Initially, he had wanted a system in which there were penetration failures but no described resistance so that the effect on papillae would not be confused with other things.

DUNKLE, mentioning that cytoplasmic streaming seems to be important in papilla formation, wondered if the cytoplasm aggregates beneath each cyst in a multiply inoculated root hair. He also asked if cytochalasin B, which inhibits cytoplasmic streaming, prevents papilla formation. AIST stated that cytoplasmic aggregates of some size almost always occur under penetrating cysts. The rare exceptions usually occur when the nucleus is blocking that site. It has not been possible to evaluate cytochalasin B as an inhibitor of papilla formation since it also has a direct effect on the fungus.

Recognition and Specificity in Plant Host-Parasite Interactions, pp. 99–112, 1979

INDUCTION OF LIGNIFICATION IN RESPONSE TO FUNGAL INFECTION

YASUJI ASADA, TOMIZO OHGUCHI, AND ISAO MATSUMOTO

College of Agriculture, Ehime University, Matsuyama, Japan

Lignification of diseased parenchyma cell wall is one of the host responses induced by host-parasite interactions. Although many reports are available with respect to the lignin formation of host plants affected by pathogenic fungi, reliable techniques for lignin identification have been used in none of them. Recently, Friend (*12*) reviewed the story of lignification in infected tissue and demonstrated that the formation of lignin-like compounds was really part of the resistance reaction in the potato tuber-*Phytophthora infestans* system. Vance and Sherwood (*19*) reported the regulation of lignin formation in reed canarygrass infected with *Helminthosporium avenae* and mentioned that lignin biosynthesis at the site of attempted fungal penetration may play an important role in the resistant response of the plant to leaf-infecting fungi. They (*18, 20, 21*) also showed that the resistance mechanism in reed canarygrass involves an induction of cathodic isoperoxidases in challenged tissue, no inducible antifungal compounds could be detected by the drop-diffusate technique, and that papilla formation appears to be a defense mechanism against fungal penetration that requires response-dependent protein synthesis. In our studies, the *Raphanus* root-*Peronospora* was selected as the host-parasite system because experimental manipulation is easy with the radish root and the downy mildew fungus is of interest in connection with long-standing question of the nature of obligate prasitism.

The results of our study so far obtained are categorized as follows:

1) Microspectrophotometric identification of lignin in fresh sections and isolation of lignin from diseased plants (*3, 4*).
2) Demonstration of difference in properties of lignins isolated from healthy and diseased plants (*5*).
3) Evidence for the presence of lignin precursors in diseased plants (*1, 7*).
4) Isolation of isoperoxidases and demonstration of their role in lignin biosynthesis (*13, 15*).
5) Presence of a lignification-inducing factor (LIF) in the homogenate of diseased plants (*8*).
6) Time course of the induction of lignification following the treatment with LIF (*14*).
7) Similarity in properties of the lignins isolated from diseased and wounded tissues (*14*).
8) Evidence for the perforation of the host plasma membrane by the haustorium (*9*).

I. MICROSPECTROPHOTOMETRIC IDENTIFICATION AND ISOLATION OF LIGNIN

Fresh sections of downy mildew-infected radish root parenchyma cell walls which were prepared on a freezing microtome had an absorption maximum of 280 nm, suggesting that the walls contained a considerable proportion of guaiacylpropane units. In contrast, an absorption maximum of 270 nm was observed in the healthy radish vessel walls, suggesting that the lignin associated with them consisted of syringylpropane units (*4, 5*). Chemical isolation of lignin was preceded by the extraction of healthy and diseased tissues with hot water, ammonium oxalate and benzene-ethanol in order to remove soluble proteins, soluble polysaccharides, pectins, fats, steroids, and phenolic substances respectively. The residue was further extracted with an amount of dioxane containing HCl, and was neutralized by adding $NaHCO_3$. The filtrate was concentrated under reduced pressure and the concentrated solutions were adjusted to pH 2 and centrifuged. The pellets material was dissolved in dioxane, and then ether was added. The suspension was centrifuged and the precipitate was washed twice with dioxane and ether. The precipitate thus obtained was designated as "dioxane lignin-like substance (DL)." The isolated DL was characterized by infrared and ultraviolet absorption, methoxyl group determination, paper chromatography of products of alkaline nitrobenzene oxidation, paper chromatography of products of ethanolysis, and also by elemental analysis (*2, 3, 5*).

II. DIFFERENCE IN PROPERTIES OF LIGNINS ISOLATED FROM HEALTHY AND DISEASED PLANTS

When DL from the healthy root was oxidized with nitrobenzene in alkaline media, syringaldehyde was derived together with *p*-hydroxybenzaldehyde and vanillin, suggesting that DL in the healthy root is composed of syringylpropane units. DL from the diseased root, however, contained more vanillin and *p*-hydroxybenzaldehyde but no syringaldedhyde. It seemed to be composed primarily of guaiacylpropane units. From elemental analyses of the isolated DL, the following empirical formulae were proposed (*5*).

Healthy lignin : $C_9H_{10.30}O_{2.20}(OCH_3)_{1.16}$
Diseased lignin : $C_9H_{8.33}O_{2.80}(OCH_3)_{0.75}$

If coniferyl alcohol is the sole precursor of the lignins, methoxyl content of the DL is expected to be 1. But the values were 1.16 and 0.75 for healty and diseased lignins, respectively. Therefore, in the healthy tissues sinapyl alcohol should be a precursor of the healthy lignin, and *p*-coumaryl alcohol should be a precursor of the diseased lignin, coniferyl alcohol being a partner in both cases. It is universally recognized that peroxidase plays a role in the dehydrogenation polymerization of *p*-hydroxycinnamyl alcohols. We then supposed that either a decrease in activity of a isoperoxidase which react to sinapyl alcohol or an increase in activity of a isoperoxidase which react to *p*-coumaryl and coniferyl alcohols occurs in the diseased tissues.

III. PRESENCE OF PHENOLIC ACIDS AS PRECURSORS OF LIGNIN IN THE INFECTED ROOT

In order to find lignin precursors in the infected root, we examined constituents of phenolic acids by gas-liquid chromatography of the extract from the infected root (*7*). Quinic, prephenic, phenylpyruvic, *trans*-cinnamic, *p*-coumaric, and caffeic acids were identified, but chorismic, *p*-hydroxyphenyl-pyruvic, ferulic, and sinapic acids were not detected in the form of free acids. Generally, the hexose monophosphate shunt seems to be the predominant pathway for glucose catabolism in diseased plants. For activation of the lignification pathway in the root, enzymes which catalyze these changes should be activated. For example, increases in activities of L-phenylalanine ammonia-lyase and peroxidase were observed in the infected roots and were shown to be due to *de novo* synthesis of the enzymes (*6*). We also examined the incorporation of L-phenylalanine-G-^{3}H into the infected cell walls by electron microscopic autoradiography. In the inoculated root, noticeable silver grains were observed first in the inner layers of cell wall and then in the middle lamella (*1*). This result is consistent with Brown and Neish's result (*10*) which showed that lignin was synthesized from phenylalanine and related aromatic monomers.

IV. ISOLATION OF ISOPEROXIDASES AND THEIR ROLE IN LIGNIN BIOSYNTHESIS

Freudenberg (*11*) suggested the mechanism for the initiation of dehydrogenation polymerization of coniferyl alcohol. Coniferyl alcohol is dehydrogenated at the phenolic hydroxyl group. A mesomeric radical is formed with limiting structures, such as aroxyl form, *p*-quinone methide form and orthoquinoid form. The combination of *p*-quinone methide and orthoquinoid forms gives a quinone methide, which is stabilized by intramolecular prototropy, giving dehydrodiconiferyl alcohol. Two *p*-quinone methide radicals give a double quinone methide, which undergoes a double prototropy, giving pinoresinol. These substances seem to be components of lignin. Thus, peroxidases which are widely distributed in the plant and are activated following fungal infection (*15*), seem to play a role in lignin biosynthesis. The physiological role of peroxidase in higher plants seems to be production of free radicals in the presence of H_2O_2.

In an attempt to determine the role of enhanced peroxidase activity in the infected root, the formation of dehydrogenation polymerization products (DHPs) from *p*-hydroxycinnamyl alcohols was investigated by using isoperoxidases isolated from the radish root (*13*). DHPs were formed from coniferyl alcohol when *p*-coumaryl or sinapyl alcohol was added to it together with crude peroxidase preparation. Characteristic properties of DHPs were similar to those of lignins isolated from the healthy and diseased roots respectively. DHP formation was also examined with peroxidase fractions obtained from the crude peroxidase preparation by carboxymethyl (CM)- and diethylaminoethyl (DEAE)-cellulose column chromatography. Of 11 fractions having peroxidase activity (A_1–A_5, B–G), Fractions D and F did not form DHP from any of the alcohols, while Fraction G only formed

DHP from *p*-coumaryl alcohol. When the substrate was mixture of sinapyl and coniferyl alcohols DHP was formed by Fractions A_1, A_3, B, and E. Each of 11 fractions was assayed for purity by polyacrylamide gel electrofocusing. Fractions E and F consisted of a single isozyme while the rest contained two or more isozymes. The crude peroxidase preparation contained 16 different isozymes. Isozyme No. 15 seemed most likely to be involved in the lignin biosynthesis, because this was the only isozyme found in Fraction E, which had a high activity with all implicated substrates. Fraction G also contained isozyme No. 15. But this lignin-forming activity was very low, probably because the isozyme content was low. Isozymes Nos. 3, 6, 11, and 16 did not seem to be involved in the lignin biosynthesis, as they were contained in Fractions D and F, which were unable to form DHP from any of the alcohols tested. The remaining isozymes were present in fractions which had previously been shown to be decreased in concentration as a result of infection (*15*). Hence these isozymes are thought unlikely to be involved in the enhanced lignin biosynthesis. Some of these isozymes, however, may possibly participate in the polymerization of sinapyl alcohol. Fraction A_2 and A_3, which had acidic property, made DHP by sinapyl alcohol in the presence of coniferyl alcohol. Thus the synthesis of guaiacyl lignin in the diseased tissue might result from the decreased concentration of the isozymes which catalyze polymerization of sinapyl alcohol and also from the increased concentration of basic isozymes which catalyze polymerization of *p*-coumaryl and coniferyl alcohols. These results coincide well with that of Vance and Sherwood (*19*).

V. PRESENCE OF A LIGNIFICATION-INDUCING FACTOR IN THE HOMOGENATE OF DISEASED ROOT

Lignin was formed not only in cell walls of root tissues infected with the fungus, but also in those of healthy tissues infiltrated with the homogenate of downy mildew-infected tissues (*8*). After the treatment with the homogenate, lignin began to be formed in cell walls in about 12 hr. Formation became rapid about 17 hr after treatment and was maintained for about 5 hr. Although lignification was also induced by treatment with the homogenate of noninoculated root tissues, formation of lignin was delayed for about 2 hr and the extent of reaction was less than with tissue treated with homogenate of diseased tissues. It is likely that some type of inducer is involved in the enhanced lignification. The inducer may either directly originate from the pathogen or be produced indirectly by the host tissues as a response to infection and/or injury.

In order to know the origin of the LIF, slices in which lignification had been induced by infiltration with the homogenate of diseased tissues were homogenized and filtered. The filtrate was used as the "second homogenate." Similarly, the filtrate obtained from the freshly prepared tissues treated with the second homogenate was used as the "third homogenate." Lignification-inducing ability of fresh tissues was assayed by using the second and third consecutive homogenates. From this "dilution experiment," the LIF must be a substance which is porduced in the tissues in response to treatment because it not only withstood massive dilution but actually increased in activity through the sequential repetition of homogenate infiltration (*14*). The LIF was presumed to be a low molecular weight compound, not larger than several thousands, as estimated from dialysis and elution profile in gel filtration chromatography. It is positive to ninhydrin and differs from monilicolin A in that it is apparently produced by host cells. Further characterization of LIF is in progress.

VI. TIME COURSE OF THE INDUCTION OF LIGNIFICATION

The homogenate-induced lignification was completely inhibited by inhibitors of nucleic acid synthesis, such as cordycepin, ethidium bromide, chromomycin A_3, and actinomycin D when they were applied within 30 min following infiltration with homogenate. When these inhibitors were applied within 2 hr after infiltration, lignification proceeded only to a limited extent. These inhibitors exerted no effect on tissue lignification when applied 3 hr or more after homogenate infiltration. Blasticidin S, a protein synthesis inhibitor, exerted a similar effect. It inhibited lignification completely when it was applied within 2 hr after homogenate infiltration and to a limited extent when applied from 2 to 6 hr after infiltration. These results may suggest that enzymatic proteins responsible for lignification were synthesized in the tissue at least 7 hr after the homogenate treatment. Lignification of root tissues was also blocked when they were exposed to a temperature of 50°C for 1 min in water or for 1 hr in air prior to homogenate infiltration. All cells in the tissues survived these heat treatment as evidenced by their ability to plasmolyze. The effect of heat shock is reversible, as the lignification could be induced when the heat-treated tissue was subjected to homogenate infiltration after incubating at 20°C for 24 hr following the heat treatment. It may be surmised that some modification of the host plasma membrane is closely associated with the induction of lignification.

Next, when root tissues were infiltrated with water *in vacuo* within 2 hr after the treatment with diseased tissue homogenate, lignification was inhibited completely, while infiltration by water later than 2 hr or more after the homogenate infiltration did not prevent lignification. Also, tissues held in water for the first 12 hr after homogenate treatment were not lignified at all, while lignification was induced when they were immersed in water later than 12 hr after the homogenate treatment. When tissue blocks were held in nitrogen gas for 2–3 hr immediately after homogenate treatment lignification was not induced, but tissues held in air for the first 12 hr were lignificed even if they were exposed to nitrogen gas for the subsequent 12 hr. This suggests that an aerobic reaction is involved in the initial induction process. Fig. 1 shows a possible model for the events during the induction of lignification in radish tissues (*14*).

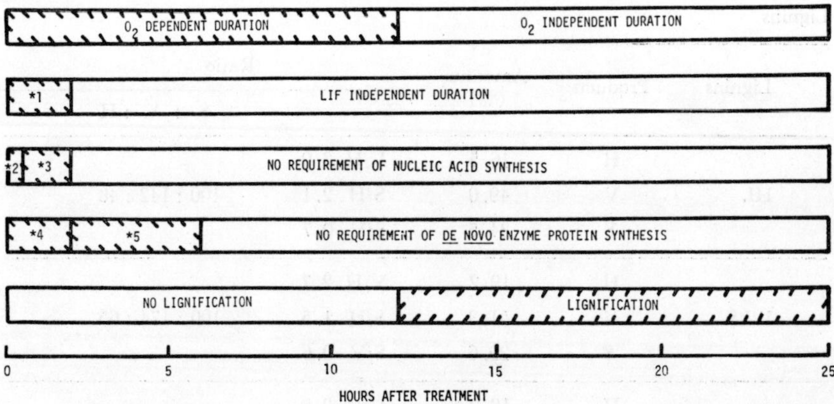

Fig. 1. Time course of induction of lignification following treatment with LIF. *[1] LIF dependent duration; *[2] complete inhibition of nucleic acid synthesis responsible for lignification; *[3] incomplete inhibition of nucleic acid synthesis responsible for lignification; *[4] complete inhibition of *de novo* enzyme protein synthesis responsible for lignification; *[5] incomplete inhibition of *de novo* enzyme protein synthesis responsible for lignification.

VII. SIMILARITY IN PROPERTIES BETWEEN DISEASED AND WOUND LIGNINS

Amounts of products from degradation by alkaline nitrobenzene oxidation of lignin isolated from root tissues which had been infiltrated with homogenates are shown in Table I. Wound lignins produced in tissues which had been infiltrated with the homogenate of healthy slices (WLS) were similar both in the amount and in the ratio of degradation products to the diseased lignins produced in tissues infiltrated with the homogenate of diseased slices (DLD). Lignins isolated from healthy tissues, however, differed from WLS and DLD in syringaldehyde content (*14*). Therefore, we concluded that there is no difference in properties between the diseased and wound lignins and both lignins have guaiacylpropane units.

TABLE I

Amounts of the Degradation Products by Alkaline Nitrobenzene Oxidation of the Isolated Lignins

Lignins	Products	Amounts (%)	Ratio	
				S : V : H
	H	16.5	V/H 3.0	
HL	V	49.0	S/H 2.1	100 : 142 : 48
	S	34.5	S/V 0.7	
	H	19.2	V/H 2.7	
WLS	V	51.3	S/H 1.5	100 : 174 : 65
	S	29.6	S/V 0.6	
	H	18.9	V/H 2.8	
DLD	V	52.5	S/H 1.5	100 : 184 : 66
	S	28.6	S/V 0.5	

HL, healthy lignin from healthy tissue; WLS, wound lignin from tissues treated with homogenate of sliced tissue; DLD, diseased lignin from tissues treated with homogenate of diseased tissue; H, *p*-hydroxybenzaldehyde; V, vanillin; S, syringaldehyde.

VIII. EVIDENCE FOR THE PERFORATION OF HOST PLASMA MEMBRANE BY THE HAUSTORIUM

We attempted to clarify by electron microscopy the presence of an injury to the host plasma membrane by the haustorium (*9*). In addition to the usual Reynolds' method (*16*), the sections were stained by alkaline bismuth method for detailed observation of the plasma membranes (*17*). At early stages of infection, the host plasma membrane was not perforated and detachment of the membrane from the host cell wall was clearly observed following treatment by a hypertonic sucrose solution. Later, however, the host plasma membrane was invaginated at the penetration site and was then perforated by the haustorium. Fig. 2 shows discontinuity and/or perforation of the host plasma membrane, and the haustorium has contacted directly with host cytoplasm. Plasmolysis of the host cell occurred even ater the haustorium had penetrated the host plasma membrane. Hence, it is suggested that the haustorium acts as a "plug" for the host plasma

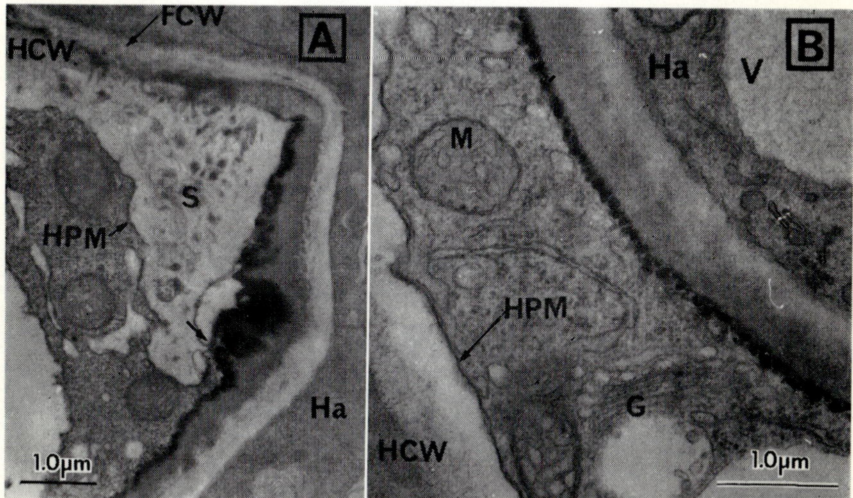

Fig. 2. Electron microphotograph of the interface of *Peronospora parasitica* on *Raphanus sativus* root.
A, by Reynolds' method; B, by alkaline bismuth method; FCW, fungal cell wall, G, Golgi body; HCW, host cell wall; Ha, haustorium; HPM, host plasma membrane; M, mitochondrion; S, sheath; V, vacuole; arrow, perforation site of HPM.

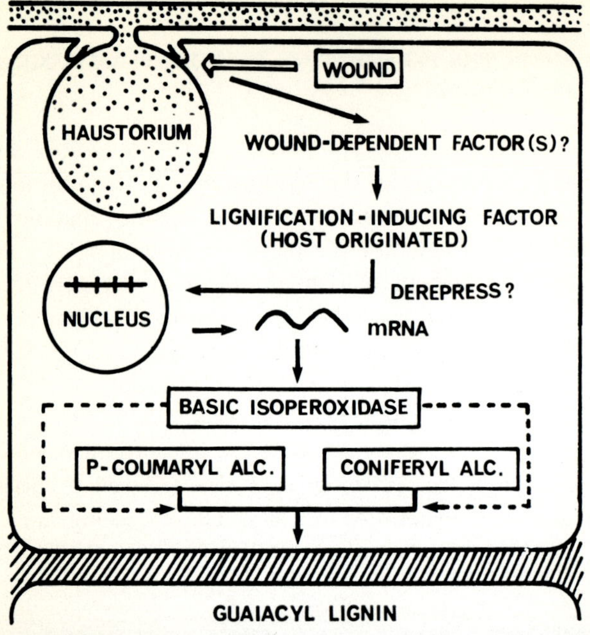

Fig. 3. Speculative diagram of the host-parasite interactions leading to lignin formation in diseased tissues.

membrane. This is important evidence in host cell-haustorium relationships and the presence of an injury of the host plasma membrane seems to lead a formation of wound-dependent elicitor(s) or first inducer(s) in the root tissues, because the LIF that described previously was a substance which apparently originates secondarily from host tissues. Guaiacyl lignin formation also takes place in wounded root tissues and LIF is formed in this tissue. Lignification of tissues, therefore, seems to be a kind of wound response.

On the basis of the results demonstrated over the eight sections, we propose the lignification process is involved in the downy mildew-infected and/or injured tissues as shown in Fig. 3.

SUMMARY

Lignin was formed in cell walls of Japanese radish (*Raphanus sativus*) parenchyma root infected with *Peronospora parasitica*. This formation also occurred in the tissue which had been infiltrated with homogenate of the diseased tissue. Chemical analysis of lignins extracted from both tissues which had been infiltrated with homogenates of diseased and sliced tissues showed that these two lignins were probably identical and had guaiacyl-propane units. Inhibitors of nucleic acid and protein synthesis applied immediately after treatment with the homogenate completely inhibited lignification. These inhibitors did not affect lignification when treated 2 or more hours with the former, 6 or more hours the latter after homogenate infiltration respectively. Lignification-inducing factor was found in the homogenate of the diseased tissue and this was a ninhydrin-positive substance which was not directly secreted by the pathogen but was indirectly formed in the tissue in response to the infection and/or injury. Presence of an injury of the host plasma membrane by the haustorium was elucidated electron microscopically.

Acknowledgments

Financial support of this study is acknowledged from the Ministry of Education, Science and Culture of Japan for research grants Nos. 86013, 586013, 936013, 136006, and 148044 in 1970, 1971, 1974, 1975, 1976, and 1977.

REFERENCES

1. Asada, Y. and T. Kugoh. 1971. Incorporation of tritiated phenylalanine into lignified cell walls of Japanese radish root infected by *Peronospora parasitica*. *Ann. Phytopathol. Soc. Japan* **37**: 311–313.
2. Asada, Y. and I. Matsumoto. 1967. Formation of lignin in the root tissues of Japanese radish affected by *Alternaria japonica*. *Phytopathology* **57**: 1339–1343.
3. Asada, Y. and I. Matsumoto. 1969. Formation of lignin- like substance in the root tissues of Japanese radish plant infected by downy mildew fungus. *Ann. Phytopathol. Soc. Japan* **35**: 160–167.
4. Asada, Y. and I. Matsumoto. 1971. Microspectrophotometric observations on the cell walls of Japanese radish (*Raphanus sativus*) root infected by *Peronospora parasitica*. *Physiol. Plant Pathol.* **1**: 377–383.
5. Asada, Y. and I. Matsumoto. 1972. The nature of lignin obtained from downy mildew-infected Japanese radish root. *Phytopathol. Z.* **73**: 208–214.
6. Asada, Y. and I. Matsumoto. 1972. *De novo* synthesis of L-phenylalanine ammonia-lyase in Japanese radish root infected by downy mildew fungus. *Mem. Coll. Agric. Ehime Univ.* **17**: 27–37.

7. Asada, Y., I. Matsumoto, and T. Tashiro. 1972. The formation of phenolic acids in the root of downy mildew-infected Japanese radish. *Ann. Phytopathol. Soc. Japan* **38**: 405–409.
8. Asada, Y., T. Ohguchi, and I. Matsumoto. 1975. Lignin formation in fungus-infected plants. *Rev. Plant Prot. Res.* **8**: 104–113.
9. Asada, Y. and M. Shiraishi. 1976. Discontinuity of the plasma membrane of *Raphanus sativus* around haustoria of *Peronospora parasitica*. *In*: K. Tomiyama, J. M. Daly, I. Uritani, H. Oku, and S. Ouchi (eds.). *Biochemistry and Cytology of Plant-Parasite Interaction*. Kodansha Ltd., Tokyo and Elsevier, Amsterdam, p. 32.
10. Brown, S. A. and A. C. Neish. 1956. Studies of lignin biosynthesis using isotopic carbon. IV. Formation from some aromatic monomers. *Can. J. Biochem. Physiol.* **34**: 769–778.
11. Freudenberg, K. 1965. Lignin: Its constitution and formation from *p*-hydroxycinnamyl alcohols. *Science* **148**: 595–600.
12. Friend, J. 1976. Lignification in infected tissue. *In*: J. Friend and D. R. Threlfall (eds.). *Biochemical Aspects of Plant-Parasite Relationships*. Annu. Proc. Phytochem. Soc. No. 13, pp. 291–303.
13. Matsumoto, I., T. Ohguchi, and Y. Asada. 1978. Induction of lignification by the homogenate of Japanese radish infected with downy mildew fungus. *Ann. Phytopathol. Soc. Japan* **44**: 22–27.
14. Ohguchi, T. and Y. Asada. 1974. Dehydrogenation polymerization products of *p*-hydroxycinnamyl alcohols by isoperoxidases obtained from the downy mildew-infected roots of Japanese radish (*Raphanus sativus*). *Physiol. Plant Pathol.* **5**: 183–192.
15. Ohguchi, T., Y. Yamashita, and Y. Asada. 1974. Isoperoxidases of Japanese radish root infected by downy mildew fungus. *Ann. Phytopathol. Soc. Japan* **40**: 519–426.
16. Reynolds, E. S. 1963. The use of lead citrate at high pH as an electron opaque stain in electron microscopy. *J. Cell Biol.* **17**: 208–214.
17. Roland, J. C., C. A. Lembi, and D. J. Morre. 1972. Phosphotungstic acid-chromic acid as a selective electron-dense stain for plasma membranes of plant cells. *Stain Technol.* **47**: 195–200.
18. Vance, C. P., J. O. Anderson, and R. T. Sherwood. 1976. Soluble and cell wall peroxidases in reed canarygrass in relation to disease resistance and localized lignin formation. *Plant Physiol.* **57**: 920–922.
19. Vance, C. P. and R. T. Sherwood. 1976. Regulation of lignin formation in reed canarygrass in relation to disease resistance. *Plant Physiol.* **57**: 915–919.
20. Vance, C. P. and R. T. Sherwood. 1976. Cycloheximide treatments implicate papilla formation in resistance of reed canarygrass to fungi. *Phytopathology* **66**: 498–502.
21. Vance, C. P. and R. T. Sherwood. 1977. Lignified papilla formation as a mechanism for protection in reed canarygrass. *Physiol. Plant Pathol.* **10**: 247–256.

Discussion of Paper by Drs. Asada et al.

KOSUGE started the discussion by asking if any other compounds have been tested to see if they can mimic the effect of the LIF. ASADA said that the same lignin can be induced by heavy metal salts such as mercuric chloride and by treatment of the tissue with acids at pH 1.

KUĆ asked what specific biosynthetic step LIF is activating or eliciting. ASADA stated that LIF increases the synthesis of phenolics as well as their polymerization; it induces phenylalanine ammonia-lyase and isoperoxidases. However, it is not clear what the initial rate-limiting step might be.

KEEN asked if some of the inhibitors, such as blasticidin S, that block lignification and response to LIF also block resistance of the tissue to the fungus. ASADA answered that he has not tested this yet and outlined the sequence of fungal development in resistant or susceptible tissue. KUĆ remarked that it appears as if lignin formation may not be responsible for resistance if the fungus is already growing more slowly in the resistant tissue before it reaches the lignin layer. ASADA explained that as *Peronospora* grows intercellularly, lignification is occurring as a continuous, extensive process. There is not a lignin layer as such, but lignification of the walls occurs throughout the infected area. In the resistant tissue the lignification is complete whereas in the susceptible tissue it is only partial.

BUSHNELL asked how extensive the evidence is for the breaks in the host plasma membranes around the haustoria. ASADA answered that he has many electron micrographs of sections of infected tissue showing the same thing. HANCEY asked if the organelles in the host cytoplasm would not be drastically disrupted or swollen if there were true holes in the plasma membrane. She suggested that the staining methods might detect certain chemical modifications of the plasma membrane in its ability to stain but that this may not necessarily mean there are ruptures at those points. ASADA said that he could not be sure that the apparent perforations of the membranes were not artifacts from the preparation procedures for electron microscopy.

NISHIMURA asked if there are differences in the mechanism of lignin induction by chemicals such as mercuric chloride and induction by LIF. Is there some type of specificity in the induction process? ASADA stated that his procedure for inducing lignification requires an incubation period of 2 hr with LIF. Lignification can be inhibited soon after initiating its induction with LIF: within 2 hr by infiltrating the tissue with water, within 3 hr by treating with inhibitors of nucleic acid synthesis, and within 6 hr by treating with inhibitors of protein synthesis. Therefore it appears that LIF is combined with some cellular component, possibly a receptor on the membrane, 2 hr after it is applied to the tissue. KUĆ asked if the lignification induced by mercuric chloride is also blocked by these inhibitors. ASADA replied that he had not tried that.

CONSTITUTIVE RECOGNITION OF SPECIFICITY

Recognition and Specificity in Plant Host-Parasite Interactions, pp. 115-131, 1979

WHAT ART THOU, O SPECIFICITY?

R. D. DURBIN AND J. A. STEELE

Plant Disease Resistance Research Unit, AR, USDA, Department of Plant Pathology, University of Wisconsin, Madison, Wisconsin, U.S.A.

The view that toxins are intimately involved in disease causation dates back to the mid-19th Century. Indeed, Gäumann (*5*) hypothesized that all plant pathogens require these substances for pathogenesis. However, as Ludwig (*7*) has stated, this concept appears to be too inclusive. Nevertheless, the participation of toxins in disease development is becoming more recognized, and experimental evidence has accumulated to show that these substances are produced by all major taxonomic groups of pathogens.

Part of the problem of accepting Gäumann's viewpoint is that, the term "toxin" has been used with such a variety of meanings that, as Dimond and Waggoner (*3*) have written, "Loose usage of the word 'toxin' has led to confusion in the study of disease causes." As a result, they, and later others, attempted to rigorously define what a toxin is, and classify them into types. In so doing they utilized the concept of specificity. It is in this connection that we would like to begin our considerations of toxin specificity.

I. OPERATIONAL DEFINITIONS

First, let us briefly review some of the past thinking on toxin terminology, especially the operational definitions as they relate to specificity. During the early period of modern interest in toxins it became apparent that some toxic substances were only cultural artifacts and had no demonstrable connection with pathogenesis whereas the experimental evidence implicating other toxins as mediators of plant disease was quite strong. Overall, the situation was chaotic. Accordingly, several workers proposed sets of terms to conceptually and operationally define toxins in relationship to disease causation. Braun and Pringle (*2*), as one example, pointed out that a toxin should exhibit some type of specificity when interacting with a host; *i.e.*, specificity as to genotype of the host affected or symptom produced. Similar views were voiced by others (*3, 11, 16, 17*). Most authors would agree with definitions which specify that toxins of the type we are considering here are synthesized by the pathogen. Also, that they are injurious to the host, and, therefore, contribute to disease development. There is less agreement, however, whether their specific effects are reflected as part of the disease syndrome or of pathogenesis. This distinction is important, since using the word syndrome would exclude substances whose effects are not visible; *viz* those that might be detectable only at the biochemical level. In our view, the definition should make no restriction as to the level at which a toxin's effect(s) is manifest. However, regardless of whose terminology is followed, it has proven difficult to experimentally satisfy the criteria for proof of complicity. The amounts of the toxins present in diseased tissues are unusually small, they are hard to isolate because of interactions with plant extracts or their chemical instability, and many times their observable effect on plants is so nonspecific that definitive conclusions cannot be drawn.

Our experimental inability to prove complicity certainly does not invalidate the criteria. But, it may well be that these criteria are not always suitable for elucidating a toxin's role in disease causation [as Wheeler and Luke (*16*) imply in their statement that the "responsibility for providing adequate evidence . . . rests with the investigator"]. To visualize why this might be so consider disease as an interaction between host and pathogen which alters the metabolic state of both organisms with the passage of time. Such a time-dependent interaction could lead to hypothetical situations in which the criteria used to demonstrate a role for a toxin in pathogenesis become inapplicable. For example, a substance which is toxic to a host following some changes resulting from the interaction may have no effect on an unaltered host plant. Also, toxins which inhibit active host resistance mechanisms, such as phytoalexin production (*9*) or cell wall thickening, will not produce observable effects in the absence of elicitors of such responses. In both cases the usual criteria fail because although the toxin is causally linked to pathogenesis, the disease syndrome cannot be reproduced by the toxin alone.

II. CHEMICAL SPECIFICITY

The actions of toxins need not necessarily be specific *biologically* but they must be *chemically* specific to some degree. The determination of this specificity encompases two interrelated, but nevertheless independent, considerations. The first is qualitative and has to do with the structural features of the toxin and the complementary region about the interaction site on the receptor molecule. Collectively they determine the specificity, or selectivity, of the interaction. Second is the quantitative aspect; *i.e.*, how intense the interaction will be between the toxin and its receptor. It is not necessary that a toxin bind tightly in order to be highly specific: toxins with low biological activity or affinity constants can still be highly specific and damaging if they occur in sufficiently high concentration in the diseased plant.

Assuming that the site of interaction is accessible, a toxin's specificity depends upon the above qualitative considerations. Nothing is specified about the receptor molecule as to its kind, where it is situated in the host, what function it might have or its taxonomic distribution. Answers to some of these questions are relevant to understanding biological specificity, but not necessarily chemical specificity. For this and other reasons it seems logical to us that we should begin to classify toxins chemically on the basis of ligand-receptor interactions. This rational system would encompass many types of specific interactions within one conceptual framework so that interrelationships might then become more apparent.

Admittedly, our understanding of the biochemical mechanisms by which pathogen-produced toxins recognize and act on their targets is very much in its infancy. The structures of known toxins (*10*) would suggest that they could interact with receptor sites in a variety of ways, ranging from covalent linkages to ones involving hydrogen bonding, electrostatic or van der Waal's interactions. Whether these potentials for interaction are ever expressed also depends upon the properties of the receptors, their surrounding environment and their compartmentation. Also, we have essentially little or no information about the actual structures of the receptors, their ability to bind toxins and toxin analogs, and in some of the more interesting host-parasite conbinations, even the structure of the toxin remains unknown.

However, from the examples we do know something of, it appears that the degree of chemical specificity varies. For example, fusicoccin, produced by the fungus *Fusicoccum amygdali*, affects membrane-bound ATPases of differing functions in various tissues of many plant species. In nature though, because of constraints imposed by host-pathogen interactions, it acts only upon an ATPase found in the guard cells of leaves from almond and peach. Tabtoxins appear to affect the same process in all plants tested to date (Durbin, unpublished data), but the pseudomonads producing them are nevertheless restricted to specific hosts. Tentoxin produced by *Alternaria alternata* is specific for a single protein species but since this receptor molecule (chloroplast coupling factor 1 (CF_1)) occurs in at least two plant-specific molecular forms, only one of which is affected, tentoxin has a broad host specificity. Finally, there are toxins, produced principally by *Helminthosporium* spp. that exhibit a high degree of host specificity and are extremely potent (*11*). Although little is known about their receptors, except for one case (*15*), they certainly appear to be highly specific chemically. Classifying these interactions on the basis of biological specificity alone leads to a confusing picture. Viewing them in the context of chemical interactions whose expression can be modified by additional variables reduces the confusion and may aid our understanding of host-parasite relations.

III. MODELING TOXIN-HOST INTERACTIONS

The dynamics of host-parasite interactions, which result in the expression of the multivariate property we call specificity, are difficult to understand qualitatively or quantitatively on either an intuitive or purely descriptive basis. To achieve such understanding, it would be useful to construct flexible, conceptual models with a mathematical basis. Any general model of host-parasite interactions which seeks to explain specificity should meet certain criteria if it is to serve as a theoretical framework to aid in the investigation of plant disease. First, factors governing specificity are multiple, so the model must deal with many variables. Second, since a static model is clearly inappropriate, the dimension of time should be incorporated. Third, such models should encompass known phenomena involving mediators of host-pathogen interactions such as toxins and specific recognition sites (consideration of other mediators such as phytoalexins and elicitors is equally appropriate). Finally, the model should provide for a broad continuous range of behaviors including, but not limited to, hypersensitivity, tolerance, mesothetic reactions, generalized resistance, and environmental predisposition. The model depicted in Fig. 1 meets many of these requirements.

Before discussing this model, it is necessary that the meanings we apply to "signal" and "channel" are clear. A signal is anything which serves to carry information from a source to one or more destinations. It is necessary that an entity or state be produced by a source and detected by a receiver if it is to serve as a signal. Thus signals may consist of patterns of matter and energy without any restriction regarding their specific forms. In biological systems we expect many signals to be joint manifestations of the genes which specify their production, detection, and disposition. Signals available to a host might include internal ATP concentration, toxin concentration, and temperature. In one system which will be discussed later, the pathogen's genetic information is transformed to a toxin (tentoxin) whose structure defines it as a signal provided that the host genome specifies a particular receptor site on chloroplast CF_1. It is the informational content of the genes which interact, not the genes themselves. A channel is an interface between systems through which many signals may pass. We emphasize that a channel may carry a multitude of signals simultaneously.

In the model illustrated, the host-pathogen system is partitioned into four interacting subsystems. The host systems are divided into a control system (HC) composed of control elements which detect signals and an effector system (HE) composed of effector elements which generate signals. The pathogen system is divided in a similar manner (PC and PE) and the subsystems are joined by the channels shown. Control elements could include such things as receptor sites for small molecules while effector elements could include enzymes which are regulated by the status of such receptor sites. These are, however, only examples; control and effector elements are not restricted to specific metabolic functions but vary with the situation under consideration. Each control system may receive signals from its own effector system, the opposing effector system, and the external environment (E). In response to this input, the functioning of the associated effector system (HE, PE), and the physiological state of the system as a whole is altered. Thus, for example, a toxin could initially reduce the host's energy resources, and thereby indirectly affect photosynthesis or lipid metabolism. Conversely, an elicitor produced by the pathogen may cause the host to produce phytoalexins which reduce the activities of the pathogen, including toxin production. These interactions may develop into very complex time-dependent patterns in which the relationship between the magnitudes of 2 (or more) signals at a certain time is critical in determining the eventual development of the disease. For example, the host's active resistance mechanisms might respond to signals produced by a pathogen but so slowly that the pathogen nevertheless overwhelms the host.

Such a model emphasizes the multideterminant nature of specificity, since each channel linking the host and pathogen can carry many signals and each signal from the control elements is potentially a function of any combination of the control system inputs. If control of the effector elements is achieved by varying the rates of their actions, then the time dimension is intrinsic. The known chemical mediators of host-pathogen relations are encompassed since they represent either signals which interact with control elements; *e.g.*, toxins, phytoalexins, elicitors, *etc.*, or specific control elements; *e.g.*, receptor sites.

If the initial states of both host and pathogen subsystems and the relationships between input and output signals are specified, then quantitative predictions of system behavior with respect to time can be made. The mathematical tools for accomplishing this are available in the form of state variable methods as applied to control system theory and realized as computer programs (*12*). Models organized in this way can exhibit an extremely wide range of behavior, including catastrophic failure (death) of either (or both) subsystem(s). A further useful feature of this kind of model is that it can be more extensively partitioned so as to include compartmentation and the additional interfaces which biological organisms typically possess.

The most immediate use one can visualize for such a model structure is to provide theoretical considerations which could aid in developing experimental strategies for studying host-parasite interactions. For example, in the context of the model presented here, it is clear that studies of host-parasite interactions could concentrate on disconnecting the interface between host and pathogen systems (along line A in Fig. 1) and determine the effects of individual pathogen or host signals upon the overall functioning of the opposing system when feedback is retained between control and effector systems. Most of the work on toxins has been either this type of study or the isolation and identification of compounds which serve as signals. However, greater experimental simplification might be obtained if the host effector feedback channel to the control system could be eliminated; *i.e.*, isolate the control system from its effector system by lines A and B of Fig. 1, so that the effect of a toxin or other identifiable disease mediators on one or more of the control elements could be examined in isolation. Only a few such studies of

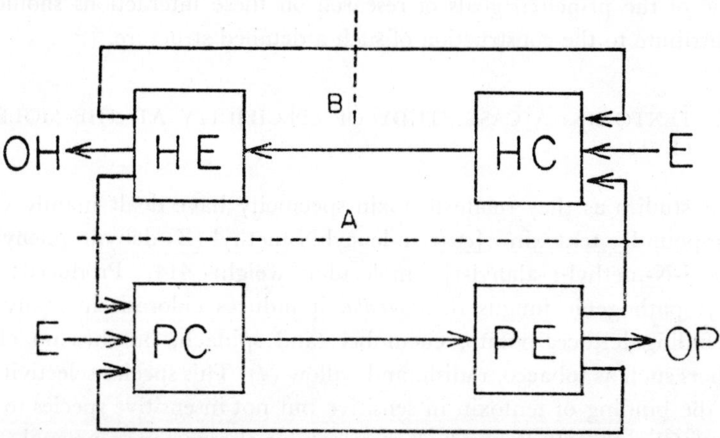

Fig. 1. A general model for host-parasite physiological interactions. The intact host-pathogen system is partitioned into host and pathogen control elements (HC, PC) and effector elements (HE, PE). Control signals are obtained from environment (E) and output of both effector systems. Development of the system in time is defined by output of the two effector systems (OP, OH). All signal paths are multiple. Most studies of toxins have cut the systems apart along line A. Some recent studies of the control elements have, in addition, partitioned the system at B.

host-parasite relations have been carried out successfully (*13, 15*), although such a partitioning approach is common practice in studying interacting systems. The advantage gained by this approach is to eliminate confusing secondary effects produced by the propagation of the original signal around the HC-HE-HC loop.

Beyond serving as a conceptual aid, the ability to predict the time-dependent behavior of a complex system, when the relevant variables and relationships are specified, provides a powerful tool for integrating our fragmentary knowledge of host-parasite interaction into a coherent structure and for developing working hypotheses by manipulating the model and examining its quantitative behavior. If experimental data is available models of moderate complexity may be studied using iterative minimization methods to obtain the most probable values for some of the parameters involved in the postulated relationships among input and output.

At present we do not know the identities of enough system signals, or enough quantitative relationships between inputs and outputs to construct an adequate operational model of any particular host-pathogen interaction.

One of the principal goals of research on these interactions should be to contribute to the construction of such a detailed structure.

IV. TENTOXIN: A CASE STUDY OF SPECIFICITY AT THE MOLECULAR LEVEL

Our studies as they relate to toxin specificity have dealt mainly with the compound tentoxin [*cyclo*(-L-leucyl-N-methyl-(*Z*)-dehydrophenylalanyl-glycyl-N-methyl-L-alanyl-)], molecular weight 414. Produced by the phytopathogenic fungus *A. alternata*, it induces chlorosis in many plants, including lettuce, potato, cucumber, and spinach, but has no effect on others such as tobacco, radish, and willow (*4*). This species selectivity is due to the binding of tentoxin in sensitive but not insensitive species to chloroplast CF_1, the effect of which is to inhibit the enzyme's normal catalytic function and its Ca^{2+}-dependent ATPase. We have examined the biological specificity of tentoxin for a broad range of plants using a combination of a seedling germination test and an ATPase activity assay. All plants tested in the *Chlorophyceae* (green algae), *Musci* (mosses), *Psilophytinae* (psilophytes), and *Equisetinae* (horsetails) were sensitive to tentoxin. Insensitivity was first encountered in the *Filicinae* (ferns) in a few of the genera tested. It is widespread within the *Cycadaceae* (cycads) and various subclasses of the *Magnoliatae* (dicots). However, the results did not reveal any broad patterns of specificity (Fig. 2). Within individual families, however, several types of responses could be distinguished. In the first type, exemplified by families 13, 30, 37, and 40, all species tested were insensitive to tentoxin. Families of the second type (numbers 4, 5, 7, 10, 14, 15, 21, 23, 24, and 33) contained both sensitive and insensitive species. In some cases, species within a genus varied in their reaction, *e.g.*, *Nicotiana*, whereas in other genera of the same family all species reacted the same, *e.g.*, *Capsicum*. In the third type all species within a family were sensitive. Regardless of the family type, all cultivars of a species have to date reacted in the same manner. At present we are testing additional groups between the lower plant forms and the angiosperms in an attempt to ascertain at what level of evolutionary development insensitivity first appears.

Recently, we genetically analyzed tentoxin response using certain *Nicotiana* spp. which are interfertile and vary in their sensitivity. Reciprocal interspecific hybrids were made using as parental material two sensitive and two insensitive species. In addition, miscellaneous interspecific crosses were

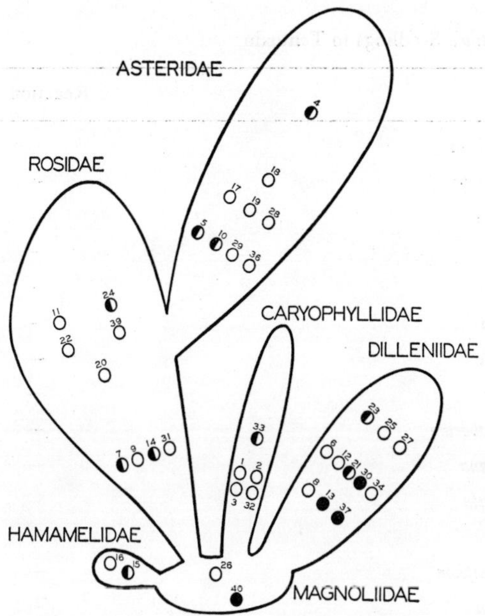

Fig. 2. Reaction of various plant families within the subclasses of *Magnoliatae* to tentoxin. Open circles represent families containing only sensitive species; half-open circles represent families containing both sensitive and insensitive species, and closed circles represent families containing only insensitive species. The families represented are: 1, *Aizoaceae;* 2, *Amaranthaceae;* 3, *Chenopodiaceae;* 4, *Compositae;* 5, *Convolvlaceae;* 6, *Cucurbitaceae;* 7, *Leguminosae;* 8, *Malvaceae;* 9, *Rutaceae;* 10, *Solanacea;* 11, *Umbelliferae;* 12, *Violaceae;* 13, *Cruciferae;* 14, *Rosaceae;* 15, *Fagaceae;* 16, *Juglandaceae;* 17, *Scrophulariaceae;* 18, *Campanulaceae;* 19, *Verbenaceae;* 20, *Vitaceae;* 21, *Salicaceae;* 22, *Balsaminaceae;* 23, *Moraceae;* 24, *Euphorbiaceae;* 25, *Primulaceae;* 26, *Piperaceae;* 27, *Cannabaceae;* 28, *Lamiaceae;* 29, *Asclepiadaceae;* 30, *Begoniaceae;* 31, *Crassulaceae;* 32, *Portulaceae;* 33, *Plumbaginaceae;* 34, *Cistaceae;* 35, *Urticaceae;* 36, *Apocynaceae;* 37, *Sterculiaceae;* 38, *Opuntiaceae;* 39, *Tropaeolaceae;* 40, *Magnoliaceae.*

tested utilizing other species with differential tentoxin reactions. Examination of 30 interspecific hybrids showed that in all cases the reaction of the female parent to tentoxin determined the reaction of the F_1 progeny (Table I). Progeny from other crosses in which the parental material had identical reactions to tentoxin, always had the same reaction as the parents. These results show that the receptor site on CF_1 for plant sensitivity to tentoxin is cytoplasmically inherited. It is tempting to speculate that the structural

TABLE I

Reaction of Interspecific *Nicotiana* Seedlings to Tentoxin

Hybrid	Reaction
benavidesii × *knightiana*	−
benavidesii × *paniculata*	−
benthamiana × *gossei*	−
bigelovii × *tabacum*	−
clevlandii × *glutinosa*	−
cordifolia × *tabacum*	−
glutinosa × *sylvestris*	−
glutinosa × *tabacum*	−
plumbaginifolia × *tabacum*	−
raimondii × *knightiana*	−
raimondii × *paniculata*	−
repanda × *sylvestris*	−
suaveolens × *megalosiphon*	−
suaveolens × *tabacum*	−
fragrans × *tabacum*	+
knightiana × *benavidesii*	+
knightiana × *raimondii*	+
paniculata × *benavidesii*	+
paniculata × *raimondii*	+
sylvestris × *tomentosiformis*	+
tabacum × *alata*	+
tabacum × *benavidesii*	+
tabacum × *cordifolia*	+
tabacum × *glutinosa*	+
tabacum × *knightiana*	+
tabacum × *longiflora*	+
tabacum × *megalosiphon*	+
tabacum × *nudicaulis*	+
tabacum × *plumbaginifolia*	+
tabacum × *sylvestris*	+

− denotes leaf chlorosis; + denotes a normal appearance.

gene(s) conditioning this reaction is located in the chloroplast, however other cytoplasmic sources cannot be disregarded at this time.

The case for tentoxin's chemical specificity is the following: tentoxin inhibits coupled electron transport to a greater extent in chloroplasts of sensitive species than in insensitive species (Fig. 3). The concentration of tentoxin required for 50% inhibition in sensitive species were: lettuce, spinach, and potato, 0.7 μM; whereas for insensitive species the values were: tobacco 13 μM, cabbage 14 μM, and radish 17 μM (*13*). The inhibition curves for the ATPase activities of solubilized lettuce and radish CF_1s are presented in Fig. 4. Tentoxin levels as high as 250 μM, which is 10,000-fold higher than that required for 50% inhibition of lettuce CF_1 (0.025 μM at equilibrium), had no effect on radish CF_1. Using equilibrium ultrafiltration, a tentoxin affinity constant of 2×10^8 M^{-1} (20°C) was measured for lettuce CF_1; for radish, the affinity constant was $< 10^4$ M^{-1}. There is no evidence that tentoxin affects any other reaction. The growth of tissue cultures from sensitive species

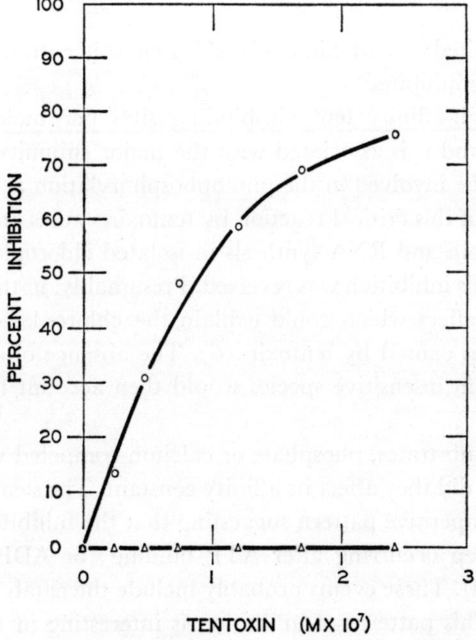

Fig. 3. Effect of tentoxin on coupled electron transport in isolated chloroplasts of lettuce (○) and radish (△). Assays done as described (*13*).

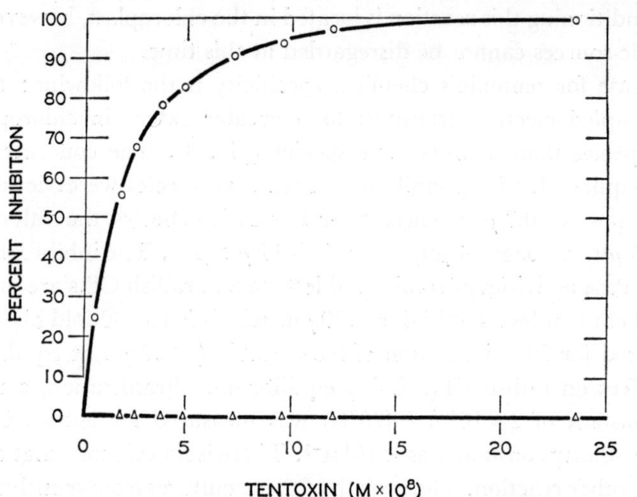

Fig. 4. Inhibition of Ca^{2+}-dependent ATPase activity of CF_1 from lettuce (○) and radish (△) after a 2-hr preincubation period. Assays done as described (*13*).

of *Nicotiana* was not inhibited by tentoxin at physiological concentrations, but greening in the light was inhibited.

The number of high-affinity tentoxin-binding sites per molecule of CF_1 appears to be one, and it is associated with the major subunits (*14*), α and β, which appear to be involved in the photophosphorylation activity of CF_1 (*8*). The inhibition of this critical reaction by tentoxin causes an inhibition of light-driven protein and RNA synthesis in isolated chloroplasts (*1*). When ATP was added this inhibition was reversed. Presumably, in the intact plant there is a similar effect which could explain the chloroplast-specific ultrastructural alterations caused by tentoxin (*6*). The absence of a strong interaction with CF_1 from insensitive species would then account for their insensitivity to chlorosis.

Neither nucleotide substrates, phosphate or calcium competed with the tentoxin binding site nor did they affect its affinity constant. The steady state kinetics best fit an uncompetitive pattern suggesting that the inhibited steps follow an irreversible step occurring after ATP binding (or ADP in the membrane-bound system). These events probably include the catalytic steps of phosphate transfer. This patterns of inhibition is interesting in that the interaction with tentoxin appears to be determined by a portion of CF_1 which is not directly concerned with its enzymatic function. A higher degree of specificity is likely to occur in such cases because the receptor site is relatively independent of the critical functional sites which have evolved over long periods of time.

Indeed, we would expect *a priori* that the regions about catalytic and control sites of enzymes at critical points in the host's metabolism would be logical candidates for receptors. What constitutes a "critical point" would be expected to vary according to the type of pathogen; *i.e.*, rusts *vs.* facultative parasites. It may be significant that already three toxins, tentoxin, fusicoccin, and helminthosporoside, of the relatively few we know something about, directly affect important bioenergetic systems, *i.e.*, ATPases. In some cases there also exists the possibility that such toxins are mimicing an endogenous substance, especially if their affinity constant is high ($>10^8$ M^{-1}). One is reminded of the opiate receptor in the brain which recently has been shown to be the receptor for a new class of endogenous neurotransmitters, the enkephalins.

We suggest that the existence of a tentoxin-binding site on CF_1 was a chance happening (insofar as tentoxin and *A. alternata* are concerned) which has been perpetuated from a very early time in the evolution of plants. At some point a random mutation in the structural gene(s) of CF_1 occurred which resulted in the elimination of the site; hence the ability of CF_1 to react with tentoxin was lost. The taxonomic distribution of insensitivity merely reflects the subsequent pathway of normal plant evolution. For this reason, tentoxin response has proven useful for determining what this pathway was in specific cases (Durbin, unpublished data). This view suggests that the receptor site arose independently from tentoxin; their union was only by biological chance. While we are not suggesting that this is a major path for the evolution of toxin specificity, it could be in the case of certain types of pathogens. Certainly the structural components of host cells are replete with potential receptors and these, together with the ability of microorganisms to synthesize and modify a great variety of small molecules, make for the critical ingredients.

SUMMARY

We are approaching a time when we should begin to use an all-encompassing biochemical basis for organizing our knowledge of toxin specificity. Realizing this goal will require a greater effort in obtaining purified components from which can come the necessary quantitative analyses. However difficult, it is a worthy goal. From it may come an understanding, at the molecular level, of the central problems of pathogenesis and resistance.

REFERENCES

1. Bennet, J. 1976. Inhibition of chloroplast development by tentoxin. *Phytochemistry* **15**: 263–265.
2. Braun, A. C. and R. B. Pringle. 1959. Pathogen factors in the physiology of disease—toxins and other metabolites. *In*: C. S. Holton *et al.* (eds.). *Plant Pathology Problems and Progress 1908–1958,* Univ. Wisconsin Press, Madison, pp. 88–99.
3. Dimond, A. E. and P. E. Waggoner. 1953. On the nature and role of vivotoxins in plant disease. *Phytopathology* **43**: 229–235.
4. Durbin, R. D. and T. F. Uchytil. 1977. A survey of plant insensitivity to tentoxin. *Phytopathology* **67**: 602–603.
5. Gäumann, E. 1954. Toxins and plant diseases. *Endeavour* **13**: 198–204.
6. Halloin, J. M., G. A. de Zoeten, G. Gaard, and J. C. Walker. 1970. The effects of tentoxin on chlorophyll synthesis and plastid structure in cucumber and cabbage. *Plant Physiol.* **45**: 310–314.
7. Ludwig, R. A. 1960. Toxins. *In*: J. G. Horsfall and A. E. Dimond (eds.). *Plant Pathology: An Advanced Treatise.* vol. 2. Academic Press, New York, pp. 315–357.
8. Nelson, N., D. W. Deters, H. Nelson, and E. Racker. 1973. Partial resolution of the enzymes catalyzing photophosphorylation. XIII. Properties of isolated subunits of coupling factor 1 from spinach chloroplasts. *J. Biol. Chem.* **248**: 2049–2055.
9. Patil, S. S. and S. S. Gnanamanickam. 1976. Suppression of bacterially induced hypersensitive reaction and phytoalexin accumulation in bean by phaseotoxin. *Nature* **259**: 486–487.
10. Rudolph, K. 1976. Non-specific toxins. *In*: R. Heitefuss and P. H. Williams (eds.). *Encyclopedia of Plant Physiology.* vol. 4. Springer-Verlag, Berlin, pp. 270–315.
11. Scheffer, R. P. and R. B. Pringle. 1967. Pathogen-produced determinants of disease and their effects on host plants. *In*: C. J. Mirocha and I. Uritani (eds.). *The Dynamic Role of Molecular Constituents of Plant-Pathogen Interaction.* Bruce Publ. Co., St. Paul, Minnesota, pp. 217–236.
12. Shinners, S. M. 1973. *Modern Control System Theory and Application.* Addison-Wesley Publ. Co., Menlo Pk., California, p. 528.
13. Steele, J. A., T. F. Uchytil, R. D. Durbin, P. Bhatnagar, and D. H. Rich. 1976. Chloroplast coupling factor 1: a species-specific receptor for tentoxin. *Proc. Natl. Acad. Sci. U.S.* **73**: 2245–2248.
14. Steele, J. A., T. F. Uchytil, and R. D. Durbin. 1977. The binding of tentoxin to a tryptic digest of chloroplast coupling factor 1. *Biochim. Biophys. Acta* **459**: 347–350.

15. Strobel, G. A. 1973. The helminthosporoside-binding protein of sugarcane. Its properties and relationship to susceptibility to the eye spot disease. *J. Biol. Chem.* **248**: 1321–1328.
16. Wheeler, H. and H. H. Luke. 1963. Microbial toxins in plant disease. *Annu. Rev. Microbiol.* **17**: 223–242.
17. Wood, R.K.S. and A. Graniti. 1976. *Specificity in Plant Diseases.* Plenum Press, New York, p. 354.

Discussion of Paper by Drs. Durbin and Steele

Ellingboe started a general discussion by noting that as Durbin had diagrammed his model of chemical interactions between pathogens and hosts (see Fig. 1 on p. 121), the potential genetic behavior would not follow the gene-for-gene relation (see Ellingboe's paper). On the other hand, if PC and PE in the diagram were reversed, the gene-for-gene relationship would hold. Durbin explained his model was developed without consideration for genetic systems and was an attempt only to formalize biochemical interactions in order to develop quantitative consideration for computer simulations capable of experimental testing. Yoder asked about the extent of variation found among sensitive and insensitive species and whether variation and sensitivity were a function of the particular bioassay of the two employed by Durbin's group. Durbin explained that in both assays the amount of tentoxin is extremely high so that all plants show little variation, that is, the response is 100% or nothing. But he pointed out that because the ATPase activity involves isolated organelles some sensitive species respond poorer in the chlorosis assay because of failure of toxin to penetrate. Kuć then asked several questions concerning the relationship between tentoxin and its ability to cause disease. Durbin summarized considerable data obtained in his laboratory: *Alternaria tennis* is not a particularly note-worthy pathogen and there are numbers of plants sensitive to toxin but which are not natural hosts; consequently, he views tentoxin as a inherited biochemical accident which only in certain biological instances becomes important as an agent in disease. In response to comments from Uritani and Keen, he indicated it certainly did not determine specificity but in cases where it is a pathogen, the toxin can be isolated from diseased tissue and thus is playing a role in symptom expression. However, his group has not looked specifically for instances of pathogenicity on plants insensitive to toxin. Day asked if chlorosis caused by tentoxin was light dependent. Durbin referred to experiments done by Bennett in which tentoxin inhibited light driven DNA and RNA synthesis of isolated chloroplasts from sensitive, but not insensitive, species. Addition of ATP abolished such effects indicating tentoxin was effectively uncoupling. He also cited experiments with heterotrophic organisms grown on various carbon sources which nullified the effects of tentoxin. Thus, it appears that the primary action is on ATP formation in the light. GRACEN asked if there was evidence that, since chloroplast DNA might be determining sensitivity, if anyone had observed segregation for sensitivity that was correlated with known differences in chloroplast genomes such as has been described by Wildman and others for tobacco. DURBIN indicated there was evidence for this and that laboratories were actively investigating the area. Finally, NISHIMURA commented that they believed some of his *A. kikuchiana* and *A. mali* isolates were producing tentoxin in addition to host-specific toxins and DURBIN noted that his model made it possible for two or more toxins to interact in producing disease.

Recognition and Specificity in Plant Host-Parasite Interactions, pp. 133–146, 1979

THE ROLE OF HOST-SPECIFIC TOXINS IN SAPROPHYTIC PATHOGENS

SYOYO NISHIMURA, KEISUKE KOHMOTO, AND HIROSHI OTANI

Faculty of Agriculture, Tottori University, Tottori, Japan

During the past ten years, the toxin concept in plant pathology has undergone a great change. It had generally been believed that phytotoxic metabolites of plant pathogens lead to visible injury on host plants, resulting in the reproduction of some disease symptoms, but are not an initial inciting agent of disease. This traditional view has, however, been challenged by host-specific toxin (HST) researchers, who are now emphasizing that such toxins are not only host-specific, but also a primary determinant for pathogenicity.

One must approve and conclude, without any universal validity, that the present status of HST research is interesting, but still restricted to relatively few plant pathogens. Actually, many questions regarding HST flash across our minds. The present knowledge of HST has come almost entirely from so-called "saprophytic pathogens." Included are familiar fungi, such as *Alternaria* and *Helminthosporium,* as well as others less well known (*9, 19*). Strangely, most of these appeared to be so-called "man-made diseases," which occur only on newly bred or introduced cultivars of crop plants. A discussion of such a specific group of fungal metabolites, and of the fungi which produce them, requires a brief introduction to the inevitability of why the finding of HST-producers has been limited to some of the saprophytic pathogens. Then, two general problems concerning HST will be discussed; the exact role of HST during fungal pathogenesis, and the host-specific mechanism of HST actions. Recently, comprehensive accounts of the HST problem have been provided by several American researchers (*17, 19–21, 26*). However, a review of the data presented would contribute little information on *Alternaria* toxins. In Japan, there are at least two host-parasite combinations known where toxins produced in culture, display the same host-specificity as that of the pathogen themselves (*9, 10*). These are *Alternaria kikuchiana* Tanaka and the Japanese pear, and *Alternaria mali* Roberts and apple. Most of this paper will be concerned with *A. kikuchiana* (AK) and *A. mali* (AM) toxins. There are many parallels between *Alternaria* HST and *Helminthosporium* HST problems. We do not attempt to make an exhaustive review of the latter ones, but instead emphasize several unique points about *Alternaria* HSTs.

I. HST-PRODUCING PATHOGENS IN THE GENUS OF *ALTERNARIA*

Before discussing the *Alternaria* HSTs, the known four examples (Table I) must be mentioned briefly. Black spot disease affecting Japanese pears suddenly appeared after widespread planting of a new natural mutant, cv. "Nijisseiki," about 70 years ago. Most of the older cultivars apparently are immune to the disease (*22*). On the other hand, in about 1956, the occurrence of Alternaria blotch of apples was noted throughout the apple-growing areas of Japan. Most cultivars, such as "Indo" and "Delicious," suffered seriously from the disease (*18*). Stem canker of fresh market tomatoes, caused by a distinct pathotype of *A. alternata*, also excited interest; it was reported recently from southern California, and "Earlypak 7" and several

TABLE I

List of Known *Alternaria* Host-specific Toxins (1977)

Pathogen and toxin	Disease	Susceptible cultivar of host
A. alternata f. sp. *lycopersici* toxin	Stem canker of tomato	Earlypak 7
A. citri toxin	Brown spot of citrus	Emperor mandarine or Dancy tangerine
A. kikuchiana toxin	Black spot of Japanese pear	Nijisseiki or Shinsui
A. mali toxin	Alternaria blotch of apple	Indo or Orei

other cultivars were highly susceptible to the disease (*3*). Still another example was shown with citrus brown spot, caused by a distinct strain of *A. citri*; it was first recorded on the Emperor mandarine of Australia in 1966 (*16*), and more recently, Whiteside (*27*) reported that since 1974 it has become prevalent on the Dancy tangerine of Florida.

However, the origin of these four fungi looks similar, and all of them may be identical morphologically with collective species *A. alternata* (Fr.) Keissler. This species has been known to be a saprophyte or a weak pathogen on a number of plants. In the case of *A. kikuchiana*, the wild type isolates often lose their specific pathogenicity and host-specific toxin productivity, and return to a state of native saprophyte. In the field, it appears that this fungus leads a dual mode of life, fluctuating between saprophytic and pathogenic. It overwinters as mycelium in pear buds and shoots, and almost loses pathogenicity during the winter season. In spring, a small number of the fungi which preserved their pathogenicity begin to attack younger pear leaves. After several infection cycles, it attacks severely, suggesting that a mass of susceptible Nijisseiki pear orchards is involved in maintaining their pathogenicity and toxin productivity. Thus, an increase in the rate of field populations of virulent *A. kikuchiana* appears to take place during the seasonal development of the disease. Besides, our recent data also indicated that, among many conidia of completely saprophytic *A. alternata* available in our collection, there exists a natural mutant which has the ability to induce specific pathogenicity on Nijisseiki pear leaves, as is the case with virulent *A. kikuchiana*. These mutants also were found to have the ability to produce AK-toxin in cultures.

A theoretical picture about the origin and appearance of HST-producing *A. alternata* is given in Fig. 1. Each of the known four HST-producers appears to arise as distinct pathotypes of *A. alternata*, *via* acquisition of each HST metabolite. We do not know how widespread such HST producers may be in nature, but it seems likely that for the development of a new HST disease, a large acreage of a certain highly susceptible crop, as well as toxin production, is necessary.

The fungi belonging to *A. alternata* have a general aggressiveness, as used by Gäumann (*2*); usually this ability can be exhibited on mature or senescent tissues of many different plants, independently of HST production. As a result, we often observe the occurrence of so-called "indefinite disease" of crops, caused by non-pathogenic *A. alternata*. Of further interest is the fact that this fungus can induce an opportunistic infection even into facial

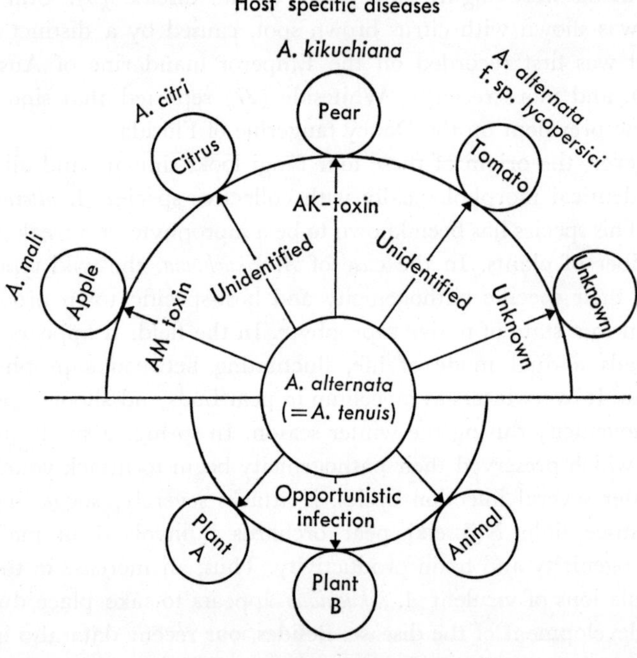

Fig. 1. Disease pattern caused by the fungi belonging to *A. alternata.*

skin tissues, as a disease of humans (unpublished). Thus, it is possible to conclude that the pathogenicity of HST-producing *A. alternata* is composed of aggressiveness, common to this species of *Alternaria*, and specific virulence, exhibited by HST productivity.

II. *ALTERNARIA KIKUCHIANA* TOXIN AND *A. MALI* TOXIN

The discovery that the culture filtrate of *A. kikuchiana* contains a host-specific factor was made by Tanaka in 1933 (*22*); this seems to be the first known report about a HST problem. Since then, several groups in Japan have challenged the role of HST (AK-toxin) in these studies. They indicate that characterization of AK-toxin is difficult, since it is unstable in a homogeneous condition. Our recent results confirmed the fact that highly virulent isolates of this fungus produce at least three HSTs in cultures. Two of these three

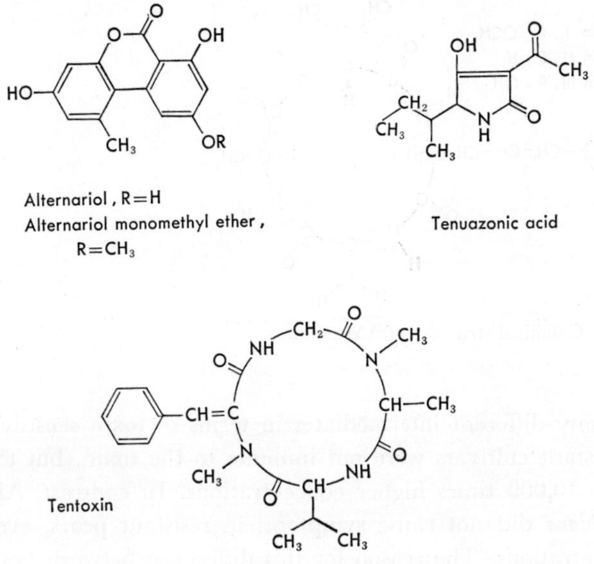

Alternariol, R=H
Alternariol monomethyl ether, R=CH_3

Tenuazonic acid

Tentoxin

Fig. 2. Phytotoxic metabolites from *A. kikuchiana*.

HSTs were isolated and shown to be pure, based on droplet countercurrent distribution and thin layer chromatography. The final products of purification produced veinal necrosis on the susceptible leaves in amounts as small as 0.01 and 0.1 μg/ml, respectively; there was little or no toxicity to resistant pears or to other non-host plants, even at 100 μg/ml (*9*). During isolation of AK-toxin, non-specific phytotoxic metabolites, such as tenuazonic acid, alternariol and its monomethylether, and tentoxin, were isolated from culture filtrates or mycelial mats (Fig. 2).

Highly virulent isolates of *A. mali*, produce several toxins (AM-toxins) in cultures, each with a high degree of host-specificity (*6*). Of these toxins, the major three have been isolated in crystalline form, AM-toxin I (*23*) (alternariolide (*12*)), AM-toxin II, and AM-toxin III. Their chemical structures have been established as depsipeptides (Fig. 3) (*12, 24, 25*).

The structure of AM-toxin I was further confirmed by chemical synthesis (*8*). AM-toxin I induced veinal necrosis within 24 hr and caused an instantaneous increase of electrolyte loss at approximately 10^{-9} M in the highly susceptible cv. "Indo" and at a concentration of over 10^{-5} M in considerably resistant cv. "Jonathan." Among collected 39 cultivars of apple,

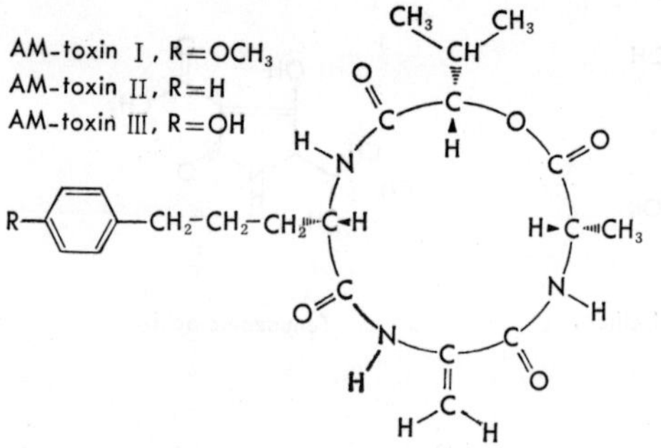

AM-toxin I, R=OCH_3
AM-toxin II, R=H
AM-toxin III, R=OH

Fig. 3. Chemical structure of AM-toxin.

there were many different intermediates in terms of toxin sensitivity (*7*). Thus, the resistant cultivars were not immune to the toxin, but tolerated approximately 10,000 times higher concentrations. In contrast, AK-toxin from *A. kikuchiana* did not cause symptoms in resistant pears, even with massive concentrations. The reason for this difference between both combinations is known from their genetic background; the susceptibility of apple to *A. mali* is controlled by multiple dominant genes, and the susceptibility of Japanese pear to *A. kikuchiana* is by a single dominant gene.

III. RELEASE OF HST FROM GERMINATING SPORES

Both AK- and AM-toxins are readily detectable in Richards' cultures of the virulent isolates of *A. kikuchiana* and *A. mali*, respectively. However, more emphasis is needed on the importance of the HSTs generated by germinating spores of virulent isolates, and not generated by avirulent spores (*14*). This finding is a significant point, for it emphasizes the importance of allelopathetic host-recognition at the site of the initial contact of the germinating spores and the host tissues.

Spore germination, mycelial growth and appressorial formation of *A. kikuchiana* were similar on both susceptible and resistant Japanese pear leaves. Fungal inhibitory or phytoalexin-like compounds were not detected in either of the leaf tissues that were previously inoculated with the spores. AK-toxin was not detected in resting spores, but was synthesized quickly and released with germination. Four hr after inoculation, one germinating spore produced approximately 10^{-6} μg toxin, which was capable of disturbing the metabolic activities of approximately 100 host cells. The first physiological event induced by germinating spores was an increased loss of electrolytes from susceptible leaves. This reaction was evident 2–6 hr after inoculation, indicating that the leakage was by AK-toxin from germinating spores prior to the host invasion. The penetration of epidermal cells was detected only in susceptible leaves 8–12 hr after inoculation with virulent spores. At this time, a second increase in the rate of electrolyte leakage occurred; this was probably induced by AK-toxin from the invading hyphae, and was caused by membrane disruption in infected host cells. When resistant tissues were inoculated with virulent spores, or when susceptible tissues were inoculated with avirulent mutant spores, there was no increase in electrolyte leakage. Visible symptoms became evident by 12–20 hr after inoculation, and they appeared as tiny, dark necrotic spots on susceptible leaves. Thus, careful determinations of electrolyte leakage after spore inoculation have shown two different phases; there is an increase in rate at the pre-penetration stage of infection, and another increase at just-penetrated stage of infection. Such step-like increases in electrolyte losses add further interest to the hypothesis that all saprophytic pathogens which produce HST, induce disease *via* its HST secretions.

A similar mode of HST secretion during spore germination has been shown in *A. mali* (*6*), *Helminthosporium carbonum* (*1*) and *H. victoriae* (*28*). The small amount of HST from a spore probably does not kill host cells at an early stage of infection, but causes sufficient disruption of host plasma membranes to aid the fungus in colonization. At present, however, the experiments give no indication of the nature of the membrane disruption that may be caused by germinating spores.

Tenuazonic acid, a phytotoxic metabolite of several *Alternaria* spp., is not thought to be a primary determinant of pathogenicity in *A. kikuchiana* and *A. mali*, since the compound is produced even by an avirulent isolate and also is not released from the germinating spores of virulent isolates.

IV. HOST-SPECIFIC MECHANISM OF AK- AND AM-TOXIN ACTIONS

Research concerning the primary site of the actions of these HSTs dominates much of the field of toxin studies, because the information about whereby the mechanism occurs, is basic to understanding the mutual recognition between host plant and pathogen. However, final proof of the identity of HST-action site in host tissues has not been completely successful in all

HSTs reported so far. What are the underlying reasons for the extremely higher tolerance to HST which the resistant cultivar displays, or, in contrast, for the extremely higher sensitivity of the susceptible cultivar?

Our still fragmentary knowledge concerning AK- and AM-toxin actions is summarized with several lines of evidence (*9, 10*), but nothing conclusive is available at this time. There is a resemblance between them in several ways; the toxins may be compared and contrasted as follows;

1) Both of the Japanese pear-AK-toxin and apple-AM-toxin systems do not appear to have a detoxification mechanism for resistance. Repeated experiments showed no measurable differences in the abilities of resistant and susceptible leaves to inactivate the toxins.

2) Tissues from all parts of susceptible pear plants were sensitive to AK-toxin (*4*). Responses which occurred after toxin exposure were; an almost instantaneous damage of the plasma membrane system in free protoplasts; rapid loss of electrolytes from many different tissues; cessation of plasma streaming in cells; loss of plasmolytic ability in cells; and visible necrosis on many tissues. Electron microscope pictures also showed that AK-toxin causes changes in plasma membrane within 1 hr after the treatment (*15*). The change was evident as a general invagination of the membrane. None of these responses were evident in tissues of toxin-treated resistant plants. The effects of AM-toxin I on apple appeared to be similar to those of AK-toxin on pear. Our estimate of importance is on the tissue universality in the distribution of target sites of HST. The cells involved in all tissues were recognizable as a sensitive site with different responses.

3) When susceptible pear leaves were given a thermal shock (*eg.*, 2 sec in 55°C water), they became almost completely insensitive to AK-toxin (*13*). However, this acquired insensitivity to the toxin was reversible; the leaf tissues regained sensitivity to toxin about 6 hr after heat treatment. Heat treatment did not affect the lack of toxin sensitivity by tissues of resistant pears. A similar situation with apple and AM-toxin I was also found (*5*). Several possible mechanisms may be involved in the heat induction of resistance to susceptible tissues. One possibility is that toxin sensitive site or closely related portion in susceptible plasma or other cellular membranes is temporarily changed by mild heat.

4) Major components of AK-toxin-induced loss of electrolytes from the susceptible pear leaves were K^+ and phosphate (*11*). The increase in efflux was detected within 5 min after the treatment, and the leaf tissues lost 40% of total K^+ by 4 hr after toxin exposure. An increase of organic materials

(*e.g.*, amino acids, reducing sugars and hydroquinone) in the ambient solution also occurred; the efflux pattern of amino acids was consistent with that of K^+, but sugar and hydroquinone began to increase after 2 hr of the toxin exposure.

5) The K^+ efflux by AK-toxin was markedly stimulated by 5 mM $MgCl_2$. The $MgCl_2$ stimulation was due to Mg^{2+} and not due to Cl^-; it could be observed immediately after adding Mg^{2+} to the toxin-treated tissues, and rapidly returned after the Mg^{2+} was removed (Fig. 4). An effect of Na^+ or Li^+ also was observed, as was the case with Mg^{2+}, but neither Mn^{2+} nor Zn^{2+} stimulated. On the other hand, AM-toxin action on the susceptible apple leaves was markedly stimulated by Ca^{2+}, rather than Mg^{2+}, at a concentration of 5 mM. The basis of such selective stimulation by certain cations is still an enigma. At least two possible mechanisms may be involved in the cation stimulation. First and less likely, it may be suggested that an abnormal increase in the activity of a certain enzyme, for which specific

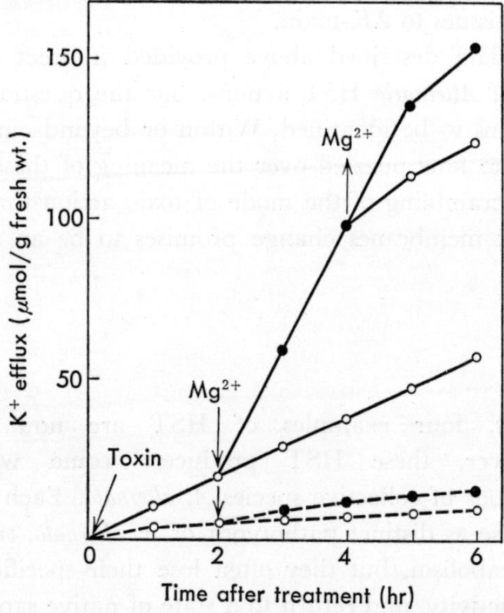

Fig. 4. Mg^{2+} stimulation on K^+ efflux induced by AK-toxin. Susceptible tissues were treated with AK-toxin, and leached in $MgCl_2$ solution (—●—) or deionized water (—○—). At times indicated, the tissues were placed in $MgCl_2$ (↓) or removed from $MgCl_2$ (↑). The K^+ efflux from $MgCl_2$ (--●--) and water (--○--) controls without toxin was also shown.

cations are essential, is an initial expression of AK- or AM-toxin action. However, the activity of membrane ATPase in susceptible pear tissues was found to be not affected by AK-toxin alone, or by AK-toxin plus magnesium chloride. A second and perhaps more likely explanation would be that by binding to toxin sensitive site in specific cation binding state, the toxin introduced into host tissues can be activated. Further work is required to distinguish between these possibilities. In either case, cation stimulation may represent an excellent start in discovering the exact mechanism of the both HST actions.

6) Pretreatments of pear leaf tissues with more than 50 different kinds of chemicals caused little decrease in sensitivity (K^+ efflux) to AK-toxin. Included were known enzyme inhibitors, such as DNP (uncoupler), oligomycin (energy transfer inhibitor), ouabain (ATPase inhibitor), quinidine (inhibitor of passive transport of K^+), nicotinic acid (adenyl cyclase inhibitor), and theophylline (phosphodiesterase inhibitor). However, pretreatment with N,N'-dicyclohexylcarbodiimide (energy transfer inhibitor), iodoacetamide (-SH binding agent) or N_2 atmosphere considerably abolished the sensitivity of susceptible tissues to AK-toxin.

Our experimental data described above provided indirect evidence concerning the nature of *Alternaria* HST actions, but the question of the exact primary site remains to be identified. Within or beyond our experimental limitations, we are now puzzled over the meaning of these events. We believe that the unscrambling of the mode of toxic action that makes the properties of plasma membranes change promises to be an arduous, but fascinating task.

SUMMARY

In *Alternaria* pathogens, four examples of HST are now known. Morphologically, however, these HST producers come within a category of the descriptions of collective species *A. alternata*. Each of toxin producers appears to arise as distinct pathotypes of *A. alternata*, *via* acquisition of each HST metabolism, but they often lose their specific pathogenicity and HST productivity, and return to a state of native saprophytic *A. alternata*. Thus, it is possible to conclude that the pathogenicity of HST-producing *A. alternata* is composed of aggressiveness, common to this species of *Alternaria*, and specific virulence, exhibited by HST productivity. These problems are discussed with a theoretical picture. Two general problems concerning HST also are discussed with AK and AM toxins; the role of HST during fungal pathogenesis, and the mode of HST actions. Although AK- and AM-toxins are readily detectable in cultures of each of virulent isolates, respectively, more emphasis is needed on the importance of the HSTs generated by germinating spores of virulent isolates, and not generated by avirulent spores. In fact, it can be recognized that primary events in the interaction between susceptible leaf tissues and virulent spores occur prior to host penetration, and are dependent upon HST produced from germinating spores. Host-specific mechanism of AK- and AM-toxin actions is discussed with several lines of evidence; the both toxins are compared and contrasted. Primary action sites of the toxins must include the drastic influence of host membrane activity, but the question of the exact mechanism remains to be determined.

REFERENCES

1. Comstock, J. C. and R. P. Scheffer. 1973. Role of host-specific toxin in colonization of corn leaves by *Helminthosporium carbonum*. *Phytopathology* **63**: 24–29.
2. Gäumann, E. 1950. *Principles of Plant Infection*. Hafner Publ. Co., New York, p. 543.
3. Grogan, R. G., K. A. Kimble, and I. Misaghi. 1975. A stem canker disease of tomato caused by *Alternaria alternata* f. sp. *lycopersici*. *Phytopathology* **65**: 880–886.
4. Kasai, T., H. Otani, K. Kohmoto, and S. Nishimura. 1975. Nature of specific susceptibility to *Alternaria kikuchiana* in Nijisseiki cultivar among Japanese pears (IV). Target tissues of AK-toxin and their characteristic responses. *J. Fac. Agric. Tottori Univ.* **10**: 6–14.
5. Khan, I. D., K. Kohmoto, and S. Nishimura. 1975. Heat-induced resistance of apple leaves against *Alternaria mali* and its host-specific toxins. *Ann. Phytopathol. Soc. Japan* **41**: 408–411.
6. Kohmoto, K., I. D. Khan, Y. Renbutsu, T. Taniguchi, and S. Nishimura. 1976. Multiple host-specific toxins of *Alternaria mali* and their effect on the permeability of host cells. *Physiol. Plant Pathol.* **8**: 141–153.
7. Kohmoto, K., T. Taniguchi, and S. Nishimura. 1977. Correlation between the susceptibility of apple cultivars to *Alternaria mali* and their susceptibility to AM-toxin I. *Ann. Phytopathol. Soc. Japan* **43**: 65–68.
8. Lee, S., H. Aoyagi, Y. Shimohigashi, N. Izumiya, T. Ueno, and H. Fukami. 1975. Symposium of AM-toxin I and its analogs. 19th Symposium on the Chemistry of Natural Products, Japan. Abstr. No. 45.

9. Nishimura, S., K. Kohmoto, and H. Otani. 1974. Host-specific toxins as an initiation factor for pathogenicity in *Alternaria kikuchiana* and *A. mali*. *Rev. Plant Prot. Res.* **7**: 21–32.
10. Nishimura, S., K. Kohmoto, H. Otani, H. Fukami, and T. Ueno. 1976. The involvement of host-specific toxins in the early step of infection by *Alternaria kikuchiana* and *A. mali*. *In*: K. Tomiyama, J. M. Daly, I. Uritani, H. Oku, and S. Ouchi. (eds.). *Biochemistry and Cytology of Plant-Parasite Interaction*. Kodansha Ltd., Tokyo and Elsevier, New York, pp. 94–101.
11. Morikawa, M., H. Otani, S. Nishimura, and K. Kohmoto. 1976. Nature of specific susceptibility to *Alternaria kikuchiana* in Nijisseiki cultivar among Japanese pears (VII). Efflux of cell constituents from pear leaves treated with AK-toxin. *J. Fac. Agric. Tottori Univ.* **12**: 1–7.
12. Okuno, T., T. Ishida, K. Sawai, and T. Matsumoto. 1974. Characterization of alternariolide, a host-specific toxin produced by *Alternaria mali*. *Chem. Lett.* **1974**: 635–638.
13. Otani, H., S. Nishimura, and K. Kohmoto. 1974. Nature of specific susceptibility to *Alternaria kikuchiana* in Nijisseiki cultivar among Japanese pears (III). Chemical and thermal protections against effect of host-specific toxin. *Ann. Phytopathol. Soc. Japan* **40**: 59–66.
14. Otani, H., S. Nishimura, K. Kohmoto, K. Yano, and T. Seno. 1975. Nature of specific susceptibility to *Alternaria kikuchiana* in Nijisseiki cultivar among Japanese pears. (V). Role of host-specific toxin in early step of infection. *Ann. Phytopathol. Soc. Japan* **41**: 467–476.
15. Park, P., M. Fukutomi, S. Akai, and S. Nishimura. 1976. Effect of the host-specific toxin from *Alternaria kikuchiana* on the ultrastructure of plasma membranes of cells in leaves of Japanese pears. *Physiol. Plant Pathol.* **9**: 167–174.
16. Pegg, K. G. 1966. Studies on a strain of *Alternaria citri* Pierce, the causal organism of brown spot of Emperor Mandarine. *Qeensl. J. Agric. Anim. Sci.* **23**: 15–28.
17. Pringle, R. B. and R. P. Scheffer. 1964. Host-specific toxins. *Annu. Rev. Phytopathol.* **2**: 133–156.
18. Sawamura, K. 1962. Studies on spotted disease of apples. I. Causal agent of Alternaria blotch. *Bull. Tohoku Natl. Exp. Stn., Japan* **23**: 163–175.
19. Scheffer, R. P. 1976. Host-specific toxins in relation to pathogenesis and disease resistance. *In*: R. Heitefuss and P. H. Williams (eds.). *Encyclopedia of Plant Physiology*. vol. 4. Springer-Verlag, Berlin, pp. 247–269.
20. Scheffer, R. P. and O. C. Yoder. 1972. Host-specific toxins and selective toxicity. *In*: R. K. S. Wood, A. Ballio, and A. Graniti. (eds.). *Phytotoxins in Plant Disease*. Academic Press, New York, pp. 251–272.
21. Strobel, G. A. 1974. Phytotoxins produced by plant parasites. *Annu. Rev. Plant Physiol.* **25**: 541–566.
22. Tanaka, S. 1933. Studies on black spot disease of the Japanese pear (*Pyrus serotina* Rehd.). *Mem. Coll. Agric. Kyoto Univ.* **28**: 1–31.

23. Ueno, T., Y. Hayashi, T. Nakashima, H. Fukami, S. Nishimura, K. Kohmoto, and A. Sekiguchi. 1975. Isolation of AM-toxin I, a new phytotoxic metabolite from *Alternaria mali*. *Phytopathology* **65**: 82–83.
24. Ueno, T., T. Nakashima, Y. Hayashi, and H. Fukami. 1975. Structure of AM-toxin I and II, host-specific phytotoxic metabolites produced by *Alternaria mali*. *Agric. Biol. Chem.* **39**: 1115–1122.
25. Ueno, T., T. Nakashima, Y. Hayashi, and H. Fukami. 1975. Isolation and structure of AM-toxin III, a host-specific phytotoxic metabolite produced by *Alternaria mali*. *Agric. Biol. Chem.* **39**: 2081–2082.
26. Wheeler, H. and H. H. Luke. 1963. Microbial toxins in plant disease. *Annu. Rev. Microbiol.* **17**: 223–242.
27. Whiteside, J. O. 1976. A newly recorded *Alternaria*-induced brown spot disease on Dancy tangerines in Florida. *Plant Dis. Rep.* **60**: 326–329.
28. Yoder, O. C. and R. P. Scheffer. 1969. Role of toxin in early interactions of *Helminthosporium victoriae* with susceptible and resistant oat tissues. *Phytopathology* **59**: 1954–1959.

Discussion of Paper by Drs. Nishimura et al.

AIST opened the discussion with several questions and comments by AIST designed to determine if the plasma membrane invagination described by NISHIMURA might instead involve wall apposition. NISHIMURA believed his observations suggested a direct effect on membranes, but stressed that he does not believe they are primary effects of toxin. He was interested only in demonstration of a change of damage to membranes which might explain other behavior of the cells such as leakage. YODER asked whether it had been possible to demonstrate different activities or effects of the individual species of host-specific toxins produced by either *A. kikuchiana* or *A. mali*. NISHIMURA reported his laboratory had this problem under study. DURBIN, SEQUEIRA, and DALY commented on NISHIMURA's intriguing interpretation of the short time (2 sec) heat treatment as causing a conformational change. NISHIMURA acknowledged that there were certainly other possible mechanisms to be considered but that his suggestion seemed feasible to test experimentally. TAKAI then summarized some of his work on Dutch elm disease which is reported elsewhere in the volume.

Recognition and Specificity in Plant Host-Parasite Interactions, pp. 147–151, 1979

SPECIAL DISCUSSION

CERATO-ULMIN, A SEMIPATHOTOXIN OF *CERATOCYSTIS ULMI*

SHOZO TAKAI,*1 W.C. RICHARDS,*1 YASUYUKI HIRATSUKA,*2 AND K.J. STEVENSON*3

*1*Department of the Environment, Canadian Forestry Service, Great Lakes Forest Research Centre, Sault Ste. Marie, Ontario,* *2*Department of the Environment, Canadian Forestry Service, Northern Forest Research Centre, Edmonton, Alberta, and* *3*Department of Chemistry, University of Calgary, Alberta, Canada*

Cerato-ulmin (CU) is a new wilt toxin produced by *Ceratocystis ulmi* (Buism.) C. Moreau, the causal fungus of Dutch elm disease (DED) (*3, 4, 5*).

CU is a small protein with a very minor carbohydrate content, the extent of which has not yet been determined. Strangely enough, it has lyotropic liquid crystalline characteristics (*2, 4*). As illustrated in Fig. 1, CU molecules assemble into "units" in an aqueous solution, and while they are in unit form the solution remains clear. These "units" then form larger assemblages such as "rods" and "fibrils," and at this time the solution turns milky. The assemblages containing "units" are all visible under a light microscope. CU also appears as "membrane," another form of assemblage, covering the entire surface of the CU aqueous solution (*4*).

Assembling and disassembling are controlled artificially by changing the physical conditions of the solution. Assembling is initiated when the solution is subjected to vacuuming or shaking, or when air is bubbled into the system, and the gaseous volume of the solution is thereby increased. Disassembling occurs when the solution with "rods" and "fibrils" is subjected to pressure or chilling. Thus, assembling and disassembling appear to be associated with the hydrophobic character and gaseous content of the solution. This observation is supported by the fact that CU loses its assembl-

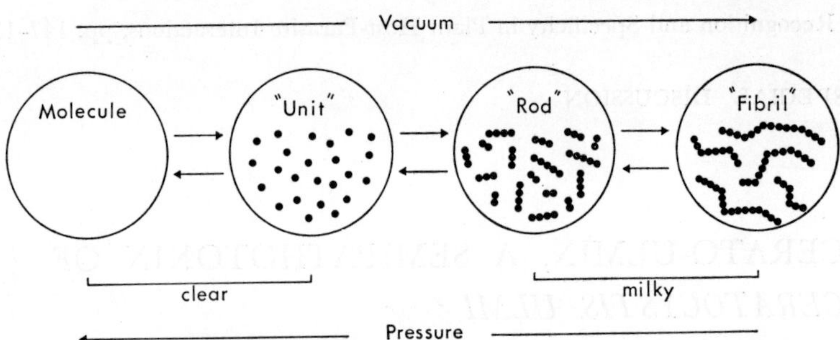

Fig. 1. Schematic diagram illustrating characteristic changes in CU structure as observed under the microscope. Application of a vacuum to the aqueous CU solution initiates assembling (shown by the arrow direction). However, application of pressure to the assembled CU causes disassembling (shown by the arrow direction). These changes are reversible. When free molecules and/or "units" are present, the solution remains clear; however, when "rods" and/or "fibrils" are formed the system turns milky.

ing capacity when it is dissolved in a 60–80% aqueous ethanol solution that appears to change the hydrophobic character of CU.

Isolating CU from the culture filtrate of *C. ulmi* (*4*) involves a novel technique, vacuum effervescence. This technique is designed to collect CU selectively as assemblages from the culture filtrate. Assembling is initiated by shaking and is developed further by vacuuming. Assemblages of CU are collected as foam which remains when the vacuum is released and the liquid is carefully drained off.

Other techniques used subsequent to vacuum effervescence are ultramolecular filtration, to confine substances to the M.W. range of 1,000–10,000, and dialysis, to retain CU selectively within the dialyzing tube. This series of treatments does not allow any peptidic substance other than CU to remain in the crude CU sample. Purification of the crude sample is done by repeating chromatography through the column of Sephadex LH 20. Column chromatography of CU is conducted with a 60% ethanol aqueous solution to prevent assembling of CU molecules, which interferes with separation. Although the degree of purity of the final product has not been confirmed yet, the sample appeared to be highly pure.

CU appears to be a specific product of *C. ulmi* (*2*). The best basal medium for *in vitro* production of CU is Salemink's medium (*1*). Replacing its carbon and nitrogen sources by D-mannose or sucrose and L-proline and increasing its inorganic salt concentration by four times the original can greatly improve the yield of CU. The highest yield, per litre of the culture filtrate, measured to date is 140 mg when sucrose is used as the carbon source (*5*).

CU as the final cell metabolic product appears to accumulate on the cell surface of *C. ulmi.* Slime containing CU, which is exuded around hyphae, fills up the interhyphal space of the synnema stalk, formed by a bundle of hyphae. It oozes up to the tip of the stalk and forms the synnema head, which resembles a water droplet.

When CU is administered to elm cuttings it displays symptoms similar to those of DED: wilting, necrosis, and chlorosis (*2*), depending on the sensitivity of the cuttings to CU. Thus far our study shows that the lowest concentration of CU that will trigger wilting is 7.5 μg/ml.* It takes a minimum of one-half hour to initiate symptom development.

Cuttings of elms and some maples are sensitive to CU, whereas tomato cuttings are insensitive. CU does not affect seed germination of white elm, radish, snapdragon, or tomato. Observed physiological effects of CU on elms are a retardation of transpiration in elm cuttings, an increase of electrolyte leakage from elm leaf cells, and an increase in respiration by elm leaf tissues.

The toxic effects of CU on elms that are mentioned above all appear to be specific to white elms, which are highly susceptible to DED. White elms are very sensitive to CU whereas Siberian and Japanese elms, which are resistant to the disease, are less sensitive. The response of white elm to CU may also vary; the growth stage of white elm cuttings that is most sensitive to CU appears to correspond to the stage that is most sensitive to normal fungus infection.

In addition, there is a correlation between the degree of CU production and pathogenicity in *C. ulmi* (*2, 3*). This observation is supported by another correlation between CU production and synnemata formation in *C. ulmi* (*3*).

Evidently CU displays indications of a pathotoxin. At the present time, however, we would classify the metabolite as a semipathotoxin, particularly if we accept the fact that some non-host maples are sensitive to it.

With respect to the 'wilt' mechanisms resulting from CU, neither plugging of vessels with CU nor restrictions in the flow rate of water due to the viscosity of CU are assumed. The low CU dosage required to trigger

---

* Even at a lower concentration of 0.002 μg/ml it is still toxic as was shown in the experiment conducted after the seminar.

symptom development eliminates these possibilities. Therefore, we think that CU triggers a host response and that it is linked to symptom expression in some manner. Increased electrolyte leakage and respiration from or in susceptible elm leaf tissues are indications of compatibility within the particular system.

REFERENCES

1. Salemink, C. A., H. Robel, L. C. P. Kerling, and V. Tchernoff. 1965. Phytotoxin isolated from liquid cultures of *Ceratocystis ulmi*. *Science* **149**: 202–203.
2. Takai, S. 1974. Pathogenicity and cerato-ulmin production in *Ceratocystis ulmi*. *Nature* **252**: 124–126.
3. Takai, S. 1974. Variation in coremium formation and cerato-ulmin production and their relation to pathogenicity in *C. ulmi*. *Proc. Can. Phytopathol. Soc.* **42**: 24.
4. Takai, S. and W. C. Richards. 1977. Studies on cerato-ulmin, a wilting toxin of *Ceratocystis ulmi* (Buism.) C. Moreau. I. Isolation and some properties of cerato-ulmin from the culture filtrate of *C. ulmi*. *Phytopathol. Z.* **91**: 129-146.
5. Takai, S. 1977. Studies on cerato-ulmin, a wilting toxin of *Ceratocystis ulmi* (Buism.) C. Moreau. II. Cultural factors affecting cerato-ulmin production by the fungus. *Phytopathol. Z.* **91**: 147-158.

Discussion of Paper by Drs. Takai et al.

According to the comments of DURBIN, in the oak wilt, WILSON has hypothesized that water disfunction occurs primarily because the parenchymatous cells next to the xylem in the tracheal elements die, and on the basis of the electrolyte leakage TAKAI found, this could be happening in this case. In response to the question on the chemistry of cerato-ulmin(CU) from KEEN, TAKAI stated that the molecular weight of CU is approximately 10,000 and that it contains at least 16 amino acids, but neither methionine nor tryptophan. He added that there is a very high concentration of L-proline, which is an excellent nitrogen source for CU production. PAXTON asked whether TAKAI specifically looked for tryptophan, which is very sensitive to degradation in protein hydrolysis treatment. Takai answered that they checked carefully for tryptophan by hydrolyzing in 4 M methane sulfonic acid containing 0.2% tryptamine, and in this analysis used a protein with a known content of tryptophan as the reference.

Recognition and Specificity in Plant Host-Parasite Interactions, pp. 153-163, 1979

ELICITORS OF INCOMPATIBLE HOST RESPONSES: THE ROLE OF HOST CELL MEMBRANES

JACK D. PAXTON

Department of Plant Pathology, University of Illinois, Urbana, Illinois, U.S.A.

The study of biochemical mechanisms whereby cells "recognize" and respond to one another is an exciting area of research that has generated increasing interest (*1, 5, 7, 14, 18, 34*). This "communication" between cells has been most intensively studied in cellular slime molds where a signal and response are necessary for cell aggregation and reproduction. Similar "communication" is now being studied in many other systems and certainly lies at the heart of the extreme specificity exhibited in the interaction of microorganisms and plant. Some form of signal, receptor for the signal, and mutual response must be the basis for the specificity demonstrated in plant-microorganism symbiosis including disease resistance or the incompatible host response. Elicitors are compounds produced by microorganisms and serve as the signals which evoke an incompatible response, including phytoalexin production, by the plant cell.

Keep in mind that most microorganisms in the plant's environment are unable to grow in the living plant even though the dead plant serves as a good substrate for growth. Many of these microorganisms, if placed in the plant, will evoke an incompatible response. This includes the production of phytoalexins (antibiotics which can stop the growth of the invading microorganism). It is not possible at this time to characterize an incompatible host response on the basis of the amount of phytoalexin produced—however this may be possible in the future. This quantitation of phytoalexin production could help in studies of the large area of intermediate plant response between immunity and total susceptibility to plant diseases.

As a working definition I will consider any plant-microorganism interaction where the microorganism stops growth with 1 to 2 days after inoculation as an incompatible interaction. This often is accompanied by rapid death of some cells in the plant and rapid accumulation of phytoalexins. Generally such a reaction is considered to be "disease resistance," however in many cases very similar responses occur in "susceptible" or "compatible" interactions. In compatible interactions these reactions generally occur over a longer period of time. The term hypersensitive reaction has been associated with disease resistance but the role of rapid cell death in plant disease resistance is far from clear (*13, 14, 16, 19, 20, 21, 24, 30, 34*).

I. ELICITORS AND THE ROLES

The term inducer or elicitor has been used to refer to compounds of fungal origin (but not necessarily restricted to fungi) which cause the production of phytoalexins (*12*) in plant tissues to which they are applied. Elicitor is a term used by Keen *et al.* (*15*) to replace the term inducer earlier used by Cruickshank and Perrin (*6*) to refer to a protein of fungal origin capable of specifically stimulating phytoalexin production in bean. Keen *et al.* felt that biochemical implications in gene activation and specific induction of plant genes were associated with the use of the term inducer. These compounds may in fact activate specific genes involved in plant disease resistance, but until this is demonstrated it is probably best to use the term elicitor. Elicitors then are compounds whereby the plant "recognizes" a potential pathogen and responds rapidly to this threat by, among other things, producing phytoalexins. The elicitor may or may not be phytotoxic. Plant cell death may actually be caused by the phytoalexin elicited by this "signal." Evidence is accumulating that the compatible or incompatible "decision" is made in the first few hours of interaction and elicitors may play a central role in this rapid "decision."

There have been numerous reports through the literature of induced resistance to various plant diseases by extracts of microorganisms or culture filtrates (*22, 25, 32*). These reports have yet to be critically studied or applied in commercial plant disease control.

II. MONILICOLIN A

The first attempt to isolate a fungal component that induced a resistance response, phytoalexin production, was the work of Cruickshank and Perrin (*6*). They isolated two compounds, probably proteins, from the mycelium of *Monilina fructicola*. These compounds actively stimulated phaseollin production when applied to bean pods. The larger compound, with a molecular weight of 21,000 daltons, was not further characterized. However the 8,000 daltons compound has an N-terminal lysine and a C-terminal alanine and is composed of 19 different, common amino acids. This compound stimulated phaseollin production in beans at 2.5×10^{-9} M but did not elicit pisatin production in peas or phytoalexin production in broad bean (*Vicia faba*) at 500 times that concentration. Interestingly this also indicates specificity of response to this elicitor. Furthermore the low molecular weight compound, Monilicolin A, did not induce necrosis in french beans, peas, or broad beans, or effect wheat seedling growth at 10^{-6} M. Paxton *et al.* (*26*) also demonstrated that 6×10^{-9} M Monilicolin A stimulated phaseollin production without any apparent ultrastructural or physiological damage to endocarp cells of french bean. The role this compound plays in host parasite interactions however remains to be demonstrated.

III. GLYCOPROTEINS, CARBOHYDRATES, AND OTHERS AS ELICITORS

The next interaction to be studied for phytoalexin inducers or elicitors was Phytophthora root rot of soybeans caused by *Phytophthora megasperma* var. *sojae*. Frans and Paxton (*10*) found a heat-stable, glycoprotein which was produced by this pathogen. This glycoprotein appeared to be differentially produced by the fungus when grown on Harosoy 63 plants or plant juice as compared to Harosoy soybean plants. It should be noted that Harosoy is susceptible to *P. megasperma* var. *sojae* race 1 whereas Harosoy 63 is resistant and that these two varieties differ in essentially the single gene Rps_1 conditioning resistance to this pathogen. Metlitskii *et al.* (*23*) proposed a similar system in the interaction of *P. infestans* with potato. They believe genes for specific resistance control the synthesis of substances stimulating the secretion of phytoalexin elicitors during growth of fungi on or in plants. The absence of receptors of the product of the resistance gene makes the pathogen insensitive to products developed by the resistance gene in the plant.

Keen *et al.* (*15*) using the soybean system, reported that elicitor production was not enhanced by exposing the pathogen to extracts of Harosoy or Harosoy 63 soybean hypocotyls. Their elicitor appeared to be a protein which was equally active on Harosoy and Harosoy 63 hypocotyls. They concluded that the Rps_1 gene is expressed only in hypocotyls, unlike the situation seen in field resistance. Further work by Keen (*14*) on this fungal metabolite indicated that in fact several elicitors are produced, however race 1 of the fungus produced one more elicitor than race 3. This difference he contended was responsible for the 2 to 5 fold difference in phytoalexin production he observed between compatible and incompatible interactions in this system.

Ayres *et al.* (*3*) further studied this host-parasite combination and concluded that no specific elicitor is present in *P. megasperma* var. *sojae.* Instead they found four non-specific, but highly potent, polysaccharide fractions which they characterized as predominantly β 1–3 linked glucans and β 1–2 and β 1–3 linked mannans. The glucan was active at 10^{-9} M which gives it hormonal level activity like Monilicolin A. These compounds appear to be normal components of this fungal cell wall (*4*). This group is further characterizing these elicitors and has been able to isolate small fragments of the elicitor that retain their phytoalexin eliciting activity. Their work also indicates that the β 1–3 linkage is not the recognition signal since natural β 1–3 glucans such as laminarin do not stimulate production of the phytoalexin glyceollin by soybean plants. Anderson-Prouty and Albersheim (*2*) also isolated a predominantly 3- and 4-linked glucan from *Colletotrichium lindemuthianum* which is active in stimulating phaseollin production in french bean plants.

Work on *P. infestans* by Tomiyama, Doke, and others (*9, 24, 29, 31*) has shown that zoospores and hyphae of this fungus contain components to which potato tuber cells respond rapidly. They showed that substances in the microsomal fraction of potato cells could bind the buffer-insoluble components of zoospore homogenates to form large complexes. There was quantitative but not qualitative specificity in this binding. The active fungal material, which may be proteinaceous, can cause intense browning in tissue carrying the *R* genes, but not in tissue lacking these genes. Doke (*8*) further showed that a high molecular weight fraction from a compatible race of *P. infestans* could prevent this hypersensitive reaction if applied to the tissue prior to inoculation; without affecting subsequent development of an incompatible race on this plant. These effects were concentration and time dependent, and restricted to the treated tissues. Chalova *et al.* (*5*) have since characterized the active fractions from this fungus as a glucan and a glycoprotein.

Research on the *Ceratocystis fimbriata*-sweet potato interaction by Kim and Uritani (*17*) demonstrated a heat stable, low molecular weight component of *C. fimbriata* is capable of stimulating phytoalexin and ethylene production in sweet potato root tissue. This material however did not show host specificity. Both compatible and incompatible strains contained this tightly-bound inducer. Kojima and Uritani (*18*) using a similar system showed that the host contained a high molecular weight glycoprotein which specifically binds to incompatible isolates of *C. fimbriata*. This may be the first isolation of a specific receptor of an elicitor.

Work by Uritani *et al.* (*33*) showed that high molecular weight, proteinaceous larval components of the sweet potato weevil also stimulated phytoalexin production in sweet potato tuber tissue. This indicates that insects also contain elicitors of phytoalexin production. It will be interesting to see if these compounds can be purified and chemically characterized.

Hadwiger and Schwochau (*11*) proposed a mechanism for gene activation where by products released from microorganisms induce host resistance by triggering the hypersensitive reaction and thereby destroying symbiosis. However this mechanism remains to be demonstrated. Daniels and Hadwiger (*7*) found at least two heterogeneous sized, proteinaceous components of *Fusarium solani* culture filtrates that could induce pisatin production in pea pods. *Fusarium solani* f. sp. *phaseoli* appeared to produce more of the same elicitors than *F. solani* f. sp. *pisi* which is a pathogen on peas. The difference was a quantitative rather than a qualitative one as far as could be determined. They indicated that an inhibitor of phytoalexin production may also be produced by these pathogens. Stekoll and West (personal communucation) have isolated a heat labile, 30,000 daltons glycoprotein from *Rhizopus stolonifer*. This compound can elicit phytoalexin production in castor bean at 0.15 μg/ml.

Now that those phenomena have been discovered and mechanisms proposed there is a definite need for careful characterization of the compounds involved and their role in recognition and the incompatible interaction.

Other work with microorganism components indicates that we may be able to protect plants from diseases with these components. For example McIntyre *et al.* (*22*) have shown that *Erwinia amylovora* DNA is able to induce resistance to fire blight in pear trees. Rohringer *et al.* (*27*) reported a RNA from *Puccinia graminis* f. sp. *tritici* as active in causing a disease resistance reaction in wheat. However this work has not been substantiated (*28*). Such work points the way toward exciting possibilities in plant disease protection and a better understanding of plant-pathogen interactions. The future for basic and applied research on elicitors and cellular recognition is bright.

SUMMARY

Elicitors of incompatible host responses that have been partially characterized are proteins, glycoproteins, or polysaccharides of fungal origin that stimulate phytoalexin production in plants. These compounds are very active and some of the better characterized compounds stimulate phytoalexin production at 10^{-9} molar concentration, which is hormonal-level activity.

These elicitors appear to be the compounds whereby plants "recognize" potential pathogens and respond to them by producing phytoalexins to restrict or prevent the pathogen's growth.

Efforts are needed to chemically characterize these elicitors and determine the structure of their active sites as well as the "receptor" of these elicitors in the plant. Lectins are one logical possibility for the plant receptor which specifically binds to the elicitor.

In addition, exciting possibilities suggest themselves for the use of these elicitors in protecting plants from various diseases and as a screening tool in plant breeding. As a protectant the elicitors should present a low level of environmental insult since they appear to be natural glycoproteins or polysaccharides which stimulate the normal plant disease resistance response. In plant breeding they would increase the speed and accuracy of population screening procedures since using this abiotic component would eliminate one source of variability in testing host-parasite interactions.

REFERENCES

1. Albersheim, P. and A. J. Anderson-Prouty. 1975. Carbohydrates, proteins, cell surfaces, and the biochemistry of pathogenesis. *Annu. Rev. Plant Physiol.* **26**: 31–52.
2. Anderson-Prouty, A. J. and P. Albersheim. 1975. Host-pathogen interactions VIII. Isolation of a pathogen-synthesized fraction rich in glucan that elicits a defense response in the pathogens hosts. *Plant Physiol.* **56**: 286–291.
3. Ayres, A. R., J. Ebel, B. Valent, and P. Albersheim. 1976. Host-pathogen interactions X. Fractionation and biological activity of an elicitor isolated from

the mycelial walls of *Phytophthora megasperma* var. *sojae*. *Plant Physiol.* **57**: 760–765.

4. Bartnicki-Garcia, S. 1966. Chemistry of hyphal walls of *Phytophthora*. *J. Gen. Microbiol.* **42**: 57–69.
5. Chalova, L. I., O. L. Ozeretskovskaya, L. A. Yurganova, V. G. Baramidze, M. A. Protsenko, Yu, T. D'Yakov, and L. V. Metlitskii. 1976. Metabolites of phytopathogenic fungi as inductors of the protective reactions of plants (illustrated by the interrelations of potatoes with *Phytophthora infestans*). *Dokl. Akad. Nauk S.S.S.R.* **230**: 722–725. in Chem Ab. **86**: 12957t.
6. Cruickshank, I. A. M. and D. R. Perrin. 1968. The isolation and partial characterization of monilicolin A, a polypeptide with phaseollin-inducing activity from *Monilinia fructicola*. *Life Sci.* **7**: 449–458.
7. Daniels, D. L. and L. A. Hadwiger. 1976. Pisatin-inducing components in filtrates of virulent and avirulent *Fusarium solani* cultures. *Physiol. Plant Pathol.* **8**: 9–19.
8. Doke, N. 1975. Prevention of the hypersensitive reaction of potato cells to infection with an incompatible race of *Phytophthora infestans* by constituents of the zoospores. *Physiol. Plant Pathol.* **7**: 1–7.
9. Doke, N., K. Tomiyama, N. Nishimura, and H.S. Lee. 1975. *In vitro* interactions between components of *Phytophthora infestans* zoospores and components of potato tissue. *Ann. Phytopathol. Soc. Japan* **41**: 425–533.
10. Frank, J. A. and J. D. Paxton. 1971. An inducer of soybean phytoalexin and its role in the resistance of soybeans to Phytophthora root rot. *Phytopathology* **61**: 954–958.
11. Hadwiger, L. A. and M. E. Schwochau. 1969. Host resistance responses—An induction hypothesis. *Phytopathology* **59**: 223–227.
12. Ingham, J. L. 1972. Phytoalexins and other natural products as factors in plant disease resistance. *Bot. Rev.* **38**: 343–424.
13. Jones, D. R., W. G. Graham, and E. W. B. Ward. 1974. Ultrastructural changes in pepper cells in a compatible interactions with *Phytophthora capsici*. *Phytopathology* **64**: 1084–1090.
14. Keen, N. T. 1975. Specific elicitors of plant phytoalexin production: Determinants of race specificity in pathogens? *Science* **187**: 74–75.
15. Keen, N.T., J.E. Partridge, and A.I. Zaki. 1972. Pathogen-produced elicitor of a chemical defense mechanism in soybeans monogenically resistant to *Phytophthora megasperma* var. *sojae*. *Phytopathology* **62**: 768 (Abstr.).
16. Khan, F. Z. and J. M. Milton. 1975. Phytoalexin production by lucerne (*Medicago sativa* L.) in response to infection by *Verticillium*. *Physiol. Plant Pathol.* **7**: 179–187.
17. Kim, W. K. and I. Uritani. 1974. Fungal extracts that induce phytoalexins in sweet potato roots. *Plant Cell Physiol.* **15**: 1093–1098.
18. Kojima, M. and I. Uritani. 1974. The possible involvement of a spore agglutinat-

ing factor(s) in various plants in establishing host specificity by various strains of black rot fungus, *Ceratocystis fimbriata. Plant Cell Physiol.* **15**: 733–737.

19. Kojima, M. and I. Uritani. 1976. Possible involvement of furanoterpenoid phytoalexins in establishing host-parasite specificity between sweet potato and various strains of *Ceratocystis fimbriata. Physiol. Plant Pathol.* **8**: 97–111.
20. Maclean, D. J., J. A. Sargent, I. C. Tommerup, and D. S. Ingram. 1974. Hypersensitivity as the primary event in resistance to fungal parasites. *Nature* **249**: 186–187.
21. Mayama, S., J. M. Daly, D. W. Rehfeld, and C. R. Daly. 1975. Hypersensitive response of near-isogenic wheat carrying the temperature-sensitive Sr6 allele for resistance to stem rust. *Physiol. Plant Pathol.* **7**: 35–47.
22. McIntyre, J. L., J. Kuć, and E. B. Williams. 1975. Protection of Bartlett pear against fire blight with deoxyribonucleic acid from virulent and avirulent *Erwinia amylovora. Physiol. Plant Pathol.* **7**: 153–170.
23. Metlitskii, L. V., Yu D'Yakov, and O. L. Ozeretskovsykaya. 1973. Binary induction—a new hypothesis concerning the immunity of plants to *Phytophthora* and similar diseases. *Dokl. Akad. Nauk S.S.S.R.* **213**: 209–212.
24. Nakajima, T., K. Yomiyama, and M. Kinukawa. 1975. Distribution of rishitin and lubinim in potato-tuber tissue infected by an incompatible race of *Phytophthora infestans* and the site where rishitin is synthesized. *Ann. Phytopathol. Soc. Japan* **41**: 49–55.
25. Oku, H., T. Nakanishi, T. Shiraishi, and S. Ouchi. 1973. Phytoalexin induction by some agricultural fungicides and phytotoxic metabolites of pathogenic fungi. *Sci. Rep. Fac. Agric. Okayama Univ.* **42**: 17–20.
26. Paxton, J., D. J. Goodchild, and I. A. M. Cruickshank. 1974. Phaseollin production by live bean endocarp. *Physiol. Plant Pathol.* **4**: 167–171.
27. Rohringer, R., N. K. Howes, W. K. Kim, and D. J. Samborski. 1974. Evidence for a gene-specific RNA determining resistance in wheat to stem rust. *Nature* **249**: 585–588.
28. Rohringer, R., N. K. Howes, W. K. Kim, and D. J. Samborski. 1977. Lack of reproducibility in bioassays for gene-specific RNA reportedly involved in the resistance response of wheat to stem rust. *Can. J. Bot.* **55**: 851–852.
29. Sato, N., K. Kitazawa, and K. Tomiyama. 1971. The role of rishitin in localizing the invading hyphae of *Phytophthora infestans* in infection sites at the cut surfaces of potato tubers. *Physiol. Plant Pathol.* **1**: 289–295.
30. Shiraishi, T., H. Oku, S. Ouchi, and M. Isono. 1976. Pisatin production prior to the cell necrosis demonstrated in powdery mildew of pea. *Ann. Phytopathol. Soc. Japan* **42**: 609–612.
31. Tomiyama, K., H. S. Lee, and N. Doke. 1974. Effect of hyphal homogenate of *Phytophthora infestans* on the potato-tuber protoplasts. *Ann. Phytopathol. Soc. Japan* **40**: 70–72.

32. Trivedi, N. and A. K. Sinha. 1976. Resistance induced in rice plants against *Helminthosporium* infection by treatment with various fungal fluids. *Phytopathol. Z.* **86**: 335–344.
33. Uritani, I., T. Saito, H. Honda, and W. K. Kim. 1975. Induction of furanoterpenoids in sweet potato roots by the larval components of the sweet potato weevils. *Agric. Biol. Chem.* **39**: 1857–1862.
34. Ward, E. W. B. and A. Stoessl. 1976. On the question of 'elicitors' or 'inducers' in incompatible interactions between plants and fungal pathogens. *Phytopathology* **66**: 940–941.

Discussion of Paper by Dr. Paxton

Following Dr. PAXTON's paper, the discussion initially focused on the specificity of elicitors. GRACEN noted that elicitors induce phytoalexin production in both susceptible and resistant plants and asked if there were any differences in the reaction between resistant and susceptible plants and if cells from resistant plants treated with elicitors die as they would eventually die in a compatible reaction. PAXTON stated that cells treated with elicitors die within 48 hr but whether they are killed by the elicitor or by products induced by the elicitor is not known. Phytoalexin production in these cells occurs within 24 hr and at this time the cells appear physiologically healthy and ultrastructurally sound. PAXTON acknowledged that most elicitors are non-specific and are more likely involved in general resistance than in gene-for-gene interaction. BELL reported that he could obtain a specific response on cotton with heat killed cells of *Verticillum* but only if intact cells were used. Specificity was lost by freezing and was dependent on the nutrition of the plants. On the other hand, cell wall preparations of *Xanthamonas malvacearum* elicited a specific response on cotton. DURBIN mentioned a possible problem with bioassay of elicitor. PAXTON applied the elicitor to the inside of a bean pod rather than to a cutinized surface normally encountered by the fungus. Could specificity be lost if the host encounters the elicitor one way in the bioassay and another way in the host-parasite interaction? PAXTON acknowledged that wounding is necessary for the application of the elicitor, however wounding itself does not elicit phytoalexin production. KUĆ then noted that since all the elicitors reported are elicitors of phytoalexin production, their role in disease can be no better than the role of phytoalexins which is not known. Although confident that disease can be controlled by methods other than chemical fungicides, KUĆ was doubtful that this could be done by applying elicitors of phytoalexin production. PAXTON agreed that so far there is only a correlation between phytoalexin production and the inability of an organism to grow, but was optimistic that elicitors of phytoalexin production could be used for disease control. He proposed that elicitors, placed on the leaf surface, could be taken inside the plant on penetration by the fungus and induce phytoalexin production. In response to general comments from SEQUEIRA and KUĆ, PAXTON stated that in an interaction the plant must recognize some component and since elicitors are active at low concentrations they probably induce a response different from the response induced by mercuric chloride. PAXTON indicated to KUĆ that he did not consider the plant as "recognizing" mercuric chloride as it recognizes an inducer since it causes cell death. KUĆ replied that since damage to cells is apparent with elicitors after 24 hr there must have been some effect on cells prior to 24 hr.

Recognition and Specificity in Plant Host-Parasite Interactions, pp. 165–179, 1979

THE RELATION BETWEEN BACTERIAL TOXIC ACTION AND PLANT GROWTH REGULATION

RYUTARO SAKAI,*1 KOUSHI NISHIYAMA,*2
AKITAMI ICHIHARA,*3 KUNIO SHIRAISHI,*3 AND
SADAO SAKAMURA*3

*1*Obihiro University of Agriculture and Veterinary Medicine, Obihiro,* *2*National Institute of Agricultural Sciences, Tokyo, and* *3*Faculty of Agriculture, Hokkaido University, Sapporo, Japan*

It is well known that various plant pathogenic microorganisms may produce specific compounds. These compounds can regulate growth of plants, but there is little evidence that this happens in plant-pathogen combinations except in the case of fusicoccin, the phytotoxic glycoside produced by submerged culture of *Fusicoccum amygdali* Del. (*2*). Fusicoccin elicits wilt and necrotic lesions similar to the symptoms caused by the fungus on its hosts (*4*). Other data have shown that fusicoccin produces a pronounced increase in the wet weight of pea internodes, an increase in the rate of tissue elongation, and enhances tissue deformability, suggesting that it may either possess auxin-like activity or promote such activity (*10*).

Pseudomonas coronafaciens var. *atropurpurea* (Reddy and Godkin) Stapp causes chocolate spot disease on Italian ryegrass (*Lolium multiflorum* Lam.). This organism resembles *Ps. coronafaciens* (Elliott) Stevens, the incitant of halo blight of oat (*Avena sativa* L.), except for host range and appearance of lesions.

During the study of bacterial physiology, we found that the virulent isolates of *Ps. coronafaciens* var. *atropurpurea* caused outgrowths on the tissues of potato tubber, a non-host plant of the bacterium. Avirulent ones did not show such activity. The same activity also was found in the filtrates of the culture fluids. The fact suggests that the activity may be one of the essential requirements for the pathogenicity of the bacterium.

In 1975, the causal substance of the activity was purified from filtrates obtained from shake-cultures of the virulent isolate (*7*). We have named the substance as "coronatine." Recently, we found and reported that coronatine was present in the leaves of Italian ryegrass diseased by the bacterium (*14*) and that diluted coronatine solution produced chlorotic halos on the leaves of Italian ryegrass (*13*).

Firstly, we would like to present our studies on the mechanisms of physiological activity of coronatine. Secondly, we would like to discuss the sensitive site for coronatine in host cells in relation to the course of disease development.

I. OUTGROWTH FORMATION ON POTATO TUBER

Irish cobbler was used as the potato cultivar. Tuber discs were 20 mm in diameter and 10 mm thick. These discs were cut from the central part of the tuber for ensuring material of high uniformity. After washing in running tap water, the discs were held in a moist condition in petri dishs. A drop of the bacterial suspension was then placed on each disc. This system was incubated at 23°C. Three days after application, a solid outgrowth with rough surface occured at the inoculation site. The outgrowths rapidly increased in size with time for several days. At six to seven days after inoculation, this outgrowth was approximately 3 to 4 mm in height and 7 to 9 mm in diameter at the maximum. At this time, the top began to turn a brownish color. The outgrowth was generally observed on the upper surface of the discs, and on rare occasion it was observed on both surfaces of the discs. Microscopic evidence clearly shows that the bacterium has markedly enhanced cell enlargement and that starch grains disappeared from the enlarged cells. The outgrowth, induced by the bacterium, resulted from marked enlargement of individual parencyma cells, that is to say, from hypertrophy, but not from cell division.

II. ABILITY OF PLANT PATHOGENIC BACTERIA TO INDUCE THE HYPERTROPHY

It is well known that various living pathogenic bacteria induce hypertrophy and galls in various plants. So, several pathogenic and saprophytic bacteria were tested for their ability to induce hypertrophy on potato tuber. One hundred eighty nine test isolates were obtained from 75 bacterial species of 11 genera. For example, the bacterial species are *Pseudomonas* (51 species, 160 isolates), *Erwinia* (5 species, 7 isolates), *Corynebacterium* (3 species, 3 isolates), *Xanthomonas* (7 species, 7 isolates), *Agrobacterium, Azotobacter* (1 species, 1 isolate), and *Bacillus* (5 species, 5 isolates). Among these bacteria, hypertrophy was induced on the potato tuber discs by 50 virulent isolates of *Ps. coronafaciens* var. *atropurpurea* and one isolate of *Ps. morsprunorum* (NCPPB 330, which was received from the National Collection of Plant Pathogenic Bacteria in England). These results indicate that the pathogenicity of *Ps. coronafaciens* var. *atropurpurea* may be related to the physiological activity of potato-tubers.

III. ISOLATION OF CORONATINE

Coronatine was isolated from the culture fluid of a virulent isolate of *Ps. coronafaciens* var. *atropurpurea.* This bacterium was incubated at 23°C for 3 days in glucose-potassium nitrate medium under aeration. The cultured cells were removed by centrifugation and the supernatant was processed as shown in Fig. 1. The supernatant and 2% activated charcol-celite (1:1 w/w) was mixed well and the adsorbent was packed in the column. The column was washed with water and eluted with acetone. The eluate was concentrated to samll volume *in vacuo,* adjusted to pH 2.5, and extracted with ethyl acetate. The extracts were concentrated to small volume. This material was chromatographed on a column containing of silicic acid and hyflosupersel (10:1 w/w). The column was first eluted with benzene, then stepwise with benzene-ethyl acetate and finally with methyl alcohol. Fractions from the column were tested for hypertrophy-inducing activity on potato tuber discs. The fractions demonstrating the physiological activity were collected and combined. The active fraction was further purified on a Kieselgel column which was eluted with isopropyl ether-acetic acid (95:5 v/v), acetone and methyl alcohol. The acetone eluate, fraction of strong hypertrophy-inducing activity, was separated by silicic acid chromatography using ether and benzene-acetone (1:1 v/v) as eluent. The active compound was detected on silicic acid TLC-plates as an yellow spot after spraying with 2,4-dinitrophenyl-hydrazine, anisaldehyde, and 10% sulfuric acid.

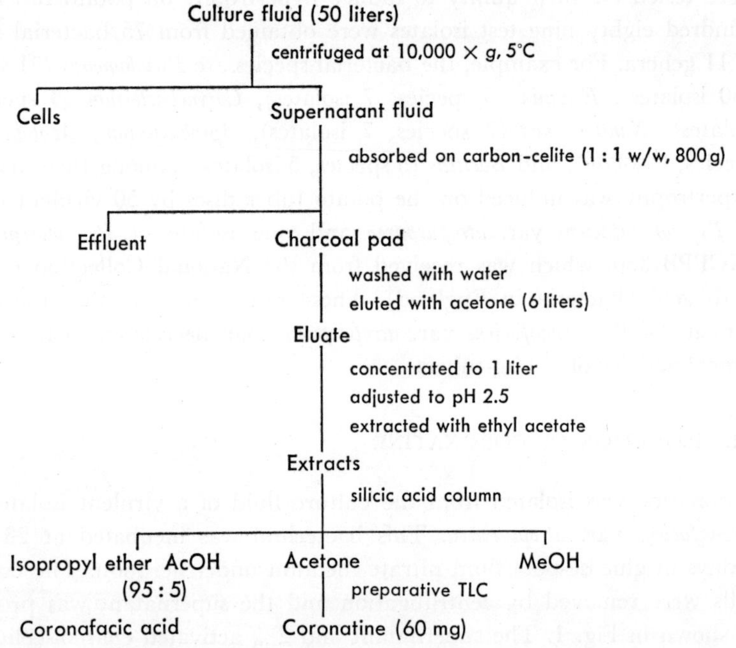

Fig. 1. Isolation procedures of coronatine and coronafacic acid.

IV. CHEMICAL STRUCTURE OF CORONATINE

The chemical structure of coronatine was determined spectroscopically on its derivatives and by crystallographic analysis by X-ray of coronafacic acid. As shown in Fig. 2 (*7, 8*). Coronatine, $[\alpha]_D^{20}+68.4°$ (c 2.2, CH_3OH), mp 151–153°C, was formulated as $C_{18}H_{25}O_4N$ (m/e M^+ found, 319.1753; calcd, 319.1731) and shows the following spectral data, UVλ_{max}^{EtOH} 208 nm (ε 8378); IRν_{max}^{KBr} 1,740 (five-membered ring C=O), 1,620 (C=C), 3,720, 1,645, and 1,525 cm^{-1} (—CONH—). The high resolution mass spectrum indicates that coronatine consists of two significant fragments $C_{12}H_{15}O_2$ and $C_6H_{10}O_2N$. These two fragments are bonded to each other by an amide linkage. In fact, hydrolysis of coronatine gave an acid and an amino acid. The R_f value of an acid on TLC was identical with that of coronafacic acid. Furthermore, the R_f value of an amino acid, an α-amino acid, was identical with that of coronamic acid.

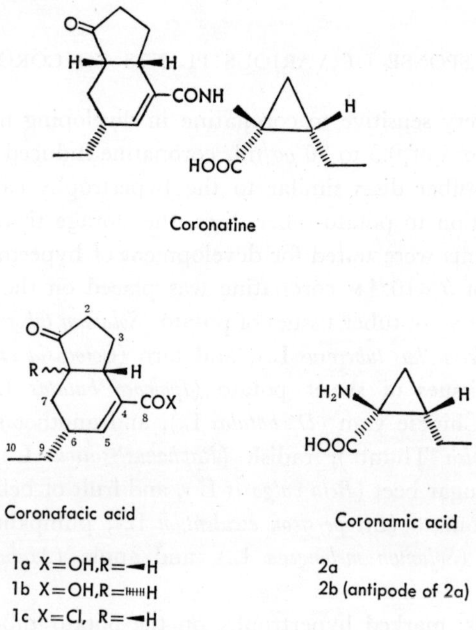

Coronatine

Coronafacic acid

Coronamic acid

1a X=OH, R=–H

1b X=OH, R=⋯H

1c X=Cl, R=–H

2a

2b (antipode of 2a)

Fig. 2. Chemical structure of coronatine and its derivatives.

V. PHYTOTOXIC EFFECTS OF CORONATINE

Coronatine produced lesions on leaves of Italian ryegrass upon the injection (1 μl) of its aqueous acetone solution at 3.2 to 3,200 ng/μl. The necrosis with chlorotic halo produced by coronatine was similar to the symptom on the leaves inoculated with the pathogenic bacterium (*13*). In addition, a substance, isolated from infected plants, had some properties identical with those of coronatine, while such substance was isolated neither from healthy nor from the bacterial cells (*14*). From the results on the phytotoxicity tests, coronatine was suggested to be a chlorosis-inducing toxin in the pathogenesis. In order to determine host-specificity, tests were carried out on many plant species, but coronatine and the bacterium did not exhibit the same host range. Therefore, coronatine is not a host-specific toxin.

VI. HYPERTROPHY RESPONSE OF VARIOUS PLANTS TO CORONATINE

Potato-tuber tissue is very sensitive to coronatine in diveloping hypertrophy. At low concentrations of 0.3 to 30 μg/ml, coronatine induced marked hypertrophy on potato-tuber discs similar to the hypertrophy caused by the bacterium. In addition to potato-tuber discs, the storage tissues of 14 species in 10 genera plants were tested for development of hypertrophy by coronatine. One drop of 5×10^{-4} M coronatine was placed on the discs of test plants. Tested plants were tuber tissues of potato (*Solanum tuberosum* L.), Jerusalem artichoke (*Helianthus tuberosus* L.), and taro (*Colocasia antiquorum* Schott), storage root tissues of sweet potato (*Ipomoea batatas* L.), yam (*Dioscorea bulbifera* L.), Chinese yam (*D. batatas* L.), and another strain of Chinese yam (*D. japonica* Thunb.), radish (*Raphanus sativus* L.), carrot (*Daucus carota* L.), and sugar beet (*Beta vulgaris* L.), and fruit of bell pepper (*Capcicum annuum* L.), tomato (*Lycopersicon esculentum* L.), pumpkin (*Cucurbita pepo* L.), eggplant (*Solanum melongena* L.), and apple (*Malus pumila* Mill.).

Among these plants, marked hypertrophy on the potato tuber tissue and a slight effect on the artichoke tuber tissue were observed, while no response was observed on other plants. These results suggest that the parenchyma cells of potato tuber may be specifically sensitive to coronatine. It is interesting to note that the parenchyma cells of potato tuber and artichoke tuber are suitable for short term auxin-induced expansion growth studies (*1*).

VII. EFFECT OF CORONATINE ON TISSUE DEFORMABILITY OF POTATO TUBER

Usually, cell enlargement in plants are considered as a minor response of some cells to auxin. In 1952, Hackett and Thimann (*5*) indicated that indolacetic acid (IAA) promotes water uptake and cell enlargement in potato tuber discs. When a thin potato tuber slice was incubated with coronatine solution at 10^{-4} M for 24 hr, it appeared to cause slight loosening in the structure of the cell wall. So, we studied the effects of coronatine on deformability of potato tuber cylinders.

Many workers have confirmed that auxin increases the irreversible deformability of plant tissues, for example, coleoptiles and storage tissues.

A primary effect of auxin on growth may therefore be to promote extensibility of the cell wall, a change which precedes cell expansion. The extensibility of cell walls can be divided into two components. They are "elasticity" and "plasticity."

In the present experiments, these two components can be determined separately by the bending method which was modified by Black *et al.* (*3*). As shown in Fig. 3A, a 10 g weight is hung at the center of a potato tuber cylinder. The increase in bending with weight hanging and recovery after the weight was removed was measured with a horizontal microscope.

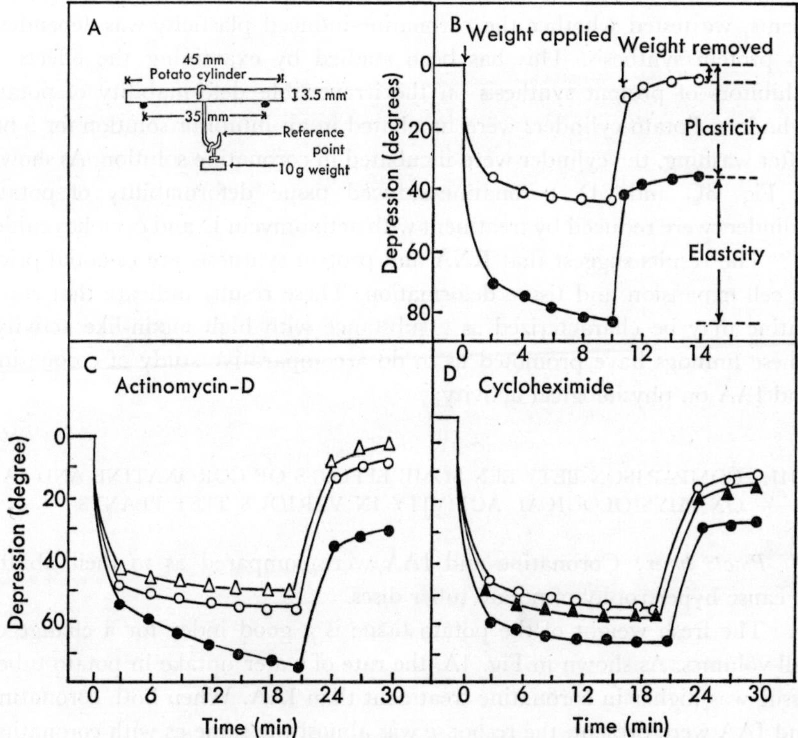

Fig. 3. Bending method used to measure the deformability of potato tuber cylinders and time course of the tissue deformation and recovery. A, bending method; B, C, and D, the arrows show the time at which the weight was applied or removed (B); ○ treatment with water; ● treatment with coronatine (10^{-4} M); △ treatment with coronatine+actinomycin D (5 ppm) (C); ▲ treatment with coronatine+cycloheximide (5×10^{-5} M) (D).

When the weight are removed, the tissue return partially but not completely back to its original form. This permanent deformation is called plastic. The reversible deformation is called elastic. The potato tuber cylinderes were incubated for 16 hr in a 10^{-4} M coronatine solution. As shown in Fig. 3B, the plasticity of treated cylinders were greater than that of the control. These results suggest that coronatine is required to increase the plasticity of the cell wall for cell expansion.

Since 1965, it has become clear that nucleic acid and protein synthesis are required for auxin-induced growth. This is suggested partly by the finding that various inhibitors on the synthesis of these macromolecules prevent the growth-promoting action of auxin (*12*). In the present experiments, we tested whether the coronatine-induced plasticity was dependent on protein synthesis. This has been studied by examining the effects of inhibitors of protein synthesis on the irreversible deformability of potato cylinders. Potato cylinders were incubated in an inhibitor solution for 5 hr. After washing, the cylinder were incubated in coronatine solution. As shown in Fig. 3C and 3D, coronatine-induced tissue deformability of potato cylinders were reduced by treatment with actinomycin D and cycloheximide.

The results suggest that RNA and protein synthesis are essential prior to cell expansion and tissue deformation. These results indicate that coronatine may be characterized as a substance with high auxin-like activity. These finindgs have promoted us to do a comparative study of coronatine and IAA on physiological activity.

VIII. COMPARISON BETWEEN SOME EFFECTS OF CORONATINE AND IAA ON PHYSIOLOGICAL ACTIVITY IN VARIOUS TEST PLANTS

1) *Potato tuber:* Coronatine and IAA were compared as to their ability to cause hypertrophy of potato tuber discs.

The fresh weight of the potato tissue is a good index for a change of cell volumes. As shown in Fig. 4A, the rate of water uptake in potato tuber tissue was higher in coronatine treatment than IAA. When both coronatine and IAA were present, the response was almost the same as with coronatine alone.

2) *Mung bean hypocotyl:* Coronatine and IAA are compared as to their ability to promote the elongation of mung bean hypocotyl segments at a concentration of 10^{-8} to 10^{-4} M. The elongation of etiolated hypocotyl segments were slightly affected by coronatine while markedly stimulated

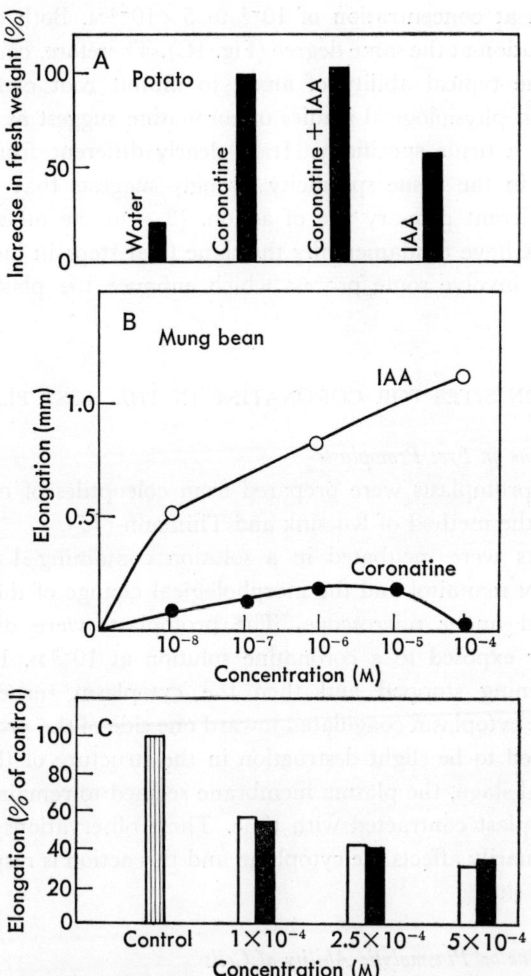

Fig. 4. Comparison between some effects of coronatine and IAA on physiological activity in different tissues from various plants species. A, effects on hypertrophy of potato tuber discs. coronatine, 5×10^{-4} M, IAA, 10^{-3} M; B, effects on elongation of mung bean hypocotyl segments. ○ IAA; ● coronatine; C, effects on elongation of wheat roots. ▨ control; □ coronatine; ■ IAA.

by IAA (Fig. 4B). Therefore, coronatine appears to lack the typical activity of auxin to elongate mung bean hypocotyl segments.

3) *Wheat root:* Coronatine and IAA showed analogous effects on root

elongation in wheat at concentration of 10^{-4} to 5×10^{-4} M. Both of them inhibited root elongation at the same degree (Fig. 4C). Therefore, coronatine appears to have the typical ability of auxin to inhibit root elongation.

These results on physiological studies of coronatine suggest as follows, (1) Coronatine has a tissue specificity. It is clearly different from IAA. (2) The difference in the tissue specificity strongly suggests that the two substances have different primary site of action. (3) On the other hand, coronatine and IAA have fundamentally the same final steps in increasing cell size. The steps involve some process which enhance the plasticity of the cell wall.

IX. INITIAL LESION SITES FOR CORONATINE IN THE HOST PLANT

1. *Effect of Coronatine on Free Protoplasts*

Cell wall free protoplasts were prepared from coleoptiles of oats and Italian ryegrass by the method of Ruesink and Thimann (*15*).

The protoplasts were incubated in a solution containing 1×10^{-3} M coronatine and 0.6 M mannitol and the morphological change of the protoplasts was observed under microscope. The protoplasts were disrupted within 30 min after exposed to a coronatine solution at 10^{-3} M. Initially, protoplasmic streaming stopped and then the cytoplasm turned light brown in color. The cytoplasm coagulated toward one side of the protoplast. Thus, there appeared to be slight destruction in the structure of the cytoplasm. At this initial stage, the plasma membrane seemed to remain intact, and then the protoplast contracted with time. These observations suggest that coronatine primarily affects the cytoplasm and this action is responsible for the initial lesion site.

2. *Effect of Coronatine on Plasmolytic Ability of Cells*

Roots of 4 day old plants of Italian ryegrass grown on wet filter paper in petri dishes were incubated in coronatine solution or water for various times. The treated roots were quickly rinsed with water, then dipped in 0.7 M mannitol solutions, and observed under a microscope. Plasmolytic ability remained normal in the epidermal root cells of Italian ryegrass at 24 and 48 hr after exposure to coronatine at 2×10^{-3} and 10^{-3} M, respectively. However, the cytoplasmic structure appeared to be disrupted. These results indicate that coronatine injures the cytoplasm before the plasmolytic ability of the plasma membrane is lost.

Through these observations, it is suggested that the most sensitive site for coronatine injury may be in the cytoplasm.

3. Effect of N, N'-dicyclohexylcarbodiimide (DCCD) on Coronatine-induced Hypertrophy

Potato-tuber discs, 3 mm thick and 11 mm in diameter, were immersed in DCCD solution for 30 min at 25°C. These discs were rinced twice with water. After discs were weighted, the discs were placed on moistened filter paper in the petri dishes. Ten microliters of coronatine solution at concentration of 5×10^{-4} M were dropped on each disc and incubated at 23°C for 5 days. Discs were weighted at the end of the incubation. The results of this experiment indicated that the coronatine-induced hypertrophy of potato tuber discs was clearly affected by 5×10^{-4} M DCCD and was markedly inhibited by 1×10^{-3} M DCCD (Fig. 5).

Recently, the role of membrane-bound ATPases has been considered in relation to the mechanisms of plant hormonal action (*6*). Marre *et al.* (*11*) reported that in pea internode segments, DCCD inhibited both auxin-induced cell enlargement and proton extrusion, suggesting the close association of auxin action and plasma membrane-bound ATPase. In fact, auxin stimulation of plasma membrane-bound ATPase has been demonstrated (*9*). Data obtained in this study showed that DCCD, an inhibitor of membrane-bound ATPases, inhibited coronatine-induced hypertrophy on potato tuber discs. This result suggests a close association between coronatine and membrane-bound ATPase.

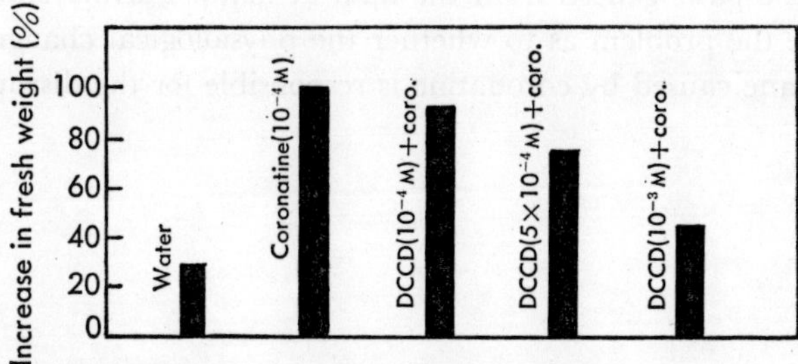

Fig. 5. Effect of DCCD on coronatine-induced hypertrophy of potato tuber discs. Pretreatment with DCCD for 30 min; post-treatment with coronatine for 5 days. Each bar represents the mean 10 sections. coro., coronatine, 10^{-4} M; DCCD, 10^{-4} M, 5×10^{-4} M, 10^{-3} M.

4. Effect of Coronatine on the Loss of Electrolytes

Change in permeability might be the initial event in pathogenesis. Several pathogens are known to produce toxins which cause a rapid increase in the loss of electrolytes from host tissues. Coronatine was tested for similar effects on potato tuber and Italian ryegrass leaves. Permeability changes were determined by the changes of the electrical conductivity of the ambient solutions in which tissues were submarged. Tissues were treated with coronatine solution (10^{-5} to 10^{-3} M) or water for 20 hr. Coronatine treated potato tuber discs and Italian ryegrass released electrolytes at a much faster rate than did the control. Potato tuber discs, 8 mm in diameter and 2 mm thick, were added with 10 μl coronatine solution at concentration range from 2.5×10^{-4} to 10^{-3} M and incubated in petri dishes. After treatment, conductance of the ambient solution containing discs treated by 1×10^{-3} M coronatine solution was two times greater than that of control. Two days after the mesurement of electrolytes, hypertrophic growth occurred on the potato discs. The result indicates that coronatine changes permeability of potato tuber discs 24–48 hr before the development of hypertrophy. These data suggest the posibility that coronatine might initially affect the plasma membrane. On the other hand, at 21 hr after treatment of 10^{-5} or 5×10^{-4} M coronatine solution, conductance of the ambient solution containing treated leaves of Italian ryegrass was two or three times higher than control tissue.

Thus, these studies of initial lesion sites for coronatine in host plant suggest that the disruption of the cytoplasm induced by coronatine may be secondary effects brought about indirectly by physiological change of the plasma membrane. But, it is premature to postulate the mode of action of coronatine in the pathogenesis from the data at hand. Further studies are needed to solve the problem as to whether the physiological change of the plasma membrane caused by coronatine is responsible for the disruption of the cytoplasm.

SUMMARY

Coronatine is an extracellular toxin produced by *Pseudomonas coronafaciens* var. *atropurpurea* (Reddy and Godkin), the incitant of the chocolate spot disease on Italian ryegrass (*Lolium multiflorum* Lam.). Coronatine induces the necrosis with chlorotic halo symptoms of the disease in host leaves as well as in nonhosts and thus is nonspecific. Coronatine, at low concentration of 0.3 to 30 μg/ml, also induces marked hypertrophy only on potato tuber tissues. When a potato tuber cylinder was incubated with coronatine before the extensibility measurement, the plasticity was greater than that of the control. The results suggest that coronatine is required to increase the plasticity of the cell wall for cell expansion. These results indicate that coronatine may be characterized as a substance with high auxin-like activity. However, physiological data show that coronatine has a tissue specificity. It is clearly different from IAA. The difference in the tissue specificity strongly suggests that the two substances have different primary sites of action. On the other hand, coronatine and IAA have fundamentaly the same final steps in increasing cell size. The steps involve some process which enhances the plasticity of the cell wall.

Histological and physiological data show that the most sensitive site for coronatine injury may be in the cytoplasm. On the other hand, coronatine-induced hypertrophy of potato-tuber tissues were markedly inhibited by N,N-dicyclohexylcarbodiimide, one of the inhibitors of membrane-bound ATPase. This results suggests a close association between coronatine and membrane-bound ATPase. In addition, coronatine changes the permeability 24–48 hr before the development of hypertrophy on potato tuber tissues. Thus, these results suggests that the disruption of the cytoplasm induced by coronatine may be due to secondaly effects brought about indirectly by physiological changes of the plasma membrane.

REFERENCES

1. Adamson, D. 1962. Expansion and division in auxin-treated plant cells. *Can. J. Bot.* **40**: 719–744.
2. Ballio, A., E. B. Chain, P. DeLeo, B. F. Erlanger, M. Mauri, and A. Tonoro. 1964. Fusicoccin: a new wilting toxin produced *Fusicoccum amygdali* Del. *Nature* **203**: 297.

3. Black, M., C. Bullock, E. N. Clarke, A. D. Hanson, and G. M. Jolley. 1967. Effect of inhibitors of protein synthesis on the plastic deformation and growth of plant tissues. *Nature* **215**: 1289–1290.
4. Chain, E. B., P. G. Mantle, and B. V. Milborrow. 1971. Further investigation on the toxicity of fusicoccins. *Physiol. Plant Pathol.* **1**: 495–514.
5. Hackett, D. P. and K. V. Thimann. 1952. The nature of the auxin-induced water uptake by potato tissue. *Am. J. Bot.* **39**: 553–560.
6. Hager, A., H. Menzel, and A. Krauss. 1971. Versuche und hypothese zur Primarwirkung des Auxin beim Streckungswachstum. *Planta* **100**: 47–75.
7. Ichihara, A., K. Shiraishi, H. Sato, S. Sakamura, K. Nishiyama, R. Sakai, A. Frusaki, and T. Matsumoto. 1977. The structure of coronatine. *J. Am. Chem. Soc.* **99**: 636.
8. Ichihara, A., K. Shiraishi, S. Sakamura, K. Nishiyama, and R. Sakai. 1977. Partial synthesis and stereochemistry of coronatine. *Tetrahedron Lett.* **3**: 269–272.
9. Kasamo, K. and T. Yamaki. 1974. Effect of auxin on Mg^{++}- activated and inhibited ATPase from mung bean hypocotyls. *Plant Physiol.* **15**: 965–970.
10. Lado, P., A. Pennachioni, F. R. Galdogno, S. Russi, and V. Silano. 1972. Comparison between some effects of fusicoccin and indole-3-acetic acid on cell enlargement in various plant materials. *Physiol. Plant Pathol.* **2**: 75–85.
11. Marre, E., P. Lado, F. Rasi-Caldogno, R. Colombo, and M. I. deMichelis. 1974. Evidence for the coupling of proton extrusion to K^+ uptake in pea internode segments treated in fusicoccin or auxin. *Plant Sci. Lett.* **3**: 365–379.
12. Morre, D. J. 1965. Changes in tissue deformability accompanying actinomycin D inhibition of plant growth and ribonucleic acid synthesis. *Plant Physiol.* **40**: 615–619.
13. Nishiyama, K., R. Sakai, A. Ezuka, A. Ichihara, K. Shiraishi, M. Ogasawara, H. Sato, and S. Sakamura. 1976. Phytotoxic effect of coronatine produced by *P. coronafaciens* var. *atropurpurea* on leaves of Italian ryegrass. *Ann. Phytopathol. Soc. Japan* **42**: 614–614.
14. Nishiyama, K., R. Sakai, A. Ezuka, A. Ichihara, K. Shiraishi, and S. Sakamura. 1977. Detection of coronatine in halo blight lesion of Italian ryegrass. *Ann. Phytopathol. Soc. Japan* **43**: 219–220.
15. Ruesink, A. W. and K. V. Thimann. 1965. Protoplasts from the avena coleoptile. *Botany* **54**: 56–64.

Discussion of Paper by Drs. Sakai et al.

In the discussion of SAKAI's paper, KOSUGE asked if coronatine had any effect on animals or microorganisms? SAKAI reported that animals had not been tested but of several fungi tested none were strongly affected. URITANI noted that since coronatine and IAA have similar activities they may have the same binding site. KEEN added that, since some plant hormones are known to bind at the plasmalemma, coronatine could be competing for the receptor site of IAA and asked SAKAI if the structure of coronatine was such that the two rings could be competing with the indole nucleus of IAA. SAKAI responded to URITANI and KEEN by stating that he did not want to speculate on the specific site of action but he thought it likely that both IAA and coronatine bound to the plasmalemma since the activites of both were inhibited by N,N′-dicyclohexyl carbodiimide. In response to Takai's question SAKAI stated that neither of the two coronatine derivatives, coronafacic acid or coronamic acid, were active. DURBIN asked if the necrosis effect was light dependent. SAKAI stated that in ryegrass the chlorotic response occurs in the dark as well as in the light. KUĆ asked SAKAI if coronatine affected leaves and roots. SAKAI responded that coronatine had been tested only on young sprouts and tissue cultures of potato tubers. However, coronatine did not induce hypertrophy on these tissues. SEQUEIRA pointed out that even though SAKAI had shown coronatine at 10^{-4} M to have analogous effects of IAA at 10^{-3} M, IAA had been reported to be active on roots at 10^{-7} M. SAKAI stated that he had used IAA only at 10^{-3} M on the tests of the hypertrophy in potato tuber discs. The effects of IAA on hypertrophy in potato tuber discs were consistently greatest at a concentration of 10^{-3} M.

Recognition and Specificity in Plant Host-Parasite Interactions, pp. 181-191, 1979

SPORE AGGLUTINATING FACTOR AND GERM TUBE GROWTH INHIBITING FACTOR IN HOST PLANT

IKUZO URITANI*[1] AND MINEO KOJIMA*[2]

*[1]*Laboratory of Biochemistry and* *[2]*Institute for Biochemical Regulation, Faculty of Agriculture, Nagoya University, Nagoya, Japan*

When plant tissues are penetrated by various kinds of parasitic fungi, bacteria, and viruses, they recoginize the foreign organisms by constitutive factors in the plants. Such a mechanism has been acquired by plant tissues in the course of evolution for a long period (*10, 11*). Some of the factors are antibiotic in nature by means of which plants recognize penetrating parasites (*4*). In fact, many kinds of higher plants contain antibiotic compounds belonging to either low molecular weight or high molecular weight components. For example, terpenes, alkaloids, flavonoids, and polyphenols belong to the former (*7, 9*), and proteinase-inhibitors (*6*) and anti-viral factors (*5*) are involved in the latter.

Thus, such constitutive factors in plants may participate not only in the recognition of parasites but also in the primary defense action on parasites. The interactions of those factors with constituents in the parasites may induce a secondary defense action involving phytoalexin production. Furthermore, the factors in plants may be more or less specific to species or cultivars of plants, and take part in the specificity of plant-parasite interactions (*2, 11*).

As the examples of the above constitutive factors, we would like to cite the spore agglutinating factor (*3, 12*) and germ-tube growth inhibiting factor (*4*) in sweet potato (*Ipomoea batatas* Lam.) root tissue, especially in the system of sweet potato and black rot fungus.

I. *CERATOCYSTIS FIMBRIATA* ELL. AND HALST

Various strains of the fungus were isolated from black-rot regions on many species of plants, including sweet potato, coffee, prune, cacao, oak, taro, and almond. Each strain from a different host species has a strict "inter-species" host specificity. For example, on sweet potato, only the sweet potato strain is pathogenic and all other strains are non-pathogenic.

II. SPORE AGGLUTINATING FACTOR

Endoconidia of each strain were collected after 2–3 days from a shaking culture at 30°C in a white potato extract medium containing 1% sucrose, and suspended in water to give a spore density of 3.0×10^7 spores per ml.

Sweet potato root tissue (250 g) was homogenized in the cold with 250 ml of 0.02 M KCl containing 0.2% ascorbic acid, and the homogenate was mixed with 25 g Polyclar AT and left to stand for 10 min. The homogenate was then squeezed through gauze and centrifuged at $8{,}800 \times g$ for 20 min to obtain the supernatant fraction. The fraction was heated at 80–90°C for 1 min, then centrifuged at $880 \times g$ for 10 min to remove any substance(s) which might interfere with spore agglutination. In some experiments, white potato tuber, taro tuber, cucumber fruit, and soaked kidney bean seed were used as materials, and the tissue extracts were prepared from them with some modifications, as the test solutions.

An endoconidial suspension (0.5 ml) was mixed with 3 ml of the above extract, and the mixture was incubated in a 10 ml flask at 25°C on a shaker at 100 strokes per min, and periodically examined under a microscope for agglutination of spores during the incubation.

When sweet potato extract was used, spores of the sweet potato strain were not agglutinated during an incubation period of over 24 hr, but spores of the other six non-pathogenic strains were agglutinated within 5 hr. Thus, there was a positive correlation between the spore agglutinations and host-parasite reactions (compatible and non-compatible reactions) in the sweet potato—*C. fimbriata* strain system. Such correlations were also observed when the other four plant materials were used, with three exceptions.

The agglutinating factor from sweet potato roots appears to be a high

TABLE I

Effects of Pronase[a] and Macerozyme[b] Treatments on the Spore Agglutinating Activity of Sweet Potato Extracts

Dilution of extracts (times)	Spore agglutinating activity[c]			
	Pronase	Boiled pronase	Macerozyme	Boiled Macerozyme
0	+3	+3	−	+3
2	+2	+2.5		
4	+1.5	+2.4		
8	−	+1.5		

[a] Extracts (10 ml) were mixed with either 1 ml of 30 mg of pronase (product of Kaken Kagaku Co. Ltd., Tokyo) in aqueous solution, or 1 ml of a boiled pronase solution, then they were incubated at 30°C for 3 hr. After incubation, the extracts were heated for 2 min in boiling water, diluted with water as shown at the first column in the table and assayed for their spore agglutinating activity. [b] Extracts (10 ml) were mixed with either 0.5 ml of 32.5 mg of Macerozyme (R-10 product of Kinki Yakult Co. Ltd., Osaka) in aqueous solution, or 0.5 ml of a boiled Macerozyme solution, then they were incubated at 20°C for 15 hr. After incubation, extracts were heated for 1 min in boiling water and assayed for their spore agglutinating activity. [c] Agglutinating activity was assayed with the coffee strain spores. Relative activity is denoted by the positive (+) figures and the negative sign (−) denotes no activity.

molecular weight substance consisting of protein and polysaccharide moieties, since it was not filtered through a Diaflo (UM-20E) membrane, and was inactivated partially by pronase treatment and completely by Macerozyme treatment (Table I). When sweet potato extract was centrifuged at $105{,}000 \times g$ for 2 hr, the factor was clearly detected in both precipitable and supernatant fractions.

III. GERM-TUBE GROWTH INHIBITING FACTOR

Endoconidial suspension of each strain was prepared as shown in the above section.

Sweet potato root tissue (100 g) was homogenized in the cold with 100 ml of distilled water, and the homogenate was squeezed through gauze and centrifuged at $2{,}200 \times g$ for 5 min to obtain the supernatant fraction (called tissue extract). In some experiments, tissue extract was prepared using 0.05 M Tris-HCl buffer, pH 7.5, containing 0.24% sodium ascorbate.

The standard assay of the inhibitory activity was carried out as follows: an endoconidial suspension (4.5×10^6 spores) was mixed with an aliquot of the sample solution to be assayed, 0.2 ml of 0.1 M O-(N-morpholino)-ethanesulfonic acid-sodium hydroxide buffer, pH 6.4, and 0.1 ml of tissue extract as the source of nutrients, in a final volume of 1.45 ml. Such a low concentration of tissue extract (0.1 ml per 1.45 ml) in the assay medium did not show any appreciable inhibitory activity toward germ-tube growth of any strains used. The mixture was incubated at 28°C for 3–4 hr on a shaker at 100 strokes per min, and periodically examined under a microscope for germination and germ-tube growth during incubation. One unit of the activity was defined as the quantity of the inhibitory factor causing 50% inhibition of germ-tube growth of control (without addition of the inhibitory factor) when the oak strain, the most sensitive one, was used.

Spores of the seven strains were incubated in the 20 fold-diluted and non-diluted tissue extracts. In the diluted tissue extract, spores of all strains germinated and developed long germ tubes without appreciable inhibition. In the non-diluted tissue extract, germ-tube growth of the sweet potato strain was scarcely inhibited, whereas that of the other six non-pathogenic strains was strongly inhibited. No inhibition of germination was observed with any of the strains used. The results suggest that tissue extract of sweet potato roots contains some factor showing differential inhibitory activity toward germ tube growth of various strains of *C. fimbriata*.

IV. BIOCHEMICAL NATURE OF GERM-TUBE GROWTH INHIBITING FACTOR

Two experiments were performed to examine whether the inhibitory factor was a high or low molecular weight substance. First, tissue extract was filtered through a Diaflo (UM-20E) membrane. All strains developed long germ tubes in the filtrate, while germ-tube growth of the incompatible strains was severely inhibited in the concentrated extract inside the filter. Secondary, tissue extract was passed through a Sephadex G-25 column. In the eluate fraction containing low molecular weight substances, spores of the incompatible strain (oak strain) germinated and developed long germ tubes. However, the growth of germ tube was strongly inhibited in the void fraction even when added with a small amount of tissue extract as nutrients (0.1 ml per 1.45 ml). These results indicated that the germ-tube growth inhibitory factor was of high molecular weight.

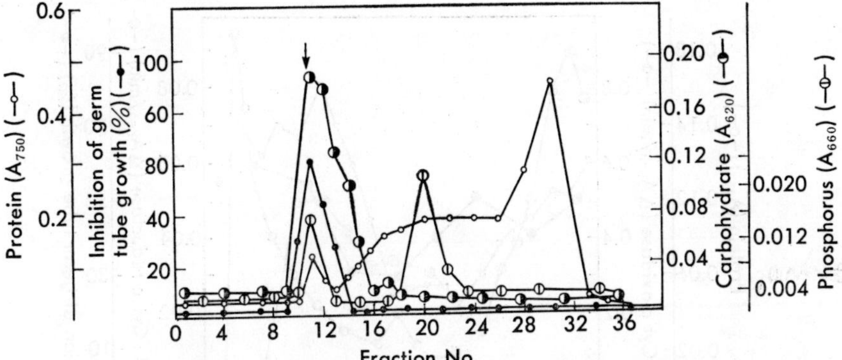

Fig. 1. Sephadex G-100 column chromatography of the supernatant fraction after centrifugation at $105{,}000 \times g$ for 2 hr. Tissue extract was centrifuged at $105{,}000 \times g$ for 2 hr, obtaining the supernatant fraction, which was concentrated using a Diaflo (UM-20E) membrane, and the concentrate was chromatographed on a column ($\phi 1.8 \times 44$ cm) of Sephadex G-100. Three ml fractions were collected, and assayed for inhibitory activity (●), and protein (○), carbohydrate (◑), and phosphorus contents (⦶). Arrow indicates the void volume of the column determined with blue-dextran (see Ref. *4*).

The void fraction of Sephadex G-25 column was centrifuged at 105,000 $\times g$ for 2 hr. Distribution of the activity in the percipitate and supernatant fractions were 54 and 33% of the original activity, respectively. Then, the supernatant fraction was chromatographed on a Sephadex G-100 column after concentration using a Diaflo (UM-20E) membrane (Fig. 1). The inhibitory activity was detected only in the void fraction, which contained protein, carbohydrate, and phosphorus. When Sepharose 6B was used for the chromatography, the inhibitory activity was also found only in the void fraction. The data suggest that the inhibitory activity is associated with some membrane or particulate with molecular weight of over 4×10^6 which remains in the supernatant fraction. The dispersed suspension of the above $105{,}000 \times g$ precipitate exhibited essentially the same differential inhibitory activity toward germ-tube growth of various strains as the non-diluted tissue extract.

The dispersed suspension of the above precipitate was subjected to a discontinuous sucrose density gradient centrifugation. According to the centrifugal distribution pattern, most of the inhibitory factor was distributed in the sucrose gradient as microsome membrane was, suggesting that the

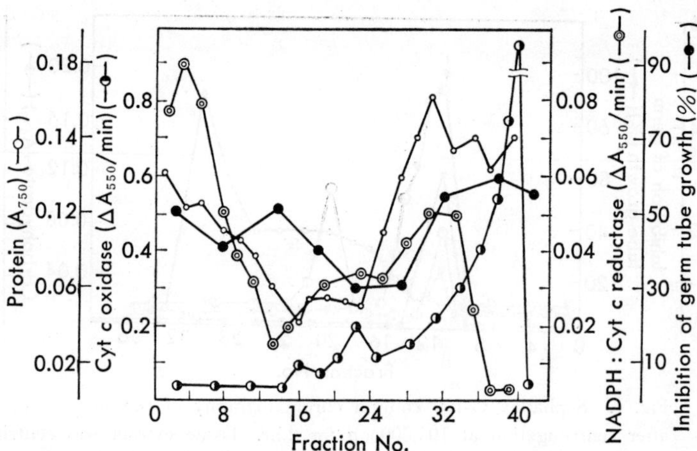

Fig. 2. Discontinuous sucrose density gradient centrifugation of the germ-tube growth inhibitory factor from sweet potato root tissue. ●, ○, ◎, and ◑ indicate inhibitory activity, protein contents, $NADPH_2$: chtochrome *c* oxidoreductase activity, and cytochrome *c*: O_2 oxidoreductase activity, respectively (see Ref. *4*).

factor had a comparable density to those of biomembranes, such as microsomal membrane (Fig. 2). The pattern showed also that the inhibitory activity was not confined to a particular fraction but distributed over various fractions. This broad distribution of the inhibitory activity might be due to the distruption of the factor during preparation.

When the inhibitory factor was treated by pronase, activity was not lost, although all proteins in the factor were digested (Table II). On the

TABLE II

Effect of Pronase Treatment of the Germ-tube Growth Inhibiting Factor on Its Activity and Content of Protein, Carbohydrate, and Phosphorus

	Control sample	Treated sample
Inhibitory activity[a] (units/ml)	1.4	1.4
Protein content[b] (μg/ml)	400	0
Carbohydrate content[b] (μg/ml)	100	108
Phosphorus content[b] (μg/ml)	7	10

[a] See the text. [b] See Ref. *4*.

TABLE III
Comparison of the Monosaccharide Composition of the Germ-tube Growth Inhibiting Factor after the Treatment by Various Enzymes

Monosaccharides[a]	Relative contents of monosaccharides	
	Non-treated	Enzyme-treated
Rhamnose	1.0	1.0
Arabinose	2.1	0
Mannose	0.3	0.2
Galactose	7.7	2.4
Glucose	9.9	3.3
Unidentified 1	1.0	0
Unidentified 2	1.5	0

[a] The content of each component was relatively estimated from the area of each peak of the corresponding alditol acetate in the gas chromatogram, when the content of rhamnose-alcohol acetate was assumed to be 1 (see text).

other hand, treatment by periodate caused inactivation of more than 50%. However, individual treatment by carbohydrate hydrolytic enzymes such as Macerozyme, cellulase, α-glucosidase, and β-glucosidase did not cause inactivation. Neither phospholipase C nor RNase treatment inactivated the activity. After the inhibitory factor was simultaneously treated by all the above enzymes, the remaining material still had activity. The substance was hydrolyzed by 2 N hydrochloric acid at 120°C for 70 min, and the monosaccharides thus obtained were analyzed by gas chromatography, after the conversion to alditol acetate. They were composed of glucose, galactose, and rhamnose in large amounts and of mannose in only small amounts (Table III).

It seems likely that the inhibitory factor is associated with a membrane fraction, and the main moiety in the factor are poly- or oligo-saccharides.

V. MODE OF INHIBITION

According to the time course of germ tube growth and germination of the oak strain in the presence and absence of the inhibitory factor, the factor did not completely stop germ tube growth, but did decrease growth rate. The factor also inhibited growth from pre-germinated spores. On the other hand, the factor had no appreciable effect on germination, as described above. The plot of percent inhibition of germ-tube growth against concentration of the factor exhibited a hyperbolic curve, which was similar to the Michaelis-Menten type curve, showing the relation of enzyme activity with concentration of the substrate.

When the germinated spores were pre-treated with pronase, they became less sensitive to the factor and developed long germ tubes. On the other hand, when they were pre-treated by boiled pronase or water, they remained sensitive to the factor. However, when the ungerminated spores were treated with pronase, the sensitivity to the factor was not changed. The results suggest that the inhibition of germ-tube growth is caused by the specific interaction of the factor with some protein- or glycoprotein-containing structure on the surface of germ tubes of the non-pathogenic strains.

VI. CONCLUDING REMARKS

There was a positive correlation between the sensitivity to spore agglutinating and germ-tube growth inhibiting factors and the specificity in sweet potato-*C. fimbriata* interaction. Thus, those two factors may participate in the recognition of incompatible parasites as foreign entities by the host cells, and in the primary defense action at the initial stage of infection. Furthermore, they may play also the role in triggering the hypersensitive reaction and successive secondary defense action in the host cells such as phytoalexin production in the host cells, and/or inducing the physiological and cytological changes in the parasite cells. It will be important to determine whether or not such factors may occur normally in other plants and take part in the recognition and primary defense action in general, in the specific relation of plant-parasite interactions.

In this context, it must be emphasized that both the spore agglutinating and germ-tube growth inhibiting factors include some carbohydrate moiety, although we think that the spore agglutinating factor is different from the germ-tube growth inhibiting factor. There are differences between them, such as sensitivity to the treatment by pronase or Macerozyme. Those factors may be related to lectin-like substances in sweet potato root tissue.

Most lectins are glycoproteins and seem to be combined with the plant cell wall to some extent. It is likely that lectins play a role in plant-cell recognition of foreign organisms such as pathogenic bacteria when they penetrate into plant cells, and the recognition may be performed by the combination of lectins with the carbohydrate moieties of parasitic organisms, with some specificity in plant-foreign organism relationship (*1, 8*).

SUMMARY

Sweet potato root tissue contained a *C. fimbriata*—spore agglutinating factor and a *C. fimbriata*—germ-tube growth inhibiting factor. The former agglutinated endoconidia of the coffee, prune, cacao, oak, taro, and almond strains, all incompatible to sweet potato, but not the sweet potato strain, compatible to sweet potato. The latter inhibited germ-tube growth of the above six incompatible strains, but scarcely inhibited the sweet potato strain.

Both factors were of high molecular weight, contained some poly- or oligo-saccharides, and appeared to be associated with membranes in sweet potato root tissue. However, both factors are different from each other, in terms of their biochemical nature.

It is very likely both factors play the role in recognizing foreign organisms as "non-self," causing the agglutination of spores of the organisms penetrating into host cells, and inhibiting germ-tube growth at the initial stage of infection. Thus, they may take part in a primary defense action.

REFERENCES

1. Albersheim, P. and A. J. Anderson-Prouty. 1975. Carbohydrates, proteins, cell surfaces, and the biochemistry of pathogenesis. *Annu. Rev. Plant Physiol.* **26**: 31–52.
2. Daly, J. M. 1976. Introduction. *In*: K. Tomiyama, J. M. Daly, I. Uritani, H. Oku, and S. Ouchi (eds.). *Biochemistry and Cytology of Plant-Parasite Interaction.* Kodansha Ltd., Tokyo and Elsevier, Amsterdam, pp. 1–10.
3. Kojima, K. and I. Uritani. 1974. The possible involvement of a spore agglutinating factor(s) in various plants in establishing host specificity by various strains of black rot fungus, *Ceratocystis fimbriata. Plant Cell Physiol.* **15**: 733–737.
4. Kojima, K. and I. Uritani. 1977. Studies on factor(s) in sweet potato which specifically inhibits germ tube growth of incompatible isolates of *Ceratocystis fimbriata. Plant Cell Physiol.* **18** (in press).
5. Loebenstein, G. 1972. Localization and induced resistance in virus-infected plants. *Annu. Rev. Phytopathol.* **10**: 177–206.

6. Ryan, C. A. 1973. Proteolytic enzymes and their inhibitors in plants. *Annu. Rev. Plant Physiol.* **21**: 173–196.

7. Schönbeck, F. and E. Schlösser. 1976. Preformed substances as potential protectants. *In*: R. Heitefuss and P. H. Williams (eds.). *Encyclopedia of Plant Physiology*. vol. 4. Springer-Verlag, Berlin, pp. 653–678.

8. Sequeira, L., G. Gaard, and G. A. De Zoeten. 1976. Interaction of bacteria and host cell walls: its relation to mechanisms of induced resistance. *Physiol. Plant Pathol.* **28**: 479–501.

9. Swain, T. 1977. Secondary compounds as protective agents. *Annu. Rev. Plant Physiol.* **28**: 479–501.

10. Tomiyama, K., J. Akai, and T. Washio. 1952. Studies on the specific affinity between the host-plant juice and parasitic fungus. I. Effect of host-plant juice on the germination of the spores of parasitic fungus. *Res. Bull. Hokkaido Natl. Agric. Expt. Sta.* **63**: 1–12.

11. Uritani, I. 1976. Protein metabolism. *In*: R. Heitefuss and P.H. Williams (eds.). *Encyclopedia of Plant Physiology*. vol. 4. Springer-Verlag, Berlin, pp. 509–525.

12. Uritani, I., K. Oba, M. Kojima, W. K. Kim, I. Oguni, and H. Suzuki. 1976. *In*: K. Tomiyama, J.M. Daly, I. Uritani, H. Oku, and S. Ouchi (eds.). *Biochemistry and Cytology of Plant-Parasite Interaction*. Kodansha Ltd., Tokyo and Elsevier Amsterdam, pp. 239–252.

Discussion of Paper by Drs. Uritani and Kojima

In response to questions from DALY, URITANI stated that, although there is yet no conclusive evidence, he believed the agglutinating factor is different from spore inhibiting factor although they both could arise from a larger protein associated with membranes. SIEGEL inquired about the enzymatic composition of the Macerozyme preparation in view of the observation that the factors were differentially resistant to it. URITANI reported it to be mainly pectinase with α-glucosidase, β-1, 3-, and β-1-4-glucosidase activity but did not believe pectinase was important in this phenomenon. In response to TAKAI's comment on the presence agglutinating and inhibitory active in ppt and supernatant, URITANI pointed out this behavior would be expected if the factors were associated with membrane and membrane fragments, but KEEN observed such a cellular location would be difficult to reconcile with its presumed biological function.

KUĆ noted the similarity between URITANI's observations and those his group has found with protected cucumbers. Factors in protected cucumbers cause spore agglutination and inhibition and asked if URITANI has observed such phenomena on the inoculated surface of tissue slices. This possibility had not yet been tested. AIST noted that agglutinating factor could act directly at wall surfaces or else cause spores to produce something that caused subsequent agglutination but URITANI indicated these possibilities had not been evaluated. DURBIN noted that the effect of pronase in reducing sensitivity of spore inhibition of the factor could be the result of an action of pronase in shortening germination but URITANI pointed out that pronase had no observable effect on germination. HANCHEY commented on the probability that lectins were involved and WHEELER asked if the agglutination factor might be a peroxidase known to increase in resistant tubers.

Recognition and Specificity in Plant Host-Parasite Interactions, pp. 193-210, 1979

THE ROLE OF HOST CELL MEMBRANES

PENELOPE HANCHEY AND HARRY WHEELER

Department of Botany and Plant Pathology, Colorado State University, Fort Collins, Colorado, and Department of Plant Pathology, University of Kentucky, Lexington, Kentucky, U.S.A.

The "hypothesis-become-dogma" (*38*) in physiological studies of diseased plants is that pathogens or their metabolic products cause disease by effects on cell permeability. This hypothesis originated with Thatcher (*56–58*) who proposed, on the basis of deplasmolysis times in urea, that susceptibility was associated with increased permeability and that decreased permeability would lead to resistance. Permeability changes would provide or withhold nutrients necessary for successful growth and parasitism. Since that time numerous papers have reported permeability changes, but it is increasingly evident that in many cases these changes do not differentiate resistance or susceptibility, but merely reflect the extent of cellular injury.

Mechanisms for specificity have been sought for many diseases and the hypothesis of a direct effect on membranes is only one of several suggested mechanisms. In this review, we will address three questions concerning the role of host membranes: (a) what is the nature of permeability changes in diseased plants? (b) what is the evidence that effects on the plasmalemma or other membranes are responsible for these permeability changes? and (c) how may effects on the plasmalemma or other membranes account for specificity?

I. NATURE OF PERMEABILITY CHANGES IN DISEASED PLANTS

Evidence of increased efflux from cells or decreased uptake into cells is frequently interpreted as an effect on plasmalemma permeability and thus upon its structure. It is important to recognize that these two effects may simply represent opposite sides of the same coin. Futhermore, such changes may not represent differences in permeation through the membrane, but may be merely reflections of partial or total disruption of the normally continuous surface. For the latter reason, it is difficult to interpret many reported cases of increased electrolyte loss in terms of membrane permeability phenomena. Permeability changes in diseased plants range from drastic nonspecific effluxes of cellular solutes to subtle selective changes in influx as well as efflux. The latter may more properly indicate changes in plasmalemma permeation.

1. Permeability Changes Induced by Victorin

Perhaps more papers have described permeability changes induced by victorin, the toxic product of *Helminthosporium victoriae*, than by any other toxin or pathogen. Electrolyte leakage, measured by conductometric methods, are detectable within 2–5 min after application of the toxin. The rates of release of electrolytes and other solutes are not identical and this suggests an early effect on permeation rather than gross disruptions of membrane structure (*3*).

Rapid losses of electrolytes, together with ultrastructural evidence of early effects on the plasmalemma and cell wall suggested that the initial effect of victorin occurred at the cell surface (*35*). This hypothesis assumed a mode of action or 'site of action' at the outer surface of the plasmalemma or at the inner surface of the cell wall. Since other effects, including those on respiration, occurred later and isolated organelles were not directly affected, they were assumed to result indirectly from effects on permeability.

Other data confirmed permeability changes and strengthened the concept of early, possibly direct, effects on the plasmalemma. Novacky and Hanchey (*37*) found a depolarization of transmembrane potentials within 1–2 min after toxin application to susceptible oat roots. A transient increase in potential followed the decrease, but after 10–20 min the potential steadily decreased. The initial decrease may be caused by effects on wall potential or temporary effects on ion permeability. Membrane potentials are composed of two components: an active component which is abolished with respiratory inhibitors and a passive component. The victorin-induced depolarization is thought to be on the passive component (*13*, Novacky, personal communication).

Keck and Hodges (*32*), studying efflux of ^{86}Rb from victorin-treated tissues, reported that leakage across the tonoplast and plasmalemma appeared to occur simultaneously. A similar result was the almost simultaneous rupture of both the tonoplast and plasmalemma when isolated protoplasts were exposed to the toxin (*45*). In both cases a lag time of approximately 20 min was required for the effects of the toxin to be manifest. Although earlier and smaller changes may have gone undetected, these results suggest that the tonoplast is affected by victorin.

2. *Permeability Changes Induced by Other Host-selective Toxins*

Alternaria mali, the causal agent of apple blotch, produces several host-selective toxins. Susceptible leaves treated with these toxins lose electrolytes rapidly and this loss has been interpreted as an initial effect on the plasmalemma (*33*).

An effect on permeability was also reported in susceptible corn treated with *H. maydis*, race T-toxin. Gracen *et al.* (*15*) found increased electrolyte leakage from several susceptible varieties, but not from resistant ones. Halloin *et al.* (*17*) confirmed the electrolyte leakage, but also found carbohydrate efflux from both susceptible and resistant plants. Pelcher *et al.* (*40*) reported that toxin-treated resistant and nontreated protoplasts gradually swelled after 24–27 hr. They suggested that the protoplast volume of susceptible treated protoplasts remained in equilibrium due to the opposing forces of uptake and leakage. Apparently contradictory results were found by Keck and Hodges (*32*) who reported that T-toxin caused similar efflux of ^{86}Rb from both resistant and susceptible plants. This efflux apparently occurred only from the cytoplasm since no effects on tonoplast permeability were observed. Recently, Tipton *et al.* (*60*) have suggested that the presence of ophiobolin A in T-toxin preparations is the cause of non-host-selective effects on carbohydrate transport.

Frick *et al.* (*10*) have reported differences in sensitivity to toxin in different root zones when K^+ uptake was measured. Basal K^+ uptake was inhibited by toxin in both normal and Tcms cytoplasms in the root midzone. However, the root apex K^+ uptake was more inhibited in Tcms than in normal cytoplasm. The development of augmented uptake ('aging') was more toxin sensitive in mature regions of roots of T-cytoplasm plants. Protein synthesis is required for augmented uptake suggesting a cytoplasmic effect of the toxin. These workers suggested that toxin sensitivity results from a complex interaction between the nucleus, cytoplasm and plasma membrane. Clearly, T-toxin induced permeability changes are complex, however since high concentrations of toxin preparations of unknown composition are required, these may be secondary effects or effects of impurities.

3. Permeability Changes in Relation to Other Diseases and Hypersensitive Reactions
Several studies have shown that disease affects both influx and efflux from cells. Gracen *et al.* (*16*) showed that treatment of susceptible oat roots with victorin before ^{86}Rb uptake resulted in a lower final ^{86}Rb content than victorin treatment after ^{86}Rb uptake. This indicates a dual, but not necessarily related effect on membrane permeability. A dual effect was also shown with *Curvularia lunata* phytotoxin on permeability of corn roots. Uptake of sulphate and ^{86}Rb was inhibited after 40 and 20 min, respectively. Leakage of these compounds occurred after 2 and 4 hr (*64*). Barley leaves infected with *Rhynchosporium secalis* lost electrolytes and carbohydrates prior to symptom development. Infection also stimulated uptake of ^{86}Rb in both susceptible and resistant varieties. In the susceptible variety, both passive and active uptake were stimulated, whereas in the resistant variety, only active uptake was stimulated (*31*). *Helminthosporium carbonum* toxin stimulated absorption of solutes by susceptible corn roots. Toxin-induced leakage was a much later effect of damage (*69, 70*). These studies suggest that electrolyte leakage is not necessarily detrimental to uptake processes and that the two processes, influx and efflux, may be affected independently. It is possible furthermore, that changes in one process may have a positive or negative effect on the other.

Thatcher (*56*) reported increased permeability within lesions and at a distance from lesions induced by *Sclerotinia sclerotium* on excised celery petioles. These results have been confirmed by others (*22, 36*). However, the nature of permeability changes is more complicated in inoculated tissues of intact plants. Tissue above lesions lost fewer electrolytes than comparable, noninoculated tissue (*22*). The rate of water loss, measured as rate of tissue weight loss in a hypertonic mannitol solution, was also lower from above-lesion tissue than from healthy tissue. Tissue dehydrated in mannitol and then rehydrated regained water more slowly and then failed to retain this water. Although interpreted in terms of reduced plasmalemma permeability to water, these results may also reflect a combination of decreased wall permeability and decreased cell viability. These data would be considered more reliable if studies were conducted on individual cells rather than on tissues. A dual carrier system for 3-O-methylglucose (MeG) was found in both healthy and diseased sunflower, but the high affinity carrier was more active in the diseased than in the healthy tissue (*22*).

Hancock reported an increased rate of amino acid leakage and an increase in apparent free space in squash lesions induced by *Hypomyces solani* f. sp. *cucurbitae* (*20*). No change in apparent free space or permeability to water, glycerol, mannitol, urea, or amino acids was found in tissue above lesions. Rates of MeG uptake suggested an inducible carrier system in tissue above the lesions (*21, 23*). Presumably, this change reflects an alteration of host physiology and not uptake by the pathogen.

Hypersensitive reactions are characterized by a higher rate of electrolyte leakage than susceptible reactions (*4, 14, 41*). Few studies, however, have determined whether leakage results from cell disruption and consequent nonspecific efflux or from changes in plasmalemma permeation. Turner (*61, 62*) considered three parameters of cell permeability in tobacco inoculated with the pathogen *Pseudomonas tabaci* or the nonpathogen *Ps. pisi*. The hydrolytic permeability coefficient, L_p, is a measure of the rate of movement of water under the influence of a pressure or osmotic gradient. This value was 1.1×10^{-11} cm^3 dyne^{-1} sec^{-1} for protoplasts of noninoculated stem parenchyma, a value close to that reported for other plant cells. Hydrolytic conductivity coefficients of tissues inoculated with *Ps. pisi* are approximately 20 times lower than controls after 2–3 hr. Tissues inoculated with *Ps. tabaci* do not show decreases until 40–50 hr after inoculation. These results were interpreted in terms of a closure of water-selective pores in the plasmalemma.

Permeability coefficients for thiourea, ethylene glycol, and propionamide increased in tobacco 42–46 hr after inoculation with *Ps. tabaci*. Permeability coefficients were less affected in *Ps. pisi*-inoculated tissues. Reflection coefficients which serve to define the degree of semipermeability, are significantly decreased in tissues inoculated with *Ps. pisi*, however this may be largely a consequence of the lower hydrolytic conductivity. The reflection coefficient to propionamide was decreased in tissue inoculated with *Ps. tabaci*, but coefficients for five other penetrating compounds did not change. These results suggest alterations in the lipid portion of the plasmalemma of plants infected with *Ps. tabaci* such that nonelectrolyte permeability is increased, results dissimilar to those of Hancock (*20*). Turner's results also show that penetrations of solute and solvent across membranes are independent and may be affected separately.

Novacky *et al.* (*39*) compared membrane potentials in susceptible and hypersensitive responses of cotton inoculated with *Xanthomonas malvacearum*. A decreased total potential occurred in 10 hr in the hypersensitive combination whereas decreases were not detected in the susceptible combination until after 96 hr. Before this change was observed, the cyanide insensitive component of the potential decreased with a corresponding increase in the cyanide sensitive component. Cyanide treatment resulted in a rapid, partial depolarization. A partial recovery in potential following cyanide treatment in healthy cotton, corn, and sugarcane leaves occurred in the light. Recovery after cyanide did not occur in the dark or in dark-grown plants and thus may depend upon photosynthetic processes. Cotton cotyledon cells lose the ability to recover potentials in the presence of cyanide when inoculated with *X. malvacearum*. This loss in cyanide recovery is evident in 3 hr after inoculation in the hypersensitive combination and after 12 hr in the susceptible combination. Although further studies on the nature of cyanide recovery are needed, the results suggest an effect on energy coupling between chloroplast and cytoplasm which alter the active component of plasmalemma potentials (*38*).

II. EVIDENCE FOR CHANGES IN MEMBRANE COMPOSITION

Since many plant pathogens produce enzymes which can degrade proteins and lipids, it is important to determine the role of these enzymes in permeability changes. The occurrence and possible role of these enzymes in pathogenesis has been reviewed recently (*1*) and at this time there is no basis for concluding that they play an early role.

Several studies have focused on lipid composition of diseased plants. There is evidence that properties of membrane permeability are dependent on the types of lipids present. Jennings *et al.* (*30*) analyzed sterol compositions in maize hybrids inoculated with *H. carbonum*. The susceptible reaction resulted in a lower total sterol content than three resistant interactions. The largest decrease was found in β-sitosterol. Decreases in sterols may be related to the degree of penetration since these were found in resistant reactions, however no changes in the proportions of various sterols was found in resistant reactions.

Hoppe and Heitefuss conducted detailed analyses of lipid metabolism in *Phaseolus vulgaris* infected with *Uromyces phaseoli*. In their experiments, chlorotic spots appeared after 4 days and this coincided with electrolyte leakage (*24*). Decreases in several predominant chloroplast lipids occurred after symptom development. Decreases in other lipids may have been masked by the presence of the fungus (*25*). Fatty acid composition of lipids changed only in the region of the pustule and probably represented the presence of fungal tissue (*26, 27*). No significant changes in sterols were found in these studies (*28*). Elnaghy and Heitefuss have shown that the occurrence of the germination self-inhibitor, methyl-3,4-dimethoxycinnamate coincides with the permeability change in susceptible, infected plants (*8*). In resistant plants, they reported that a permeability change occurs earlier than in susceptible plants and suggested that phaseollin accumulation may be responsible for this permeability change (*9*). Phaseollin has been shown to cause permeability changes in bean hypocotyls (*63*). An effect of pisatin (*48*) and α-tomatine (*43*) on higher plant cell permeability has also been demonstrated. These studies demonstrate that the fungitoxic phytoalexins may also play an important role in symptom development in the host.

Zeller *et al.* (*72*) reported marked decreases in chloroplast lipids in *Beta vulgaris* treated with *Ps. phaseolicola* toxin. Changes in other lipids did not seem sufficient to explain the effect of the toxin on decreased permeability.

Other studies have provided evidence for changes in membrane components, but such evidence is, at best, indirect and could reflect changes at any number of alternative sites. Huang *et al.* (*29*) reported that 'structural proteins' isolated from chloroplasts of tobacco inoculated with the non-pathogen, *Erwinia amylovora*, failed to form membrane-like structures when mixed with lipids of healthy chloroplasts. Whether this change is causally related to the hypersensitive response and permeability change or whether it is a secondary response is not known.

The suppressive effect on disease and permeability by calcium and other divalent cations has been shown in victorin-treated oats (*7, 18*) and the hypersensitive reaction to *X. vesicatoria* in pepper (*5*), but not in corn treated with T-toxin (*16*). α-Tomatine induced permeability changes could also be reversed by calcium (*43*). Several compounds which can bind to carbonyl or sulfhydril groups protected against victorin-induced permeability changes, but had no effect against *Periconia circinata* toxin on susceptible sorghum (*11*). Damage by *P. circinata* toxin was reduced by uranyl salts, which did not complex with the toxin, and by phospholipase D and cycloheximide (*11*).

Oats treated with cycloheximide 12 hr before victorin treatment were also protected against electrolyte loss (*12*). Tissues regained sensitivity when removed from cycloheximide solutions and this suggests that victorin sensitivity requires protein synthesis, although other explanations are also possible. Cycloheximide pretreatment also protects against protoplast lysis and victorin-induced decreases in leucine incorporation (*42*).

III. CELL MEMBRANES AS SITES FOR SPECIFICITY

Helminthosporium sacchari produces a host-selective toxin, reported to be 2-hydroxy-cyclopropyl-α-D-galactopyranoside (helminthosporoside) (*50*). One of the first visible symptoms on susceptible leaves treated with the toxin is water clearing and the exudation of water droplets. These symptoms suggested that the toxin affects plasmalemma permeability (*52*). According to Strobel, susceptible clones contain a plasmalemma-bound protein which binds the toxin, whereas resistant clones do not (*51, 52*). α-Galactosides were reported to confer protection against the toxin and reduce toxin-binding protein activity. Strobel proposed that the binding protein functions in α-galactoside transport (*53*). Furthermore, he discounts other sites of action since the binding protein conferred susceptibility (toxin-induced lysis) when added to otherwise resistant protoplasts (*55*).

Questions have been raised concerning the variability of the toxin bioassay and the calculation of the binding constant for helminthosporoside. The binding constant is apparently not 6.8×10^{-5} as originally reported (*52*), but instead is closer to 2×10^{-4} (Strobel, personal communication, *6, 66*). This value is unlike the binding constants of other α-galactosides and is possibly too low to permit consistent detection of differences in binding to resistant or susceptible plants. Thom *et al.* (*59*) have also reported toxin binding to membranes from susceptible plants, especially to fractions enriched in plasma membranes. However, they did not try binding studies on resistant plant membranes. It would be desirable to repeat the binding experiments using a toxin preparation with higher specific activity.

How interference with α-galactoside transport could lead to toxicity has not been explained. Strobel reported that plasmalemma ATPase activity and K^+-^{86}Rb uptake were stimulated in toxin-treated susceptible clones (*53*). These changes were thought to be secondary effects of toxin binding, and Strobel hypothesized that they were lethal effects. Novacky *et al.* (*38, 39*) predicted that such stimulation should result in a change in the active component of the membrane potential. Helminthosporoside caused a decreased membrane potential, but unlike the depolarization observed with victorin, this new potential was maintained. This suggested that the extent of leakage from cells was limited. The magnitude of cyanide sensitivity was also not altered by helminthosporoside, suggesting that the level of energy supply was not altered (*38*). However, they showed that the toxin did prevent recovery of potential in the presence of cyanide. If cyanide recovery is related to ion transport across the chloroplast envelope, this result suggests an early effect of the toxin on the structure or function of the chloroplast. This hypothesis is supported by ultrastructure studies which indicate that the earliest effects in toxin-treated susceptible leaves are in chloroplast structure, whereas other changes occurred later (*54*). Clearly, further studies on the mechanisms of helminthosporoside sensitivity are warranted.

The early effect of victorin on cell permeability, together with ultrastructure studies suggested that the primary effect of victorin was on the cell membrane. Hanchey *et al.* (*19*) suggested that ultrastructural effects of victorin treatment resembled calcium deficiency. Calcium is essential for normal permeability through the plasmalemma and is thought to stabilize the membrane by interacting with anionic sites. Doupnik (*7*) found that calcium salts suppressed victorin-induced leakage and visible symptoms when applied simultaneously with the toxin. There is also evidence that a susceptible oat variety was more sensitive to calcium deficiency than a resistant variety (*34*). Hanchey (*18*) reported that uranyl salts, which presumably do not penetrate cells also suppressed victorin-induced electrolyte leakage and visible symptoms when applied simultaneously or as pretreatments. Uranyl also binds to anionic sites. However, drastically high concentrations of both calcium and uranyl were required for the protective effects and evidence suggests that both ions bind to the toxin (*12, 44, 46*). Such binding does not imply inactivation, however.

Saftner *et al.* (*44*) used the binding of ^{45}Ca to victorin to obtain a radioactive product which they could follow in resistant and susceptible plants. Interestingly, in their work victorin eluted from columns as one relatively narrow peaks, a result not found in the experience of these writers. Labeled calcium eluted with victorin and thus was presumed to bind to the toxin.

The ^{45}Ca-victorin complex bound to membrane preparations, which included the plasmalemma, equally well in resistant and susceptible cultivars. Binding was decreased in the presence of unlabeled calcium or victorin, but not by deactivated victorin. The resistant cultivar had a higher calcium content and a higher affinity for calcium than did the susceptible cultivar. Saftner *et al.* hypothesized that victorin or a victorin-calcium complex may compete for calcium binding sites in susceptible plants, thus removing calcium from its normal stabilizing location. According to this hypothesis, much higher concentrations of victorin would be necessary to affect resistant plants, a result in fact found in other studies (*42, 68*). Much more detailed kinetic analyses are needed to confirm or deny this hypothesis. However, it seems doubtful that this mechanism solely could explain the extreme specificity of victorin for only certain lines of oats.

In related studies, Scheffer (*47*) treated membranes isolated from susceptible or resistant cultivars with victorin and separated 'bound' from 'free' toxin by Sephadex column chromatography. He found that resistant and susceptible membrane preparations bound equal amounts of victorin. However, preparations containing toxin and detergent contained as much 'bound' toxin as did preparations with membranes. These results suggest that if victorin-induced permeability changes are caused by direct interaction with the membrane, any binding is easily reversible. An alternative explanation is that victorin does not bind to the membrane, but instead causes the removal of some essential component from the membranes. The latter hypothesis may be tested by reconstituting membranes in experiments similar to those performed by Huang *et al.* (*29*).

Wheeler (*65, 66*) has pointed out a consistent 20 min lag period which preceded toxic effects of victorin. Increases in respiration are not detected until about 30 min after toxin treatment. Victorin-induced elongation of susceptible coleoptiles begins after 5 min but persists for only 30 min. Electrolytes are rapidly lost during the first 5 min after victorin treatment. The rate then decreases for 20–30 min, followed by another rapid rate of loss. The early membrane deplolarization is followed by an initial recovery and a second depolarization occurs after 20 min. These results are consistent with an early effect of victorin on permeability, but also suggest that this toxin may have more than one site of action. An additional site may be intracellular and could explain the consistent lag found with many effects of this toxin.

The mode of action of *H. maydis*, race T-toxin is at present confusing. Not only is permeability affected, but also mitochondria are affected selectively *in vitro*. In a recent study, an effect of T-toxin on the density of the mitochondrial matrix was reported (*71*). Whether T-toxin has more than one cellular site of action remains to be determined (*10*). However, a firm association with a binding site was not found (*2*).

The only case in which binding to a specific receptor site also explains the symptoms induced by a toxin is the binding of tentoxin, produced by *Alternaria tenuis*, to chloroplast coupling factor 1 (CF_1) of sensitive species (*49*). This toxin induces chlorosis in many plants. Toxin binding to CF_1 results in inhibition of ATPase and photophosphorylation. Radish, an insensitive species, binds less toxin and the toxin has little or no effect on ATPase or photophosphorylation. Other species, such as corn, may be insensitive to the toxin because of permeation barriers or toxin-degradation.

SUMMARY

The hypothesis that plants are susceptible to certain disease agents because they possess sites which are sensitive to pathogen products is a logical, but at present, mostly unsubstantiated hypothesis. Searches for specific sites have implicated the plasmalemma (*33, 35, 53*), mitochondria (*40*), and chloroplasts (*49*). Although such sites may be found for some diseases, it is important to recognize that other mechanisms to explain specificity have also been proposed (*34*).

REFERENCES

1. Bateman, D.F. and H. G. Basham. 1976. Degradation of plant cell walls and membranes by microbial enzymes. *In*: R. Heitefuss and P. H. Williams (eds.). *Encyclopedia of Plant Physiology*. vol. 4. Springer-Verlag, Berlin, pp. 316–355.
2. Bednarski, M.A., S. Izawa, and R. P. Scheffer. 1977. Reversible effects of toxin from *Helminthosporium maydis* race T on oxidative phosphorylation by mitochondria from maize. *Plant Physiol.* **59**: 540–545.
3. Black, H. S. and H. Wheeler. 1966. Biochemical effects of victorin on oat tissues and mitochondira. *Am. J. Bot.* **53**: 1108–1112.
4. Cook, A. A. and R. E. Stahl. 1968. Effect of *Xanthomonas vesicatoria* on loss of electrolytes from leaves of *Capsicum annum*. *Phytopathology* **58**: 617–619.
5. Cook, A. A. and R. E. Stahl. 1971. Calcium suppression of electrolyte loss from pepper leaves inoculated with *Xanthomonas vesicatoria*. *Phytopathology* **61**: 484–487.
6. Daly, J. M. 1976. *In*: R. K. S. Wood and A. Graniti (eds.). *Specificity of Plant Diseases*. Summary of points from contribution and discussions, by S. S. Patil. Plenum Press, New York and London, pp. 231–234.

7. Doupnik, B., Jr. 1968. The suppression of victorin-induced disease by calcium. *Phytopathology* **58**: 215–218.
8. Elnaghy, M. A. and R. Heitefuss. 1976. Permeability changes and production of antifungal compounds in *Phaseolus vulgaris* infected with *Uromyces phaseoli*. I. Role of the spore germination self-inhibitor. *Physiol. Plant Pathol.* **8**: 253–268.
9. Elnaghy, M. A. and R. Heitefuss. 1976. Permeability changes and production of antifungal compounds in *Phaseolus vulgaris* infected with *Uromyces phaseoli*. II. Role of phytoalexins. *Physiol. Plant Pathol.* **8**: 269–278.
10. Frick, H., L. F. Bauman, R. L. Nicholson, and T. K. Hodges. 1977. Influence of *Helminthosporium maydis*, Race T, toxin on potassium uptake in maize roots. II. Sensitivity of development of the augmented uptake potential to toxin and inhibitors of protein synthesis. *Plant Physiol.* **59**: 103–106.
11. Gardner, J. M., I. S. Mansour, and R. P. Scheffer. 1972. Effects of the host-specific toxin of *Periconia circinata* on some properties of sorghum plasma membranes. *Physiol. Plant Pathol.* **2**: 197–206.
12. Gardner, J. M. and R. P. Scheffer. 1973. Effects of cycloheximide and sulfhydril-binding compounds on sensitivity of oat tissues to *Helminthosporium victoriae* toxin. *Physiol. Plant Pathol.* **3**: 147–157.
13. Gardner, J. M., R. P. Scheffer, and N. Higinbotham. 1974. Effects of host-specific toxins on electropotentials of plant cells. *Plant Physiol.* **54**: 246–249.
14. Goodman, R. N. 1968. The hypersensitive reaction in tobacco: a reflection of changes in host cell permeability. *Phytopathology* **58**: 872–873.
15. Gracen, V. E., C. O. Grogan, and M. J. Forster. 1972. Permeability changes induced by *Helminthosporium maydis*, race T. toxin. *Can. J. Bot.* **50**: 2167–2170.
16. Gracen, V. E., H. H. Luke, S. H. West, and A. T. Wallace. 1976. The use of labeled cations to measure victorin-induced permeability changes. *Can. J. Bot.* **54**: 395–398.
17. Halloin, J. M., J. C. Comstock, C. A. Martinson, and C. L. Tipton. 1973. Leakage from corn tissues infected by *Helminthosporium maydis*, race T. toxin. *Phytopathology* **63**: 640–642.
18. Hanchey, P. 1969. Suppression of victorin toxicity in oats by uranyl salts. *Phytopathology* **59**: 1960–1962.
19. Hanchey, P., H. Wheeler, and H. H. Luke. 1968. Pathological changes in ultrastructure: effects of victorin on oat roots. *Am. J. Bot.* **55**: 53–61.
20. Hancock, J. G. 1968. Effect of infection by *Hypomyces solani* f. sp. *cucurbitae* on apparent free space, cell membrane permeability and respiration by squash hypocotyls. *Plant Physiol.* **43**: 1666–1672.
21. Hancock, J. G. 1969. Uptake of 3-O-methylglucose by healthy and *Hypomyces*-infected squash hypocotyls. *Plant Physiol.* **44**: 1267–1272.
22. Hancock, J. G. 1972. Changes in cell membrane permeability in sunflower hypocotyls infected with *Sclerotinia sclerotiorum*. *Plant Physiol.* **49**: 358–364.

23. Hancock, J. G. 1975. Influence of *Hypomyces* infection and excision on amino acid and 3-O-methylglucose uptake by squash hypocotyls. *Physiol. Plant Pathol.* **6**: 65–73.

24. Hoppe, H. H. and R. Heitefuss. 1974. Permeability and membrane lipid metabolism of *Phaseolus vulgaris* infected with *Uromyces phaseoli*. I. Changes in the efflux of cell constituents. *Physiol. Plant. Pathol.* **4**: 5–9.

25. Hoppe, H. H. and R. Heitefuss. 1974. II. Changes in lipid concentrations and ^{32}P incorporation into phospholipids. *Physiol. Plant Pathol.* **4**: 11–23.

26. Hoppe, H. H. and R. Heitefuss. 1974. III. Changes in relative concentrations of lipid bound fatty acids and phospholipase activity. *Physiol. Plant Pathol.* **4**: 25–35.

27. Hoppe, H. H. and R. Heitefuss. 1975. IV. Phospholipids and phospholipid fatty acids in healthy and rust-infected bean leaves resistant and susceptible to *Uromyces phaseoli*. *Physiol. Plant Pathol.* **5**: 263–271.

28. Hoppe, H. H. and R. Heitefuss. 1975. V. Sterols in healthy and rust-infected bean leaves resistant and susceptible to *Uromyces phaseoli*. *Physiol. Plant. Pathol.* **5**: 273–281.

29. Huang, J. S., P-Y. Huang, and R. N. Goodman. 1974. Ultrastructural changes in tobacco thylakoid membrane protein caused by a bacterially induced hypersensitive reaction. *Physiol. Plant Pathol.* **4**: 93–97.

30. Jennings, P. H., F. P. Zscheile, Jr., and B. L. Brannaman. 1970. Sterol changes in maize leaves infected with *Helminthosporium carbonum*. *Plant Physiol.* **45**: 634–635.

31. Jones, P. and P. G. Ayres. 1972. The nutrition of the subcuticular mycelium of *Rhynchosporium secalis* (barley leaf blotch): permeability changes induced in the host. *Physiol. Plant Pathol.* **2**: 383–392.

32. Keck, R. W. and T. K. Hodges. 1973. Membrane permeability in plants: Changes induced by host-specific pathotoxins. *Phytopathology* **63**: 226–230.

33. Kohmoto, K., I. D. Khan, Y. Renbutsu, T. Taniguchi, and S. Nishimura. 1976. Multiple host-specific toxins of *Alternaria mali* and their effects on the permeability of host cells. *Physiol. Plant Pathol.* **8**: 141–153.

34. Luke, H. H. and V. E. Gracen, Jr. 1972. *Helminthosporium toxins*. *In*: S. Kadis, A. Ciegler, and S.J. Ajl (eds.). *Microbial Toxins*. vol. 8. Academic Press, New York and London, pp. 139–168.

35. Luke, H. H., H. E. Warmke, and P. Hanchey. 1966. Effects of the pathotoxin victorin on ultrastructure of root and leaf tissue of *Avena* species. *Phytopathology* **56**: 1178–1183.

36. Newton, H. C., D. P. Maxwell, and L. Sequeira. 1973. A conductivity assay for measuring virulence of *Sclerotinia sclerotiorum*. *Phytopathology* **63**: 424–428.

37. Novacky, A. and P. Hanchey. 1974. Depolarization of membrane potentials in oat roots treated with victorin. *Physiol. Plant Pathol.* **4**: 161–165.

38. Novacky, A. and A. L. Karr. 1977. Pathological alterations in cell membrane

bioelectrical properties. *In*: E. Marre and O. Cifferi (eds.). *Regulation of Cell Membrane Activities in Plants.* Elsevier/North-Holland Biomedical Press, Amsterdam, pp. 137–144.

39. Novacky, A., A. L. Karr, and J. W. Van Sambeek. 1976. Using electrophysiology to study plant disease development. *Bioscience* **26**: 499–504.
40. Pelcher, L. E., K. N. Kao, O. L. Gamborg, O. C. Yoder, and V. E. Gracen. 1975. Effects of *Helminthosporium maydis,* Race T, toxin on protoplasts of resistant and susceptible corn (Zea mays). *Can. J. Bot.* **53**: 427–431.
41. Pellizzari, E. D., J. Kuć, and E. B. Williams. 1970. The hypersensitive reaction in *Malus* species: changes in the leakage of electrolytes from apple leaves after inoculation with *Venturia inaequalis. Phytopathology* **60**: 373–376.
42. Rancillac, M., R. Kaur-Sawhney, B. Staskawicz, and A. W. Galston. 1976. Effects of cycloheximide and kinetin pretreatment on responses of susceptible and resistant *Avena* leaf protoplasts to the phytotoxin victorin. *Plant. Cell Physiol.* **17**: 987–995.
43. Roddick, J. G. 1975. Effect of α-tomatine on the permeability of plant storage tissues. *J. Exp. Bot.* **26**: 221–227.
44. Saftner, R. A., M. L. Evans, and P. B. Hollander. 1976. Specific binding of victorin and calcium: evidence for calcium binding as a mediator of victorin activity. *Physiol. Plant Pathol.* **8**: 21–34.
45. Samaddar, K. R. and R. P. Scheffer. 1968. Effect of the specific toxin in *Helminthosporium victoriae* on host cell membranes. *Plant Physiol.* **43**: 21–28.
46. Samaddar, K. R. and R. P. Scheffer. 1971. Early effects of *Helminthosporium victoriae* toxin on plasma membranes and counteraction by chemical treatments. *Physiol. Plant Pathol.* **1**: 319–328.
47. Scheffer, R. P. 1975. Fungal toxins as determinants of host specificity. *Proc. First Intersectional Congress of IAMS.* vol. 3, Science Council of Japan, Tokyo, pp. 12–21.
48. Shiraishi, T., H. Oku, M. Isono, and S. Ouchi. 1975. The injurious effect of pisatin on the plasma membrane of pea. *Plant Cell Physiol.* **16**: 939–942.
49. Steele, J. A., T. F. Uchytil, R. D. Durbin, D. Bhatnager, and D. H. Rich. 1976. Chloroplast coupling factor 1: a species-specific receptor for tentoxin. *Proc. Natl. Acad. Sci. U.S.* **73**: 2245–2248.
50. Steiner, G. W. and G. A. Strobel. 1971. Helminthosporoside, a host-specific toxin from *Helminthosporium sacchari. J. Biol. Chem.* **246**: 4350–4357.
51. Strobel, G. A. 1973. Biochemical basis of the resistance of sugarcane to eyespot disease. *Proc. Natl. Acad. Sci. U.S.* **70**: 1693–1696.
52. Strobel, G. A. 1973. The helminthosporoside-binding protein of sugarcane. *J. Biol. Chem.* **248**: 1321–1328.
53. Strobel, G. A. 1974. The toxin-binding protein of sugarcane, its role in the plant and in disease development. *Proc. Natl. Acad. Sci. U.S.* **71**: 4232–4236.

54. Strobel, G. A., W. M. Hess, and G. W. Steiner. 1972. Ultrastructure of cells in toxin-treated and *Helminthosporium sacchari*-infected sugarcane leaves. *Phytopathology* **62**: 339–345.

55. Strobel, G. A. and K. D. Hapner. 1975. Transfer toxin susceptibility to plant protoplasts via the helminthosporoside binding protein of sugarcane. *Biochem. Biophys. Res. Commun.* **63**: 1151–1156.

56. Thatcher, F. S. 1939. Osmotic and permeability relations in the nutrition of fungus parasites. *Am. J. Bot.* **26**: 449–458.

57. Thatcher, F. S. 1942. Further studies of osmotic and permeability relations in parasitism. *Can. J. Res., Sect. C.* **20**: 283–311.

58. Thatcher, F. S. 1943. Cellular changes in relation to rust resistance. *Can. J. Res., Sect. C.* **21**: 151–172.

59. Thom, M., W. M. Laetsch, and A. Meretzki. 1975. Isolation of membranes from sugarcane cell suspensions: evidence for a plasma membrane enriched fraction. *Plant Sci. Lett.* **5**: 245–253.

60. Tipton, C. L., P. V. Paulsen, and R. E. Betts. 1977. Effects of ophiobolin A on ion leakage and hexose uptake by maize roots. *Plant Physiol.* **59**: 907–910.

61. Turner, J. G. 1976. The nonelectrolyte permeability of tobacco cell membranes in tissues inoculated with *Pseudomonas pisi* and *Pseudomonas tabaci*. Ph. D. dissertation. University of Missouri, 154 pp.

62. Turner, J. G. and A. Novacky. 1976. Effect of *Pseudomonas tabaci* and *P. pisi* on permeability of tobacco protoplasts to nonelectrolytes. *Phytopathology* (Suppl.) **3**: 260.

63. VanEtten, H. D. and D. F. Bateman. 1971. Studies on the mode of action of the phytoalexin phaseollin. *Phytopathology* **61**: 1363–1372.

64. Vianello, A., F. Macri, and C. Passera. 1976. Effect of *Curvularia lunata* phytotoxin on membrane permeability of corn roots. *Can. J. Bot.* **54**: 2918–2923.

65. Wheeler, H. 1975. *Plant Pathogenesis*. Springer-Verlag, Berlin, 106 pp.

66. Wheeler, H. 1976. The role of phytotoxins in specificity. *In*: R.K. S. Wood and A. Graniti (eds.). *Specificity in Plant Disease*. Plenum Press, New York and London, pp. 217–230.

67. Wheeler, H. and H. S. Black. 1963. Effects of *Helminthosporium victoriae* and victorin upon permeability. *Am. J. Bot.* **50**: 686–693.

68. Wheeler, H. and B. Doupnik, Jr. 1969. Physiological changes in victorin-treated, resistant oat tissue. *Phytopathology* **59**: 1460–1463.

69. Yoder, O. C. and R. P. Scheffer. 1973. Effects of *Helminthosporium carbonum* toxin on nitrate uptake and reduction by corn tissues. *Plant Physiol.* **52**: 513–517.

70. Yoder, O. C. and R. P. Scheffer. 1973. Effects of *Helminthosporium carbonum* toxin on absorption of solutes by corn roots. *Plant Physiol.* **52**: 518–523.

71. Yoder, O. C. 1976. *In*: R. K. S. Wood and A. Graniti (eds.). *Specificity in Plant*

Diseases. Summary of points from contributions and discussions, by J. L. Gay. Plenum Press, New York, pp. 146–150.

72. Zeller, W., K. Rudolph, and H. H. Hoppe. 1976. Effect of the *Pseudomonas phaseolicola* toxin on the composition of lipids in leaves of Swiss Chard (*Beta vulgaris,* L.) I. Changes in concentrations of phospholipids and glycolipids. *Phytopathol. Z.* **86**: 205–214.

Discussion of Paper by Drs. Hanchey and Wheeler

The discussion opened with several comments on sites-of-action of toxins. SCHEFFER indicated that a distinction must be made between firm binding of toxin to a receptor and binding which is easily dissociated. In mitochondria sensitive to toxin from *H. maydis* race T, it is easy to dissociate the toxin from a possible binding site. He suggested that *in vivo*, mitochondria of corn susceptible to *H. maydis* race T contain a significant site for *H. maydis* race T-toxin; there is no conclusive evidence for a toxin-sensitive site other than in the mitochondrion. GRACEN agreed and stated that recent evidence suggested that the apparent effects of toxin on the plasma membrane could be explained by impure toxin preparations. In response to questions and comments from KEEN, PAXTON, and SEQUEIRA, GRACEN suggested that first effects of purified toxin are seen ultrastructurally in the mitochondrial matrix and cristae, with little or no effect on the outer mitochondrial membrane. DALY suggested there might be several sites of action, at different locations in the cell, which are concentration dependent. Some sites saturate quickly at low toxin concentrations and other sites (like the mitochondria) saturate at higher concentrations and cause different effects. It may be misleading to consider only the site that is most sensitive to toxin. NISHIMURA expressed concern that most people working with race T-toxin use high concentrations of very impure preparations. Impure preparations of AK-toxin or AM-toxin are known to contain organic acids and tentoxin which can complicate experimental results.

KUĆ asked for elaboration on alternate explanations for the activity of toxin other than binding at a specific rate. HANCHEY cited WHEELER's induced self-repair hypothesis which states that susceptible plants are unable to repair damage caused by toxin. WHEELER commented on the tendency of most investigators to assume that the cellular site affected most rapidly is the site of toxin action. Rapid responses, however, are obtained by using high, unphysiological concentrations of toxin. TOMIYAMA observed that for a complex phenomenon such as disease or hypersensitive reaction more than one compound may be required. We should not draw premature conclusions on the mechanism of host-parasite interaction from experiments done using unphysiologically high concentrations of a compound. In response to URITANI, SCHEFFER indicated that about 12 hr treatment with cycloheximide is needed for maximum protection against victorin. One idea is that cycloheximide inhibits the synthesis of a proteinaceous toxin receptor that has a short half-life or a fast turnover.

DAY viewed phytotoxins from a genetical perspective. There is no case known in which a toxin-producing pathogen has modified its toxin to cope with the evolution of a resistant plant. Perhaps pathogenicity based on toxin production is not a major mechanism at all but rather an evolutionary fluke. SCHEFFER cited the example of *H. carbonum* race 1 on corn as an alternative to DAY's point of view. Resistance to *H. carbonum* race 1-toxin and to the fungus is controlled by the same dominant genes. There are two genes for resistance to *H. carbonum* race 1 on separate chromosomes and at least two additional alleles that give intermediate levels of resistance. Various combinations of these genes can provide corn with at least 10 different levels of resistance to the fungus. Some of these have been tested and found to have the same levels of resistance to the toxin as they do to the fungus. If studies of the mechanism of disease initiation had been started with such intermediates, the toxin would not have been detected. GRACEN agreed and stated that disease in which host-specific toxins are involved represent genetic changes which resulted in major effects that are easily studied. If there is anything unusual about these diseases, it is that molecular basis of pathogenicity is understood, at least in part. SCHEFFER summarized with the observation that all evolutionary changes are based on flukes which are either major or minor.

Recognition and Specificity in Plant Host-Parasite Interactions, pp. 211–227, 1979

THE NATURE OF BASIC COMPATIBILITY: COMPARISONS BETWEEN PISTIL-POLLEN AND HOST-PARASITE INTERACTION*[1]

W.R. BUSHNELL*[2]

Department of Agriculture, University of Minnesota, St. Paul, Minnesota, U.S.A.

The compatibility systems which operate between pistil and pollen offer several close parallels to those which operate between host and parasite, particularly to those which operate in biotrophic associations such as the rusts and powdery mildews. Close similarities exist in genetics, structural relationships, physiology, and possibly in triggering mechanisms. This is true for interactions both within species and between species. Thus within species, self-incompatibility between pistil and pollen closely resembles the race specificity that is conditioned by corresponding genes in host and parasite ("gene-for-gene" specificity); and between species, pistil-pollen incompatibility resembles the incompatibility that is present between species of host and parasite that are inappropriate for one another. Furthermore, pistil-pollen incompatibility between species offers insight into the nature of basic compatibility; *i.e.*, into those aspects of the morphology and meta-

---

*[1] Cooperative investigations, Agricultural Research, Science and Education Administration, U.S. Department of Agriculture, and Department of Plant Pathology, University of Minnesota. Paper No. 1682, Misc. Journal Series, Minnesota Agricultural Experiment Station.

*[2] Research Plant Physiologist, Cereal Rust Laboratory, Agricultural Research Science and Education Administration, U.S.

bolism of two species that make it possible for one to live in intimate association with the other, even though pairings of certain individuals or subpopulations within the species may be incompatible.

Pistil-pollen compatibility will be discussed here first as it occurs within species and second as it occurs between species. My objectives are first, to compare pistil-pollen interaction to host-parasite interaction; and second, to show what the comparison suggests about the nature of basic compatibility.

I. SELF-INCOMPATIBILITY IN ANGIOSPERMS

Selfing is prevented in many species of angiosperms by the operation of an allelomorphic series of genes (S_1-S_n) such that the growth of a pollen tube carrying one allele is inhibited in a pistil carrying the same allele (*18*). In the presence of matching S-alleles, growth of the pollen tube is stopped either on the stigma surface or within the style so that the tube usually fails to reach the ovary and effect fertilization. A plant species may have 100–200 different S-alleles so that the chance is low that alleles will be identical in pistil and pollen in a freely interbreeding population. The result is an efficient system which forces outbreeding.

The discussion here will be restricted to the most common type of self-incompatibility in which all S-alleles are located at one locus. Single locus self-incompatibility systems in the angiosperms are of two types: the sporophytic type in which the specificity of pollen is determined by the diploid anther tissue in which it is produced; and the gametophytic type in which the specificity of pollen is determined by its own haploid genotype. In both types, the S-alleles are co-dominant in that both are expressed in diploid tissue. Thus whenever any one S-allele is present in pistil and pollen (or pistil and anther tissue in the sporophytic system), the two are incompatible.

The S-allele pistil-pollen self-incompatibility system is much like the "gene-for-gene" host-parasite system in that matched dominant genes confer incompatibility in both types of associations (Tables I and II). In the S-allele system, identical genes occur in both partners, the genes are allelic, and usually only one locus is involved. In the host-parasite system, different genes occur in host and parasite, genes are allelic only in the host, and several loci are involved in both partners (*14*).

The "gene-for-gene" system for incompatibility between host and parasite is often expressed as the "quadratic check" (Table III) (*14*), which serves to show that, usually, only matched corresponding dominant genes

TABLE I
Incompatibility as Conditioned by Matching Dominant Genes in Pistil and Pollen

Pollen genotype	Pistil genotype		
	S_1	S_2	S_3
S_1	−	+	+
S_2	+	−	+
S_3	+	+	−

Genes are allelic and identical in pistil and pollen. +, compatible interaction; −, incompatible interaction.

TABLE II
Incompatibility as Conditioned by Matching Dominant Genes in Host and Parasite

Parasite genotype	Host genotype		
	H_1	H_2	H_3
P_1	−	+	+
P_2	+	−	+
P_3	+	+	−

Host genes can be allelic, the corresponding parasite genes are not. +, compatible interaction; −, incompatible interaction.

TABLE III
Incompatibility as Conditioned by Dominant and Recessive Genes in Host and Parasite

Parasite genotype	Host genotype	
	H_1	h_1
P_1	−	+
p_1	+	+

+, compatible interaction; −, incompatible interaction.

condition an incompatible interaction, whereas all other combinations of dominant and/or recessive genes condition compatible interactions. Since the S-allele genes are usually co-dominant, pistil-pollen self-incompatibility genes do not have simple dominant-recessive relationships. However, in some species, spontaneous or induced deletion mutations have occurred, giving inactive genes at the S-locus (*32, 43*) which condition a compatible interaction much like that conditioned by recessive genes in host-parasite systems.

1. Physiology of Sporophytic Self-incompatibility

The stigma surface in species with sporophytic self-incompatibility is suspected to carry determinants of self-recognition (*18*). Stigmas of these species have a relatively dry surface without copious fluid exudate. The stigma surface is usually "papillate" in that the ends of individual cells project out from the stigma surface. The cuticle on the surface of these cells is covered with what appears to be a dried secretion layer containing lipids, protein, and nonspecific esterase activity (*38*). The stigma surface is the principal self-incompatibility barrier in sporophytic systems, at least in the *Cruciferae*. Pollen cells germinate poorly and pollen tubes develop abnormally on the incompatible stigma surface so that the intact stigma surface is not usually penetrated by selfing pollen tubes. However, if the cuticle on the stigma surface is breached artificially, pollen tubes can grow to the embryo sac and fertilize it (*19*). In all cases, the pollen tube grows between the stigma cell wall and the cuticle and thus never becomes intracellular as do most fungal parasites.

The stigma surface was implicated in the induction of sporophytic self-incompatibility by Kroh (*28*), who transferred individual pollen grains with a micromanipulator from one stigma to another. Development of pollen in a selfing stigma-pollen combination was enhanced if the pollen were first kept for 4–30 min in a crossing combination. Kroh speculated that the crossing combination activated cutinase presumed necessary for penetration of the stigma surface. The effectiveness of short exposures of pollen to stigma suggested that substances on the stigma surface had a role in the recognition process. In other experiments, diffusates from stigmas have blocked incorporation of ^{14}C-labeled leucine into protein and blocked germination in selfing, but not crossing, pollen (*16*), further implicating substances on the stigma surface in self-incompatibility.

The pollen grain surface is also suspected to carry determinants of self-recognition. The outer layers of the pollen grain wall (the exine) have a complex architecture forming embayments in which materials derived from the parental tapetum are trapped. Since these substances are produced by sporophytic diploid tissues, they are likely to have a role in the sporophytic type of self-recognition. Furthermore, cytochemical and immunological procedures have shown that exine substances migrate from the pollen wall to the stigma within a few minutes after pollination, as the pollen grain wall rapidly hydrates (*18*). The timing of this wall-protein emission, and the rapidity of normal stigma penetration, led Heslop-Harrison *et al.* (*18*) to conclude that the recognition events and the decision to accept or reject take place within 10 min after pollination. Cuticle penetration and entry of the pollen tube into the stigma can occur within 30 min in compatible pistil-pollen combinations.

Several lines of experimental evidence have further implicated pollen wall substances in self-recognition. Using *Cosmos bipinnatus*, Howlett *et al.* (*24*) found that the incompatibility of normal selfing pollen was reduced if the pollen were first mixed with compatible crossing pollen which had been treated with gamma irradiation, or if a diffusate from the crossing pollen were brushed on the stigma surface 1–2 min before the selfing pollen was applied.

In some cases of incompatibility a "reaction body" is deposited within stigma cells near pollen tubes, a response which has been used as a bioassay for determinants of specificity in pollen grains (*12, 20*). The reaction bodies are localized in callosic deposits which are identical in ultrastructure and in staining properties to the "papillae" that are deposited by higher plant cells in response to attempted wall penetration by fungal pathogens (*2*). Substances on the outer surface of pollen grains (*12, 13*) or leachates from pollen grains (*20*) have induced the response in greater amounts in incompatible pollen-stigma combinations than in compatible ones. The active substances are probably proteins, but they have not been identified. Furthermore, the role of the reaction body in the development of incompatibility is not clear. In host-parasite associations, the papilla is not a major factor in "gene-for-gene" incompatibility, but is instead, a more general response to attack by parasites or wounding (*2, 8, 9*).

2. *Physiology of Gametophytic Self-incompatibility*

Self-incompatibility is generally expressed later in gametophytic than in sporophytic systems. Pollen tubes enter stigmas and start to grow down the style where growth of the tube is either retarded or stopped before the tube can traverse the entire style and enter the ovary (*18*).

In contrast to the sporophytic system, no direct evidence exists for activity of determinants of specificity on pollen or stigma surfaces in gametophytic systems. The cuticle may be ephemeral or missing entirely from the surface of the stigma (*11, 46*), and the surface of the stigma is usually covered with exudate, especially after pollination. The exudate does not appear to have a role in pistil-pollen specificity (*5, 17*).

Gametophytic self-incompatibility produces a variety of abnormalities in pollen tube growth within the style. Depending on the species involved, the tube can be branched or swollen, have thickened walls, or have unusually large deposits of internal callose (*46*). The pollen tube tip bursts (*41*), tubes degenerate without bursting (*52*), or tubes stop growing without gross abnormalities (*46*).

Some lines of evidence suggest that the pollen tube suffers from nutritional deficiencies as a result of gametophytic self-incompatibility (*11, 29, 46*). Other lines of evidence suggest that incompatibility is associated with enhanced synthetic activity within pollinated stigmas (*34*). Thus self-incompatibility is prevented or weakened by heat treatments (*ca* 50°C) (*17, 23*) and by inhibitors of RNA synthesis (*10*). It has been argued that compatibility involves the retardation of a normal rejection response (*35*) or that incompatibility is due to a repressor which prevents a switch from slow to fast pollen tube growth in the style (*4*).

The gametophytic self-incompatibility reactions are generally reminiscent of host-parasite interactions conditioned by corresponding genes in host and parasite. For the gametophytic system, Heslop-Harrison (*18*) suggested that a continuing "dialogue" takes place between pistil and pollen tube (in contrast to rapid rejection in sporophytic systems), apparently involving a progressive dislocation of the metabolism of the incompatible tube (*19*). Such descriptions could be applied accurately to incompatibility in rusts and mildews in which interactions frequently continue for several days during which fungus growth is retarded (*7, 39, 49*).

3. *Specific Proteins Associated with S-alleles*

Substances which are specifically associated with the presence of individual S-alleles have been demonstrated immunologically to be present in stigmas or pollen of certain plant species with either sporophytic or gametophytic self-incompatibility (*18*). Identical antigens were found in both pollen and stigmas of *Petunia hybrida* by Linskens (*33*). In the case of stigmas of *Brassica oleracea*, unique S-allele proteins detected by gel electrophoresis proved to be the same as those detected immunologically (*40*).

The function of these S-allele-specific substances is not known, but based on Linskens' results with petunia and the fact that identical S-alleles in pistil and pollen confer self-incompatibility, identical or nearly identical determinants of specificity are generally postulated to be produced in both pistil and pollen.* The binding together of the substances from the two sources presumably triggers recognition of self. Burnet (*6*) has proposed that the like substances bind because each carries both positive and negative receptor sites whose configurations are specific for a given S-allele. By carrying both the "lock" and the "key," one molecule can bind specifically with another identical molecule. Others (*3, 31*) have proposed that like substances in pollen and pistil are subunits of proteins which combine to form dimers or tetramers. Having like molecules initiate recognition processes is a special property of self-recognition and not one encountered in host-parasite associations where the interaction is conditioned by corresponding, but probably different, genes in the two organisms concerned.

Implicit in most theories of S-gene incompatibility is the concept that the S-genes directly or indirectly govern production of substances which actively interact to trigger incompatibility. Compatibility is passive in that it proceeds if the incompatibility trigger is not released. This parallels the conclusion reached by Ellingboe (*15*) from convincing genetic evidence that the incompatibility in "gene-for-gene" host-parasite associations is the active result of interaction between corresponding genes of host and parasite. Once the trigger is released, however, we do not know if incompatibility is caused by promotion of new processes or the inhibition of existing ones in either pistil-pollen or host-parasite associations.

II. INTERSPECIFIC INCOMPATIBILITY IN ANGIOSPERMS

Pistil-pollen incompatibility has a major role in limiting interbreeding between species, although other mechanisms, operating either before pollination or at fertilization and thereafter, also have major roles (*50*). The mechanisms limiting interspecific crosses have an effect opposite to that of the S-allele system. S-allele self-incompatibility forces outbreeding among individuals within a species; interspecific incompatibility limits outbreeding and serves to protect the genetic integrity of a species.

Crosses between species belonging to different genera or families are

* Mutations at the S-locus usually are expressed only in the pollen or the pistil (*30, 43*), which suggests that the determinants of specificity for a given S-allele may differ in pollen and pistil. However, Lewis (*30*) postulates, instead, that the S-locus has two parts, one part governing specificity which is identical in pistil and pollen, the other part governing activity in pistil and pollen.

generally unsuccessful (*51*) and such wide crosses have received little attention. The data of Martin (*36*) show that pollen rarely germinates on stigmas of distantly related species. Of 254 crosses involving 24 species in 16 families, pollen germinated in only 11 crosses. Pollen of each species germinated on stigmas of the same species, although pollen of some species did not germinate on an artificial medium. Thus, the lack of germination could have been due to a lack of germination promoters in some cases, and to inhibitors in others, but the reasons for the absence of germination have not been determined (*37*).

Pollen germinates more frequently in crosses within a genus. In studies with *Solanum*, for example, pollen germinated in about 40% of crosses made among 15 species (*36*). After germination, pollen tubes of *Solanum* vary in amount of development within pistil tissues (*48*). A similar range in amount of development occurs when a given species of pathogen is placed on inappropriate host species, as illustrated by the data of Johnson (*25*) for a powdery mildew fungus (Table IV). Here, spore germination was reduced in all inappropriate host families, and germination was nearly absent in some

TABLE IV

Development of *Erysiphe cichoracearum* on an Appropriate Host Species and on Inappropriate Host Species in Six Families of Angiosperms

	Percentage of spores (%)						
	Appropriate host	Inappropriate hosts					
	Cucurbitaceae	*Leguminosae*	*Compositae*	*Solanaceae*	*Polypodiaceae*	*Gramineae*	*Liliaceae-Iridaceae*
No. of species per family	1	1	6	2	3	10	9
Development of fungus							
Germ tube	65	54	41	44	39	22	2
Appressorium	62	18	27	24	32	5	0
Penetration peg	59	10	19	20	21	1	0
Haustorium	55	7	10	14	0	0	0
Hypha	54	6	5	7	0	0	0
Colony	54	2	0	0	0	0	0

Data selected from Johnson (*25*).

families. At each subsequent stage of development, the fungus population was reduced, so that in most families the parasite was unable to colonize the host. Failure to germinate on inappropriate hosts is probably less common for fungus spores than for pollen grains, but in both cases, the early stages of development tend to be severely limited.

1. *Interspecific Pistil-pollen Recognition*

How does a pollen grain or tube recognize that it is on the pistil of its own species? Knox and co-workers (*26*) have taken the view that substances on the surfaces of pollen grains and stigmas are involved in recognition much as has been proposed for sporophytic self-incompatibility, except that self-recognition promotes pollen tube growth instead of inhibiting it. They found that gamma-irradiated or methanol-treated selfing pollen applied to a pistil would promote development of crossing pollen applied to the pistil in crosses between *Populus deltoides* and *P. alba.* Crude preparations of protein from the pollen inner wall (the intine) were also effective in promoting crossing. Such experiments suggest that specific substances promote *compatiblity* within a species. On the other hand, Willing and Pryor (*53*) found that they could promote the same cross by applying traces of hexane or ethyl acetate with a camel's hair brush to the surface of either the stigma or the pollen. This suggested that specific factors, some on the pollen and some on the stigma, promoted *incompatibility* between the two species.

In studies with *Gladiolus gandavensis* (which is self-compatible), Knox *et al.* (*27*) found that conconavalin A would bind to the stigma surface and that the bound lectin prevented stigma penetration by *Gladiolus* pollen. They also found that *Gladiolus* pollen did not germinate on *Gladiolus* stigmas if the stigmas were first washed with 0.5% sodium deoxycholate. They speculated that the treatments interfered with or removed substances which are specifically required for compatiblity between pistil and pollen of *Gladiolus.*

Such preliminary experiments serve to implicate substances on the surfaces of pollen and stigmas in the self-recognition that allows pollen of one species to be accepted by the stigma of its own species, but to be rejected by stigmas of other species. Similar experiments should be conducted on the effect of altering plant surfaces on the species specificity of plant pathogens.

2. *The Origin of Basic Compatibility*

In one form or another, several authors have suggested that basic compatibility between pistil and pollen must arise by co-evolution within a species, that basic compatibility is probably governed by many genes, and that the S-allele system of self-incompatibility is superimposed on this basic compatibility* (*18, 45, 47*). Somewhat similar views have been expressed regarding basic compatibility in relation to race specificity in plant disease (*14, 54*). For pistil-pollen interactions, the clearest and most useful explanation of basic compatibility was developed by Hogenboom (*21, 22*). In studies of crosses between species of *Lycopersicon*, he found several genes, unrelated to S-alleles, which governed interspecific incompatibility. To provide a theoretical basis for these results, he constructed a "model for incongruity in intimate partner relationships." Incongruity refers to what is here termed basic incompatibility.

Hogenboom's model is based on the divergence of two species from one another. As one part of a species population undergoes change as a consequence of geographic isolation or other factors, a change may develop in the pistil (through mutation and natural selection) in response to external environmental factors—a change which presents a partial barrier to pollen tube development. This produces incongruity between pistil and pollen which is then repaired by the emergence of a corresponding ability in the pollen to overcome the barrier. For convenience, Hogenboom terms all genes which impede pollen tube growth as "barrier" genes, all genes in pollen which overcome such barriers as "penetration" genes. After a series of corresponding barrier and penetration genes evolve, the pollen of the original species is no longer compatible with the pistil of the newly emerging species, and the two species are effectively isolated from each other. Hogenboom considers the pistil as a complex of barriers and promoters such that, "For a normal progress of the fertilization process, as a counterpart of each barrier and promotion process in the pistil, the potential for the corresponding penetration and reaction process must be present in pollen and become operative at the right moment." He concludes that many barrier and penetration genes must be matched in pistil and pollen for congruity to exist. The absence of one or more of these genes in either partner renders the relationship non-functional (incompatible).

Hogenboom's model closely parallels the "gene-for-gene" hypothesis of host-parasite race specificity, but contains the major difference that cor-

---

* S-alleles apparently are involved in incompatibility between certain closely related species (*18*), especially in combinations of self-compatible species with self-incompatible ones in which "unilateral incompatibility" is found (*1, 42, 44*).

TABLE V

Compatibility as Governed by Dominant and Recessive Genes as Predicted by Hogenboom's (*21, 22*) Model for Incongruity

Pollen genotype	Pistil genotype	
	B	b
P	+	+
p	−	+

The pistil contains "barrier" genes, the pollen contains "penetration" genes (see text). +, compatible; −, incompatible.

responding dominant genes in pistil and pollen condition compatibility (Table V) instead of incompatibility (Table III). Furthermore, the presumed origin of the genes differs between the incongruity model and the "gene-for-gene" hypothesis. The changes postulated to occur in the pistil are not a consequence of the presence of pollen, whereas host resistance genes are thought to appear as a result of selection pressure from a virulent parasite.

Hogenboom's model can be applied to basic compatibility in host-parasite systems with only slight modification, by starting with a disease in a given host species caused by a given species of prasite. As the host species develops new characters in response to external forces, a new "barrier" to the pathogen could occur, not as a response to pathogen pressure, but from the external forces directing speciation of the host population. The pathogen then could develop a corresponding "penetration" gene to overcome the "barrier" (in Hogenboom's terminology). As the new host species becomes more divergent, numerous "barrier" genes would accumulate which are matched by corresponding "penetration" genes. The parasite might be sufficiently changed to become a new species in some cases. In all cases basic compatibility between the newly emergent host species and the parasite would consist of many corresponding genes. The absence of one or more would confer incompatibility.

SUMMARY

The nature of the basic compatibility that enables two species to form an intimate partner relationship is poorly understood, partly because genetic studies between species are difficult or impossible to do, and partly because incompatibility between inappropriate species has been studied only infrequently. However, pistil-pollen incompatibility between species is usually expressed very early in pollen tube development, much like the reduced development of fungal germ tubes and infection structures that can occur on highly inappropriate host species. Basic compatibility requires that pollen or parasite react suitably to the physical and chemical properties of the pistil or host surface, and that they produce structures appropriate for penetrating pistil or host tissues. Available evidence suggests that substances on the surfaces of pollen and stigma have a major role in species discrimination in pistil-pollen associations and similar substances could have a role in the species specificity of host and parasite.

Basic compatibility may also require that the metabolic systems of the two participating organisms be suitably matched as suggested by Ellingboe (*14*). However, cytoplasmic processes and metabolic regulation tend to be similar among taxonomically divergent organisms, and the cytoplasm from one species is usually compatible with cytoplasm from another species (*8*). Thus processes at the metabolic level probably have a lesser role in determining basic compatibility than do the physical and chemical properties of the pistil-pollen or host-parasite interface.

Hogenboom's model for incongruity suggests that basic compatibility evolves by production of a series of matching genes in the two partners of an intimate association, much as has been suggested by the "gene-for-gene" hypothesis for race specificity in host-parasite interaction. In his model, matching dominant genes condition compatibility instead of incompatibility, and the formation of such genes is a result of species divergence in the host instead of a direct response of one partner to attack by the other.

Race specific incompatibility in host-parasite associations and S-allele self-incompatibility in pistil-pollen associations both appear to be superimposed on basic compatibility. The S-allele system has much in common, both genetically and physiologically, with "gene-for-gene" conditioned race specificity. Proteins on the surfaces of pollen and stigmas have been implicated as determinants of S-allele specificity. Although the surfaces of pollen and stigmas have unique structural and chemical features, analagous surface features may determine race specificity in host-parasite associations.

Acknowledgment

The author gratefully acknowledges discussions related to this paper with A.H. Ellingboe and P.D. Ascher.

REFERENCES

1. Abdalla, M. M. F. and J. G. T. Hermsen. 1972. Unilateral incompatibility: hypotheses, debate and its implications for plant breeding. *Euphytica* **21**: 32–47.
2. Aist, J. R. 1976. Papillae and related wound plugs of plant cells. *Annu. Rev. Phytopathol.* **14**: 145–163.
3. Ascher, P. D. 1966. A gene action model to explain gametophytic self-incompatibility. *Euphytica* **15**: 179–183.
4. Ascher, P. D. 1975. Special stylar property required for compatible pollen-tube growth in *Lilium longiflorum* Thunb. *Bot. Gaz.* **136**: 317–321.
5. Ascher, P. D. and L. W. Drewlow. 1971. Effect of stigmatic exudate injected into the stylar canal on compatible and incompatible pollen tube growth in *Lilium longiflorum* Thunb. *In*: J. Heslop-Harrison (ed.). *Pollen: Development and Physiology*. Appleton-Century-Crofts, New York, pp. 267–272.
6. Burnet, F. M. 1971. "Self-recognition" in colonial marine forms and flowering plants in relation to the evolution of immunity. *Nature* **232**: 230–235.
7. Bushnell, W. R. 1972. Physiology of fungal haustoria. *Annu. Rev. Phytopathol.* **10**: 151–176.
8. Bushnell, W. R. 1976. Reactions of cytoplasm and organelles in relation to host-parasite specificity. *In*: R. K. S. Wood and A. Graniti (eds.). *Specificity in Plant Diseases*. Plenum Press, New York, pp. 131–150.
9. Bushnell, W. R. and S. E. Bergquist. 1975. Aggregation of host cytoplasm and formation of papillae and haustoria in powdery mildew of barley. *Phytopathology* **65**: 310–318.
10. Campbell, R. J. and P. D. Ascher. 1976. Incorporation of label from radioactive uridine into the stylar nucleic acids of *Lilium longiflorum* Thunb. as affected by heat, 6-methylpurine and actinomycin D. *Theor. Appl. Genet.* **47**: 215–226.
11. Dickinson, H. G. and J. Lawson. 1975. Pollen tube growth in the stigma of *Oenothera organensis* following compatible and incompatible intraspecific pollinations. *Proc. Roy. Soc. (London) B* **188**: 327–344.
12. Dickinson, H. G. and D. Lewis. 1973. The formation of the tryphine coating the pollen grains of *Raphanus*, and its properties relating to the self-incompatibility system. *Proc. Roy. Soc. (London) B* **184**: 149–165.
13. Dickinson, H. G. and D. Lewis. 1975. Interaction between the pollen grain coating and the stigmatic surface during compatible and incompatible intraspecific pollinations in *Raphanus*. *In*: J. G. Duckett and P. A. Racey (eds.). *The*

Biology of the Male Gamete. vol. 7, Suppl. No. 1, Biol. J. Linnean Soc., pp. 165–175.

14. Ellingboe, A. H. 1976. Genetics of host-parasite interactions. *In*: R. Heitefuss and P. H. Williams (eds.). *Encyclopedia of Plant Physiology*. vol. 4. Springer-Verlag, Berlin, pp. 761–778.
15. Ellingboe, A. H. 1977. A genetic analysis of host-parasite interactions. *In*: D. M. Spencer (ed.). *The Powdery Mildews*. Academic Press, New York (in press).
16. Ferrari, T. E. and D. H. Wallace. 1976. Pollen protein synthesis and control of incompatibility in *Brassica*. *Theor. Appl. Genet.* **48**: 243–249.
17. Fett, W. F., J. D. Paxton, and D. B. Dickinson. 1976. Studies on the self-incompatibility response of *Lilium longiflorum*. *Am. J. Bot.* **63**: 1104–1108.
18. Heslop-Harrison, J. 1975. Incompatibility and the pollen-stigma interaction. *Annu. Rev. Plant Physiol.* **26**: 403–425.
19. Heslop-Harrison, J., Y. Heslop-Harrison, and J. Barber. 1975. The stigma surface in incompatibility responses. *Proc. Roy. Soc. (London) B* **188**: 287–297.
20. Heslop-Harrison, J., R. B. Knox, and Y. Heslop-Harrison. 1974. Pollen-wall proteins: exine-held fractions associated with the incompatibility response in *Cruciferae*. *Theor. Appl. Genet.* **44**: 133–137.
21. Hogenboom, N. G. 1973. A model for incongruity in intimate partner relationships. *Euphytica* **22**: 219–233.
22. Hogenboom, N. G. 1975. Incompatibility and incongruity: two different mechanisms for the non-functioning of intimate partner relationships. *Proc. Roy. Soc. (London) B* **188**: 361–375.
23. Hopper, J. E. and S. J. Peloquin. 1976. Analysis of stylar self-incompatibility competence by use of heat induced inactivation. *Theor. Appl. Genet.* **47**: 291–297.
24. Howlett, B. J., R. B. Knox, J. D. Paxton, and J. Heslop-Harrison. 1975. Pollen-wall proteins: physiochemical characterization and role in self-incompatibility in *Cosmos bipinnatus*. *Proc. Roy. Soc. (London) B* **188**: 167–182.
25. Johnson, L. E. B. 1977. Resistance mechanisms to powdery mildew fungi (Erysiphaceae) in nonhost and inappropriate host plants. M.S. Thesis, University of Minnesota, St. Paul, 180pp.
26. Knox, R. B., R. R. Willing, and A. E. Ashford. 1972. Role of pollen-wall proteins as recognition substances in interspecific incompatibility in poplars. *Nature* **237**: 381–383.
27. Knox, R. B., A. Clarke, S. Harrison, P. Smith, and J. J. Marchalonis. 1976. Cell recognition in plants: determinants of the stigma surface and their pollen interactions. *Proc. Natl. Acad. Sci. U.S.* **73**: 2788–2792.
28. Kroh, M. 1966. Reaction of pollen after transfer from one stigma to another. *Züchter* **36**: 185–189.
29. Kroh, M., C. Labarca, and F. Loewus. 1971. Use of pistil exudate for pollen

tube wall biosynthesis in *Lilium longiflorum*. *In*: J. Heslop-Harrison (eds.). *Pollen: Development and Physiology*. Appleton-Century-Crofts, New York, pp. 273–278.

30. Lewis, D. 1960. Genetic control of specificity and activity of the S antigen in plants. *Proc. Roy. Soc. (London) B* **151**: 468–477.
31. Lewis, D. 1965. A protein dimer hypothesis on incompatibility. *Genet. Today* **3**: 657–663.
32. Lewis, D. and L. K. Crowe. 1954. Structure of the incompatibility gene. IV. Types of mutations in *Prunus avium* L. *Heredity* **8**: 357–363.
33. Linskens, H. F. 1960. Zur Frage der Entstehung der Abwehr-körper bei der Inkompatabilitäts reaction von Petunia. III. Mitteilung: Serologische Teste mit Leitgewebs—und Pollen—Extrakten. *Z. Bot.* **48**: 126–135.
34. Linskens, H. F. 1975. Incompatibility in *Petunia*. *Proc. Roy. Soc. (London) B* **188**: 299–311.
35. Linskens, H. F. 1976. Specific interactions in higher plants. *In*: R. K. S. Wood and A. Graniti (eds.). *Specificity in Plant Diseases*. Plenum Press, New York, pp. 311–326.
36. Martin, F. W. 1970. Pollen germination on foreign stigmas. *Bull. Torrey Bot. Club* **97**: 1–6.
37. Martin, F. W. and J. L. Brewbaker. 1971. The nature of the stigmatic exudate and its role in pollen germination. *In*: J. Heslop-Harrison (ed.). *Pollen: Development and Physiology*. Appleton-Century-Crofts, New York, pp. 262–266.
38. Mattsson, O., R. B. Knox, J. Heslop-Harrison, and Y. Heslop-Harrison. 1974. Protein pellicle of stigmatic papillae as a probable recognition site in incompatibility reactions. *Nature* **247**: 298–300.
39. Mayama, S., D. W. Rehfeld, and J. M. Daly. 1975. A comparison of the development of *Puccinia graminis tritici* in resistant and susceptible wheat based on glucosamine content. *Physiol. Plant Pathol.* **7**: 243–257.
40. Nasrallah, M. E., J. T. Barber, and D. H. Wallace. 1970. Self-incompatibility proteins in plants: detection, genetics, and possible mode of action. *Heredity* **25**: 23–27.
41. Nettancourt, D. de, M. Devreux, A. Bozzini, M. Cresti, E. Pacini, and G. Sarfatti. 1973. Ultrastructural aspects of the self-incompatibility mechanism in *Lycopersicum peruvianum* Mill. *J. Cell. Sci.* **12**: 403–419.
42. Nettancourt, D. de, M. Devreux, F. Carluccio, U. Laneri, M. Cresti, E. Pacini, G. Sarfatti, and A. J. G. van Gastel. 1975. Facts and hypotheses on the origin of S mutations and on the function of the S gene in *Nicotiana alata* and *Lycopersicum peruvianum*. *Proc. Roy. Soc. (London) B* **188**: 345–360.
43. Pandey, K. K. 1962. A theory of S gene structure. *Nature* **196**: 236–238.
44. Pandey, K. K. 1968. Compatibility relationships in flowering plants: role of the S-gene complex. *Am. Nat.* **102**: 475–489.
45. Pandey, K. K. 1969. Elements of the S-gene complex V. Interspecific cross-

compatibility relationships and theory of the evolution of the S complex. *Genetica* **40**: 447–474.

46. Rosen, W. G. 1971. Pistil-pollen interactions in *Lilium*. *In*: J. Heslop-Harrison (ed.). *Pollen: Development and Physiology*. Appleton-Century-Crofts, New York, pp. 239–254.
47. Sampson, D. R. 1962. Intergeneric pollen-stigma incompatibility in the Cruciferae. *Can. J. Genet. Cytol.* **4**: 38–49.
48. Sams, D. W., P. D. Ascher, and F. I. Lauer. 1977. Crossability of some green-peach-aphid-resistant tuber-bearing *Solanums*, potential bridging species, and *Solanum tuberosum*. *Am. Potato J.* **54**: 355–364.
49. Skipp, R. A. and D. J. Samborski. 1974. The effect of the *Sr6* gene for host resistance on histological events during the development of stem rust in near-isogenic wheat lines. *Can. J. Bot.* **52**: 1107–1115.
50. Stebbins, G. L., Jr. 1950. *Variation and Evolution in Plants*. Columbia University Press, New York, 643pp.
51. Stebbins, G. L. 1974. *Flowering Plants—Evolution Above the Species Level*. Belknap Press, Cambridge, Mass., 399pp.
52. Van der Pluijm, J. and H. F. Linskens. 1966. Feinstruktur der Pollenschläuche im Griffel von *Petunia*. *Züchter* **36**: 220–224.
53. Willing, R. R. and L. D. Pryor. 1976. Interspecific hybridisation in Poplar. *Theor. Appl. Genet.* **47**: 141–151.
54. Wood, R. K. S. 1976. Specificity—an assessment. *In*: R. K. S. Wood and A. Graniti (eds.). *Specificity in Plant Diseases*. Plenum Press, New York, pp. 327–338.

Discussion of Paper by Dr. Bushnell

The generalization that spores of many fungi germinate and penetrate leaves of most plants was questioned by KUĆ. BUSHNELL replied that the evidence supporting the notion is not satisfactory and should be reevaluated. Most data are qualitative and based on only the portion of the pathogen population that is successful; the number and type of hosts used is usually limited.

J. VANETTEN described an experiment done in his laboratory which bears on the sequence of biochemical events that leads to spore germination and germ tube growth. *Rhizopus stolonifer* sporangiospores were harvested dry and compared with spores harvested in water and then dried. Both sets of spores were stored at room temperature for one year. After this time period the dry-harvested spores germinated and the fungus grew normally; in contrast, the wet harvested spores formed germ tubes and then stopped growing. Thus some unknown event must occur in the germ tube which allows the fungus to continue growing. Also certain inhibitors will permit germ tube formation but prevent further growth. The events which are required for continued growth may have some relevance to penetration of hosts by fungi.

WHEELER noted similarity between the manner in which a pollen tube grows down a style and the way that *H. maydis* penetrates a leaf, although *H. maydis* causes more swelling of the host wall. This is one of the few cases among host-parasite interactions where the fungus grows intercellularly for at least 24 hr and is encased in host cell wall material.

INDUCTION OF HOST RESPONSES FOR INCOMPATIBILITY AND COMPATIBILITY

Recognition and Specificity in Plant Host-Parasite Interactions, pp. 231-251, 1979

THE ACQUISITION OF SYSTEMIC RESISTANCE BY PRIOR INOCULATION

LUIS SEQUEIRA

Department of Plant Pathology, University of Wisconsin, Madison, U.S.A.

For decades, plant pathologists have been attracted to the possibilities that plants could be actively or passively immunized by procedures similar to those that are successful in animals. The first observations were those of Smith *et al.* (*48*), who reported in 1911 that Paris daisies which had been inoculated with *Agrobacterium tumefaciens*, with the production of tumors, became refractory to subsequent infection. Although these early observations could not be confirmed, Brown in 1923 (*3*) was successful in attempts to "vaccinate" plants using dead *A. tumefaciens*; plants inoculated with such cells failed to form tumors when inoculated one day later at the same location with live cells. Although similar observations followed, it soon became apparent that these responses were nonspecific and very different from antigen-antibody reactions in animals. Interest in plant immunization waned.

Resurgence of interest in plant immunization was due very largely to two important discoveries: "cross protection" in virus diseases, and "phytoalexin" accumulation in fungal diseases (*35, 36*). Cross-protection reactions occur in plants inoculated with closely related viruses. Generally, the phenomenon can be demonstrated readily in cases when the first virus multiplies systemically and the second virus causes necrotic lesions. The second virus usually cannot be reisolated; unrelated viruses do not cross protect. A variety of mechanisms has been proposed to explain cross protection, including the formation of inhibitors, depletion of essential metabolites required for the second virus, and capture of the RNA of the superinfecting strain by the coat protein of the original virus (*8*). It is clear, however, that cross protection is a limited, specialized reaction that has no comparable counter-part in diseases caused by other plant pathogens.

The concept that antibiotic compounds were formed in plant tissues in response to fungal infection was first expressed in concrete fashion as the "phytoalexin theory" by Müller and co-workers (*36*). The theory was formulated on the basis of experiments in which potato tubers acquired resistance when exposed to avirulent forms of *Phytophthora infestans*. A primary conclusion, however, was that the toxic principle that was formed remained confined to the tissues colonized by the fungus and to those in the immediate neighborhood.

It is evident that viruses, fungi, and bacteria also induce systemic, nonspecific, protective reactions, generally referred to as "interference" (*40*). This paper will be concerned almost exclusively with these types of reactions. In general, they can be demonstrated by challenge inoculation at a point distant from that initially inoculated. The initial inoculation may involve: a) the same pathogen used in the challenge inoculation, b) avirulent or incompatible forms of the same organism, c) heat-killed or other inactive forms of the same organism, d) cell wall or other constituents of the same or different organisms, and e) other pathogens or saprophytes. In general, the protective reaction cannot be induced by mechanical or chemical injury to plant cells.

It is unfortunate that the term cross protection has been used very loosely to describe phenomena that should have been termed interference more properly. That interference is of common occurrence and of wide interest to pathologists is evidenced in the extensive reviews by Ross (*40*) and Matta (*32*). It is significant that, in spite of this wide interest, we are no closer today to an explanation of the nature of the phenomenon than we were nearly 70 years ago when the first observations were reported.

The main purpose of this paper is to describe various systems that have been used to demonstrate systemic disease resistance, and to examine them for common features that may lead us to a better understanding of the mechanisms that induce, and of those that result in, the protective response. In our laboratories, we have examined different aspects of the acquisition of disease resistance by prior treatment of tobacco leaves with heat-killed cells of *Pseudomonas solanacearum* E. F. Sm. For this reason, this particular system will be used extensively to illustrate some of the more important aspects of inducible, protective phenomena in plants.

I. CHARACTERISTICS OF THE PROTECTION PHENOMENON

Because of the varied nature of the host and pathogen combinations used, as well as of the conditions under which acquired resistance has been demonstrated, it is difficult to determine the characteristics that the phenomenon has in common. There are relatively few common threads, and there are enough exceptions in each instance as to prevent establishment of any general rules. The following points are perhaps the most obvious and of more general value.

1. *Time-dependence*

A fundamental characteristic of induced resistance is its absolute dependence on a time interval between the intial and the challenge inoculations. With any system employed, protection is not immediate, but can be demonstrated only after an adequate response period. This time dependence indicates that specific changes in the host, perhaps involving the synthesis or accumulation of metabolites, are of particular importance in the resistance phenomenon.

The period necessary for initiation of the resistance response is: a) a function of the concentration of inocula used in both initial and challenge inoculations, b) dependent on the sensitivity of the assay used to detect resistance, and c) markedly influenced by the location of, and distance between, the initial and challenge inoculations. The examples cited below illustrate these points.

Goodman (*11*) has reported that for protection of apple stem tissue against *Erwinia amylovora*, populations of the protecting bacteria (avirulent strains of *E. amylovora, Ps. tabaci, etc.*) approximately 100 times that of the virulent pathogen were required. When this numerical advantage was reduced, suppression of the virulent pathogen was delayed and became less pronounced. In tobacco leaves, infiltration with 10^5 and 10^7 heat-killed cells of *Ps. tabaci* resulted in partial protection against live cells of the same bacterium, but at higher populations (10^9 cells/ml) protection was complete if sufficient time elapsed between inoculations (*28*).

When tobacco leaves are infiltrated with heat-killed cells of *Ps. solanacearum* and challenged immediately with an incompatible strain (B-1) of the bacterium, a normal hypersensitive response (HR) is obtained. However, as the period of incubation increases from 6 to 12 hr, the HR becomes less marked and, by 18 hr, the leaves are completely protected. Protection results from rapid reduction of the challenge inoculum below the level necessary to induce confluent cell collapse. Generally, there is complete prevention of the HR on those leaf panels where the concentration of heat-killed cells is equal to or higher than that of the live cells in the range of 9.2×10^7 to 450×10^7 cells/ml (*30*). When crude bacterial extracts, rather than heat-killed cells, are used at 0.1 mg protein/ml, partial protection is obtained with in 2 hr, and full protection within 7 hr (*45*).

These few examples suffice to illustrate the point that rapidity and intensity of the plant's protective response are quantitative phenomena directly related to the number of host cells that come in contact with the initial inoculum. The intensity of the response is also reflected in the total area of the plant that becomes resistant. If the challenge inoculation is carried out at a point far removed from the initial inoculation, the protective response may not be detectable for many days. For instance, when tobacco plants were stem-inoculated with *Peronospora tabacina*, a full protective response in the foliage was not evident until 28 days after the initial inoculation (*6*).

2. *Light-dependence*

Since protective responses probably involve synthesis and/or movement of metabolites, and these are energy-requiring processes, it is not surprising that light is an absolute requirement in several systems that have been studied. At least part of the ATP requirement probably is derived from photophosphorylation. Action spectra determined for the protective response elicited by heat-killed *Ps. solanacerum* cells in tobacco leaves indicate that the effective wavelengths are in two areas of the spectrum, 450–500 and 600–660 nm (Kraus, unpublished). It is likely that the effective receptor is chlorophyll *b* (absorption peaks at 453 and 642 nm). The minimum energy levels required to elicit protection are in the order of 5 uw/cm^2 for 12 hr. The relatively high and stringent light requirements were demonstrated also with tobacco leaves infiltrated with heat-killed bacterial cells, exposed to increasing periods of illumination (1,800 ft-c), and then challenged 24 hr after infiltration. No protection was obtained in leaves maintained in the dark, but progressive levels of protection were obtained in direct relation to the length of the photoperiod. Complete protection, in the treated panels only, was obtained with 12 hr of light; a 24-hr exposure to light resulted in complete protection in both treated and untreated panels of the same leaf (*30*).

A light requirement for acquired resistance to bacterial plant pathogens is not universal, however. In alfalfa leaflets inoculated with avirulent mutants of *Corynebacterium insidiosum*, resistance to virulent strains of the bacterium developed regardless of whether the leaflets were covered with aluminum foil for 24 hr prior to or following the challenge inoculation (*4*).

3. Temperature-dependence

Resistant responses elicited by prior inoculation appear to be extremely sensitive to temperature, but this interesting property has not been explored to any extent. The resistance that develops in tobacco as a result of local lesion formation by strains of tobacco mosaic virus (TMV) is at a maximum in plants grown at 20–24°C, but does not occur in plants grown at 30°C. Similarly, the protective response elicited by heat-killed cells of *Ps. solanacearum* is inhibited at temperatures above 32°C. This may be related to the fact that the hypersensitive response in tobacco is inhibited if plants are maintained at 36°C immediately after inoculation (*20*).

Unlike systemic resistance, phytoalexin accumulation is not affected by temperatures in the range of 30–36°C. For instance, pisatin accumulation in pea pods following inoculation with *Monilinia fructicola* was eliminated only at an incubation temperature of 45°C for 2 hr (*7*).

4. Systemic Involvement

An important characteristic of acquired resistance in many host-parasite systems is the fact that it spreads from the site of the initial inoculation. In particular, the tobacco plant shows a remarkable ability to respond in this manner to inoculation with a wide variety of pathogens. The elegant work of Ross and co-workers (*41*) has shown that in varieties of tobacco which are hypersensitive to TMV, or other viruses, the induction of necrotic local lesions results in systemic effects that move both up and down the stem. The level and extent of resistance depend upon the interval between the initial and the challenge inoculation. The effects can be measured in terms of both size and number of lesions that result from the challenge inoculation. Resistance becomes detectable by 2–3 days, and rises to a maximum at about 7 days; leaves that develop resistance are free of the virus at the time of the challenge inoculation.

That resistance may be due to translocation of a protection factor was shown clearly by experiments in which the vascular system was severed; cutting the midvein of a leaf, for instance, prevented development of resistance at a point distal to the cut (*40*).

Results very similar to those reported for viruses have been obtained with fungal and bacterial pathogens of tobacco. Stem lesions caused by either *Thielaviopsis basicola* or *P. tabacina* increased resistance in the upper leaves to TMV and other pathogens (*15, 31*). The effect was most pronounced on the first few leaves closest to the point of initial inoculation. When the two bottom leaves of a tobacco plant were infiltrated with heat-killed cells of *Ps. solanacearum* and the plant was exposed to continuous light for 24 hr, the three leaves immediately above the infiltrated one showed partial protection when challenged with live cells of the bacterium. On plants similarly treated, visible local lesion development by strains of TMV did not occur over the entire leaf surface of the plant (Lozano, unpublished). Similar, nonspecific, systemic resistance has been reported in cucumber inoculated with two fungal pathogens (*14*).

Systemic resistance is certainly not the rule, however, in many other host-parasite combinations. The numerous instances of phytoalexin induction, resulting from prior inoculation with saprophytic or pathogenic fungi, give very substantial evidence for localized effects (*7*). Bacterial infection also may result in localized resistance responses, as in the case of alfalfa leaflets inoculated with avirulent mutants of *C. insidiosum* (*4*).

5. *Persistence*

One of the most remarkable characteristics of induced resistance phenomena is the long-lasting protective effect of the initial inoculation. In cucumber plants repeatedly inoculated with *Colletotrichum lagenarium*, for instance, a systemic, resistant response against the same fungus lasted for 10 weeks (*22*). In tobacco, stem injection with *P. tabacina* resulted in a protective response in the foliage against *P. tabacina* which was not fully evident until 28 days had elapsed after injection (*6*). In these and in other cases of persistent systemic protection, the phenomenon is dependent on the fact that the pathogen in the initial inoculum remains alive and active, thus allowing for cumulative response. In those instances when the pathogen dies or is severely limited by an initial necrotic response, the protective response may be more transient. Nevertheless, induction of a hypersensitive response in flax by avirulent flax rust strains, or by alien rusts, resulted in a localized, protective response that was effective 7 days after inoculation (*24*). In tobacco varieties that are hypersensitive to TMV, inoculation with this virus results in systemic resistance that rises to a maximum in 7 days and persists for about 20 days (*40*).

6. *Nonspecificity*

A major feature that distinguishes acquired resistance in plants from that in animals is the general lack of specificity of the former as opposed to the highly specific antigen-antibody reactions of the latter. Although terms such as "immunity" and "premunity" are commonly used in the plant pathological literature, they should be avoided because they imply similarity to processes in animals which are not equivalent in plants.

The lack of specificity of protective responses in plants is reflected not only in terms of the organisms that induce the response, but of the wide range of potential pathogens that the plant is protected against as well. For instance, in tobacco, almost any virus that induces necrotic local lesions will induce systemic resistance, and this resistance is equally effective against different viruses (TMV, tobacco necrosis virus (TNV), tobacco ring spot virus (TRSV), *etc.*) (*40*). For this reason, Ross (*41*) has formulated the hypothesis that local lesion formation in the initial inoculation results in the formation of substances that move systemically to uninoculated plant parts and there activate mechanisms that normally restrict lesion size.

Initial experiments by Lovrekovich and Farkas (*28*) demonstrated that infiltration of tobacco leaves with heat-killed cells of *Ps. tabaci, Ps. syringae,* and *C. flaccumfaciens* induced a time-dependent protective reaction against infection by *Ps. tabaci.* Inoculation with similar preparations from *Ps. solanacearum, Ps. lachrymans,* and *Xanthomonas axonopodis* induced protection against *Ps. solanacearum* (*30*). The protection afforded by heat-killed bacteria in tobacco is equally effective against bacterial and viral infection (*26*), suggesting that, as in the case of resistance induced by local-lesion-inducing viruses, the resistance depends on activation of general mechanisms that normally restrict movement and/or establishment of pathogens.

Phytoalexins are generally associated with localized responses to fungi, bacteria, and even viruses, and have a relatively wide spectrum of toxicity against fungi and bacteria. The rapidity of phytoalexin accumulation is an important feature of incompatible host-parasite combinations, but compounds such as phaseollin accumulate in bean hypocotyls inoculated with either cultivar-pathogenic and cultivar-nonpathogenic races of *Colletotrichum lindemuthianum* (*38*). Compounds other than "traditional" phytoalexins appear to be involved in cases of specific protection reactions that occur distant from the site of initial inoculation with this pathogen (*9*). Berard *et al.* (*2*) have described the production of a diffusible factor from incompatible combinations, and capable of protecting only the bean cultivar from which it was obtained. This is one of the few instances in which the specificity of the response corresponds to that described under "cross-protection" in viral systems.

It is apparent that resistance acquired by prior inoculation usually is nonspecific because it may be related to recognition by the host of compounds of general occurrence in cell walls of plant pathogens. Pathogens appear able to prevent this general resistance response by means that are not entirely understood at present, or alternatively, they may be insensitive or unaffected by metabolites produced as a result of the response.

II. NATURE OF THE INDUCER

The acquisition of resistance appears to result from reactions that occur at the interface between host and parasite. It has been postulated that outer cell wall constituents, or virus coat proteins, are "recognized" by host cell wall receptor proteins. This hypothesis is in concert with recognition phenomena in mating reactions in yeasts (*5*), algae (*51*), and higher plants (*16*) where surface-localized, complementary macromolecular mechanisms have been demonstrated. In general, these mechanisms involve carbohydrate-containing surface molecules in one member, and protein receptor molecules (lectins) in the other.

The search for inducers of phytoalexin production has been complicated by the nonspecific nature of the phenomenon; it can be induced by metal ions as well as by various constituents and metabolic products of plant pathogens. Claims that such products exhibit the specificity of different races of a pathogen on particular cultivars have not been substantiated. In 1975, Keen proposed that *Phytophthora megasperma* var. *sojae* produced a specific elicitor of glyceollin production in soybean. The accumulation of this phytoalexin elicited by extracts from race 1 of the pathogen was more intense in incompatible (Harosoy 63) than in compatible (Harosoy) cultivars (*19*).

The nature and specificity of the "elicitor" described by Keen has been questioned by Albersheim and co-workers. They have described a glucan with many terminal mannose residues that does promote the accumulation of glyceollin in microgram quantities, but, on the basis of extraction from different compatible and incompatible races of the fungus, they concluded that this elicitor was not specific (*1*).

In our laboratories, emphasis has been given to the nature of the elicitor of disease resistance produced by *Ps. solanacearum* and other Gram-negative bacteria. With the exception of compatible bacteria, introduction of many types of bacteria, whether avirulent, alien, saprophytic, live, or heat-killed, into tobacco leaves results in a resistant response that varies in intensity and degree of systemic involvement. These bacteria are rapidly attached to and enveloped by the host cell wall (*46*) and these processes are thought to initiate the resistant response. If live, incompatible strains are infiltrated, the process ultimately results in the HR and subsequent collapse of the host cell. When heat-killed cells of the same bacterial strain are used, however, their attachment results in a systemic resistant response that inhibits multiplication of both compatible and incompatible bacteria, and of other pathogens. Initial experiments with crude bacterial extracts indicated that the inducer was associated with a specific constituent of the bacterial cell wall, but not involving the peptidoglycan layer (*49*). Recent work has established definitely that the lipopolysaccharide (LPS) of the outer bacterial membrane is the inducer of disease resistance in tobacco (*13*).

Purified LPS, extracted from whole cells, isolated cell walls, or culture filtrates from virulent (smooth) or avirulent (rough) strains of *Ps. solanacearum* induced disease resistance in tobacco. Lipopolysaccharide, obtained by extraction with phenol-water, phenol-chloroform-petroleum ether (for rough forms), and other methods, was effective in inducing disease resistance at concentrations as low as 50 μg/ml. The fact that Gram-positive, heat-killed bacteria (*i.e.*, *Bacillus polymyxa*, *B. subtilis*, *Staphylococcus aureus*, *Lactobacillus plantarum*) are ineffective as inducers of disease resistance, and that all Gram-negative bacteria tested so far (including several species of plant pathogenic *Pseudomonas*, *Xanthomonas*, *Erwinia*, and *Agrobacterium*, and saprophytes such as *Escherichia coli* and *E. aurescens*) are active inducers, is consistent with the hypothesis that LPS is the active component.

The fact that the active cell wall component from *Ps. solanacearum* that induces resistance was heat stable at temperatures up to 180°C at pH 7.0, but was unstable at lower pH values, is as expected for LPS. Inducer activity of crude preparations was not affected by proteases (trypsin, chymotrypsin, pepsin, papain, pronase), nucleases (ribonuclease, deoxyribonuclease), and phosphatases, but was destroyed by almond emulsin, a preparation that contains a nonspecific mixture of β-glycosidases. These, and previous findings, confirmed the carbohydrate nature of the inducer. Also, chromatographic separations indicated inducer activity in fractions with apparent molecular weights ranging from 20,000 to several Mdaltons. Such molecular weight heterogeneity would be expected for LPS, since it is known to aggregate readily. Further, the active fraction was found to contain fatty acids, keto-deoxy-octonoate (KDO), and heptose, all components of LPS.

Of the various components of LPS, *i.e.*, lipid A, core oligosaccharide, and O-specific polysaccharide, it is evident that the latter is not necessary for inducer activity. The B-1 mutant of *Ps. solanacearum* is a rough strain and lacks the O-polysaccharide portion of LPS, yet LPS from this strain is as active as that from smooth strains. When the linkage between lipid A and the core oligosaccharide was broken by mild acid hydrolysis, no activity could be detected in the free portions of the molecule. Thus, this linkage is required for activity, probably because the core oligosaccharide acts as a solubilizing carrier. Deacylation of the lipid A section by treatment with mild alkali resulted in total loss of activity. The results suggest that the lipid A section constitutes the active component of LPS, but must be present in a form sufficiently soluble to attach to a putative receptor on the host cell wall.

Of particular interest is the recent report by Mazzuchi and Pupillo (*33*) who indicate that protein-LPS complexes from *E. chrysanthemi* prevent confluent hypersensitive necrosis in tobacco leaves. These results are similar to ours, except that we did not find that the protein associated with LPS was necessary for activity. Because the core-lipid A section of LPS is fairly constant among Gram-negative bacteria (as opposed to the O-specific polysaccharide which is highly variable), this is consistent with the fact that LPS from a wide variety of Gram-negative bacteria will induce resistance in tobacco. This does not exclude the possibility that other cell wall components, such as those found in Gram-positive bacteria, could be effective inducers of disease resistance as well (*10*).

In keeping with the work that implicates external cell wall constituents of pathogens as inducers of disease resistance, Loebenstein (*25*) has reported that partial protection of *Nicotiana glutinosa* leaves could be obtained following treatment with dilute solutions of TMV protein. As with whole TMV, the resistance induced with TMV protein was systemic, even though there was no indication of translocation of the protein *per se*. Since protection was obtained in the absence of necrotization, Ross' hypothesis (*41*) that local lesion formation is essential for induction of systemic resistance either is not correct or refers to a different type of resistance.

In contrast with these reports, McIntyre *et al.* (*34*) have presented evidence for the possible involvement of bacterial DNA, rather than cell wall constituents, in the protection of pear shoots and seedlings against *E. amylovora.* Since deoxyribonuclease, but not ribonuclease, destroyed the protective activity, the possibility that contaminants of the DNA were involved does not appear likely. There was no indication that DNA preparations were toxic to the bacterium used in challenge inoculations, and the time-dependence and systemic nature of the response suggest a protective mechanism similar to that described previously for bacterial cell wall preparations.

III. NATURE OF THE MECHANISM OF PROTECTION

The nature of the systemic protective response has remained virtually unknown. A different mechanism has been postulated for almost every host-parasite system that has been described. In systems involving induction of localized resistance, on the other hand, the accumulation of phytoalexins does provide a reasonable explanation for the protective response against fungi. Numerous questions remain, however, and these are being discussed elsewhere in this symposium. Therefore, I shall limit this discussion to systemic resistance mechanisms.

Of particular interest are the observations of Loebenstein (*27*) concerning the possible involvement of an interferon-like substance in acquired resistance against viruses. In animals, acquired immunity following viral infection appears to depend on two general mechanisms; early in infection, a nonspecific antiviral protein, called interferon, is produced, whereas, somewhat later, antibodies with specific activity against the virus are produced. The data presented by Loebenstein indicate that the first mechanism may operate in plants. In leaves of *Datura stramonium* inoculated with TMV or TNV, noninfected parts contain a proteinaceous antiviral agent. This substance has a molecular weight in the range of 20,000 to 30,000 daltons and does not inactivate the virus *in vitro*, but, when mixed with inocula, it will reduce the number of lesions obtained. In contrast with these reports, Sela *et al.* (*42*) have implicated an RNA fraction as the protection factor in uninfected leaves of *N. glutinosa* plants previously infected on their lower leaves with TMV. It is unfortunate that the nature and function of these antiviral systemic factors remain unconfirmed.

Kassanis *et al.* (*18*) have reported that systemic resistance in tobacco leaves inoculated with several different viruses was correlated with the appearance of at least three proteins not present in healthy plants. The proteins themselves are not responsible for the resistant response, however. Injection of preparations containing these proteins into tobacco plants did not increase their resistance to TMV.

In tobacco plants that acquire resistance by prior inoculation with viruses and/or heat-killed bacteria, peroxidase increases substantially (*29, 39, 47*). This appears to depend on a light-dependent transfer of proteins from the leaf cell to the intercellular fluid. Although this may be due in part to leakage of cellular contents into the intercellular spaces due to injury, the active transfer of proteins only in illuminated leaves indicates that the cells must be metabolically active (*39*). It is not clear, however, how peroxidase is involved in generalized resistance responses. Increases in peroxidase activity can be detected in tissues distant from the site of initial inoculation and are correlated with the appearance of resistance (*47*), but these changes may have been triggered by translocatable substances, such as ethylene (*37*). Peroxidase may be involved, however, in formation of the antiviral or antibacterial compounds through synthesis of lignin-related compounds.

Rathmell and Sequeira (*39*) reported the presence of antibacterial substances in the intercellular fluid of protected tobacco leaves. These compounds were secreted only under light conditions that result in the development of resistance, are heat-stable, and of low molecular weight. One of the active compounds appears to be a terpenoid (Kraus, unpublished). A terpenoid inhibitor of germination of *P. tabacina* has been isolated from leaves of tobacco plants previously stem-inoculated with the fungus (*23*).

Of recent interest has been the possible involvement of agglutinating factors in induced resistance against bacterial plant pathogens. Many plants contain lectins that can bind to specific carbohydrates present in bacterial cell walls. For instance, agglutination of Gram-negative bacteria *in vitro* by potato lectin, which binds specifically to the internal N-acetyl glucosamine groups present in bacterial LPS, has been reported (*43*). Goodman and coworkers (*12*) have reported that, within the xylem vessels of apple petioles, avirulent cells of *E. amylovora* are clumped by granules that are thought to be lectin-like. Similarly, agglutinating factors were recovered from fluids of tobacco leaves previously infiltrated with *P. pisi*. Horino (*17*) provided evidence for similar phenomena in rice leaves protected by inoculation with incompatible strains of *X. oryeae*. Although it was suggested that lectins are involved in these agglutination reactions, the nature of these phenomena remains obscure.

Evidence from both ultrasturctural and biochemical studies of protection induced in tobacco leaves by heat-killed bacterial cells suggests that lectins are involved in the process that initiates the resistance response (*43, 46*). A lectin which binds LPS from *Ps. solanacearum* can be extracted from tobacco leaves by infiltration with saline and, thus, is presumed to be loosely attached to the host cell wall. Purified LPS clearly binds to the tobacco cell wall. Lectin concentration increases following infiltration of tobacco cells with heat-killed bacteria. Granular material can be seen surrounding the bacterium at the point of attachment, and also in the space between the

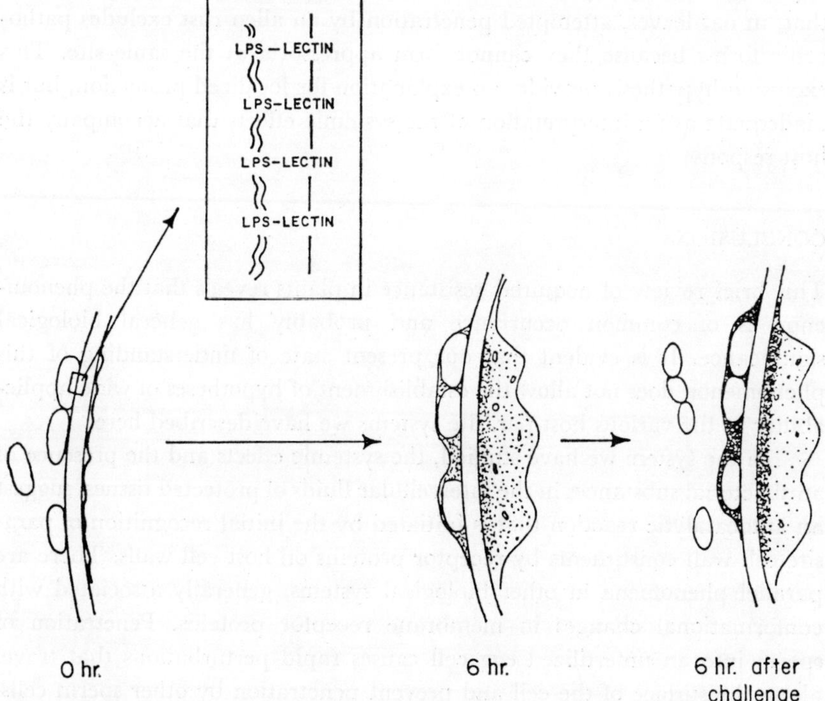

Fig. 1. Mechanism for induced resistance that results from attachment of heat-killed bacteria on the cell walls of tobacco mesophyll cell walls.

plasmalemma and the host cell wall. This host reaction extends for several micrometers beyond the site of attachment, but the granular material surrounding the bacterium remains contained by a membrane or "pellicle" and does not diffuse throughout the intercellular spaces. Challenge inoculation of protected leaves does not reveal extensive agglutination and/or attachment of the superinfecting bacteria (*46*), although bacterial populations are reduced (*44*). Thus, lectins may be involved in the initial recognition phenomenon that results in a protective response, but do not appear to be involved in the protection phenomenon itself (Fig. 1).

A possible explanation of these phenomena involves the saturation of available attachment sites following inoculation with avirulent or heat-killed bacteria, or LPS. This has been proposed for the protective effects against *Agrobacterium tumefaciens* infection in Pinto beans obtained by prior treatment with avirulent forms (*50*). The principle of exclusion may be applicable to fungal systems as well. Kochman and Brown (*21*) have shown that, in oat leaves, attempted penetration by an alien rust excludes pathogenic forms because they cannot form appressoria at the same site. This exclusion hypothesis provides an explanation for localized protection, but is inadequate as an interpretation of the systemic effects that accompany the host response.

CONCLUSIONS

This brief review of acquired resistance in plants reveals that the phenomenon is of common occurrence and probably has general biological significance. It is evident that our present state of understanding of this phenomenon does not allow the establishment of hypotheses of wide applicability to the various host-parasite systems we have described here.

In the system we have studied, the systemic effects and the presence of antibacterial substances in the intercellular fluids of protected tissues, suggest an autocatalytic reaction that is initiated by the initial recognition of parasite cell wall constituents by receptor proteins on host cell walls. There are parallel phenomena in other biological systems, generally associated with conformational changes in membrane receptor proteins. Penetration of sperm into an unfertilized egg cell causes rapid perturbations that travel along the surface of the cell and prevent penetration by other sperm cells. Mating reactions in *Chlamydomonas* and *Hansenula* are accompanied by rapid loss of surface components responsible for initial recognition. One can speculate that similar, long-lasting perturbations may be responsible for the inability of pathogens to establish themselves in tissues previously exposed to other pathogens.

SUMMARY

Many plant pathogens induce systemic, nonspecific, protective reactions in tissues of potential hosts. These reactions can be demonstrated by challenge inoculation at a point distant from that initially inoculated, and cannot be induced by chemical or mechanical injury to plant cells. Induced resistance is dependent on a) the time interval between the initial and the challenge inoculations, b) temperature, and c) light, in most of the systems that have been studied. As opposed to localized resistance, which appears to be the result of phytoalexin induction, systemic resistance spreads from the site of initial inoculation and may involve the entire plant. In the tobacco-*Ps. solanacearum* system, the systemic effects and the presence of antibacterial substances in the intercellular fluids of protected tissues suggest an autocatalytic reaction that is initiated after recognition of parasite cell wall constituents by receptor proteins on host cell walls. The LPS of the outer bacterial membrane appears to be the inducer of disease resistance in tobacco. Alteration of LPS by chemical treatments suggest that the lipid A (endotoxin) portion constitutes the active portion of LPS. The receptors for LPS appear to be lectins on the surface of tobacco mesophyll cell walls. The nature of the systemic protective response has remained virtually unknown. In the case of acquired resistance against viruses, the involvement of interferon-like proteins and of peroxidases has been suggested. In systems involving bacteria, the presence of agglutinins and of low-molecular weight inhibitors of bacterial growth has been demonstrated in protected tissues. It is evident that long-lasting perturbations of host cell metabolism are responsible for the inability of pathogens to establish themselves in tissues previously exposed to other pathogens.

REFERENCES

1. Ayers, A. R., B. Valent, J. Ebel, and P. Albersheim. 1976. Host parasite interactions. XI. Composition and structure of wall-released elicitor fractions. *Plant Physiol.* **57**: 766–774.
2. Berard, D. F., J. Kuć, and E. B. Williams. 1972. A cultivar specific protection

factor from incompatible interactions of green bean with *Colletotrichum lindemuthianum. Physiol. Plant Pathol.* **2**: 123–128.

3. Brown, N. A. 1923. Experiments with paris daisy and rose to produce resistance to crown gall. *Phytopathology* **13**: 87–99.
4. Carroll, R. B. and F. L. Lukezic. 1972. Induced resistance in alfalfa to *Corynebacterium insidiosum* by prior treatment with avirulent cells. *Phytopathology* **62**: 555–563.
5. Crandall, M. A. and J. H. Caulton. 1975. Induction of haploid glycoprotein mating factors in diploid yeasts. *In*: D. M. Prescott (ed.). *Methods in Cell Biology*. vol. XII. Academic Press, New York, pp. 186–207.
6. Cruickshank, I. A. M. and M. Mandryk. 1960. The effect of stem infestation of tobacco with *Peronospora tabacina* Adam. on foliage reaction to blue mould. *J. Aust. Inst. Agric. Sci.* **26**: 369–372.
7. Cruickshank, I. A. M. and D. R. Perrin. 1965. Studies on phytoalexins. VIII. The effect of some further factors on the formation, stability, and localization of pisatin *in vivo*. *Aust. J. Biol. Sci.* **18**: 817–828.
8. de Zoeten, G. A. and R. W. Fulton. 1975. Understanding generates possibilities. *Phytopathology* **65**: 221–222.
9. Elliston, J., J. Kuć, and E. B. Williams. 1976. Protection of *Phaseolus vulgaris* against anthracnose by *Colletotrichum* species nonpathogenic to bean. *Phytopathol. Z.* **86**: 117–126.
10. Gianinazzi, S. and C. Martin. 1976. Nouvelles connaissances sur l'immunité acquise chez les végétaux. *Physiol. Veg.* **14**: 133–139.
11. Goodman, R. N. 1967. Protection of apple stem tissue against *Erwinia amylovora* infection by avirulent strains and three other bacterial species. *Phytopathology* **57**: 22–24.
12. Goodman, R. N., P. Y. Huang, J. S. Huang, and V. Thaipanich. 1976. Induced resistance to bacterial infection. *In*: K. Tomiyama, J. M. Daly, I. Uritani, H. Oku, and S. Ouchi (eds.). *Biochemistry and Cytology of Plant-Parasite Interaction.* Kodansha Ltd., Tokyo and Elsevier, New York, pp. 35–42.
13. Graham, T. L., L. Sequeira, and T. R. Huang. 1977. Bacterial lipopolysaccharides as inducers of disease resistance in tobacco. *Appl. Environ. Microbiol.* **34**: 424–432.
14. Hammerschmidt, R., S. Acres, and J. Kuć. 1976. Protection of cucumber against *Colletotrichum lagenarium* and *Cladosporium cucumerinum*. *Phytopathology* **66**: 790–793.
15. Hecht, E. I. and D. F. Bateman. 1964. Nonspecific acquired resistance to pathogens resulting from localized infections by *Thielaviopsis basicola* or viruses in tobacco plants. *Phytopathology* **54**: 523–530.
16. Heslop-Harrison, J. 1975. Incompatibility and the pollen-stigma interaction. *Annu. Rev. Plant Physiol.* **26**: 403–425.

17. Horino, O. 1976. Induction of bacterial leaf blight resistance by incompatible strains of *Xanthomonas oryzae* in rice. *In*: K. Tomiyama, J. M. Daly, I. Uritani, H. Oku, and S. Ouchi (eds.). *Biochemistry and Cytology of Plant-Parasite Interaction.* Kodansha Ltd., Tokyo and Elsevier, New York, pp. 34–55.

18. Kassanis, B., S. Gianinazzi, and R. F. White. 1974. A possible explanation of the resistance of virus-infected tobacco plants to second infection. *J. Gen. Virol.* **23**: 11–16.

19. Keen, N. T. 1974. Specific elicitors of plant phytoalexin production: determinants of race specificity in pathogens. *Science* **187**: 74–75.

20. Klement, Z. and R. N. Goodman. 1968. The hypersensitive reaction to infection bacterial plant pathogens. *Annu. Rev. Phytopathol.* **5**: 17–44.

21. Kochman, J. K. and J. F. Brown. 1975. Studies on the mechanism of cross-protection in cereal rusts. *Physiol. Plant Pathol.* **6**: 19–28.

22. Kuć, J., G. Shockley, and K. Kearney. 1975. Protection of cucumber against *Colletotrichum lagenarium* by *Colletotrichum lagenarium. Physiol. Plant Pathol.* **7**: 195–200.

23. Leppik, R. A., D. W. Hallomon, and W. Bottomly. 1972. Quiesone: an inhibitor of the germination of *Peronospora tabacina* conidia. *Phytochemistry* **11**: 2055–2063.

24. Littlefield, L. J. 1969. Flax rust resistance induced by prior inoculation with an avirulent race of *Melampsora lini. Phytopathology* **59**: 1323–1328.

25. Loebenstein, G. 1962. Inducing partial protection in the host plant with native virus protein. *Virology* **17**: 574–581.

26. Loebenstein, G. and L. Lovrekovich. 1966. Interference with tobacco mosaic virus local lesion formation in tobacco by injecting heat-killed cells of *Pseudomonas syringae. Virology* **30**: 587–591.

27. Loebenstein, G., S. Rabina, and T. van Praagh. 1966. Induced interference phenomena in virus infections. *In*: A. B. R. Beemster and J. Djikstra (eds.). *Viruses of Plants.* North-Holland Publ., Amsterdam, pp. 151–157.

28. Lovrekovich, L. and G. L. Farkas. 1965. Induced protection against wildfire disease in tobacco leaves treated with heat-killed bacteria. *Nature* **205**: 823–824.

29. Lovrekovich, L., H. Lovrekovich, and M. A. Stahmann. 1968. The importance of peroxidase in the wildfire disease. *Phytopathology* **58**: 193–198.

30. Lozano, J. C. and L. Sequeira. 1970. Prevention of the hypersensitive reaction in tobacco leaves by heat-killed cells of *Pseudomonas solanacearum. Phytopathology* **60**: 875–879.

31. Mandryk, M. 1963. Acquired systemic resistance to tobacco mosaic virus in *Nicotiana tabacum* evoked by stem injection with *Peronospora tabacina* Adam. *Aust. J. Agric. Res.* **14**: 315–318.

32. Matta, A. 1971. Microbial penetration and immunization of uncongenial host plants. *Annu. Rev. Phytopathol.* **9**: 387–410.

33. Mazzuchi, U. and P. Pupillo. 1976. Prevention of confluent hypersensitive

necrosis in tobacco leaves by a bacterial protein-lipopolysaccharide complex. *Physiol. Plant Pathol.* **9**: 101–112.

34. McIntyre, J. L., J. Kuć, and E. B. Williams. 1975. Protection of Bartlett pear against fire blight with deoxyribonucleic acid from virulent and avirulent *Erwinia amylovora*. *Physiol. Plant Pathol.* **7**: 153–170.
35. McKinney, H. H. 1929. Mosaic diseases in the Canary Islands, West Africa and Gibraltar. *J. Agric. Res.* **39**: 557–578.
36. Müller, K. and H. Börger. 1940. Experimentelle Untersuchungen uber die *Phytophthora*-resistenz der Kartoffel. *Arb. Biol. Reichsanst. Land Forstwirtsch. (Berlin)* **23**: 189–231.
37. Pritchard, D. W. and A. F. Ross. 1975. The relationship of ethylene to formation of tobacco mosaic virus lesions in hypersensitive responding tobacco leaves with and without induced resistance. *Virology* **64**: 295–307.
38. Rahe, J. E., J. Kuć, C. M. Chuang, and E. B. Williams. 1969. Induced resistance in *Phaseolus vulgaris* to bean anthracnose. *Phytopathology* **59**: 1641–1645.
39. Rathmell, W. G. and L. Sequeira. 1975. Induced resistance in tobacco leaves: the role of inhibitors of bacterial growth in the intercellular fluid. *Physiol. Plant Pathol.* **5**: 65–73.
40. Ross, A. F. 1961. Systemic acquired resistance to plant virus infection in hypersensitive hosts. *Virology* **14**: 329–339.
41. Ross, A. F. 1965. Systemic effects of local lesion formation. *In*: A. B. R. Beemster and J. Djikstra (eds.). *Viruses of Plants.* North-Holland Publ., Amsterdam, pp. 127–150.
42. Sela, I., I. Harpaz, and Y. Birk. 1966. Identification of the active component of an antiviral factor isolated from virus-infected plants. *Virology* **28**: 71–78.
43. Sequeira, L. and T. L. Graham. 1977. Agglutination of avirulent strains of *Pseudomonas solanacearum* by potato lectin. *Physiol. Plant Pathol.* **11**: 43–54.
44. Sequeira, L. and L. M. Hill. 1974. Induced resistance in tobacco leaves: the growth of *Pseudomonas solanacearum* in protected tissues. *Physiol. Plant Pathol.* **4**: 447–455.
45. Sequeira, L., S. Aist, and V. Ainslie. 1972. Prevention of the hypersensitive reaction in tobacco by proteinaceous constituents of *Pseudomonas solanacearum*. *Phytopathology* **62**: 536–542.
46. Sequeira, L., G. Gaard, and G. A. de Zoeten. 1977. Attachment of bacteria to host cell walls: its relation to mechanisms of induced resistance. *Physiol. Plant Pathol.* **10**: 43–50.
47. Simons, T. J. and A. F. Ross. 1970. Enhanced peroxidase activity associated with induction of resistance to tobacco mosaic virus in hypersensitive tobacco. *Phytopathology* **60**: 383–384.
48. Smith, E. F., N. A. Brown, and C. O. Townsend. 1911. Crown gall of plants: its cause and remedy. *U. S. Dept. Ag. Bur. Plant Indus. Bull.* 213.

49. Wacek, T. J. and L. Sequeira. 1973. The peptidoglycan of *Pseudomonas solanacearum*: chemical composition and biological activity in relation to the hypersensitive reaction in tobacco. *Physiol. Plant Pathol.* **3**: 363–369.
50. Whatley, M. H., J. S. Bodwin, B. B. Lippincott, and J. A. Lippincott. 1976. Role for Agrobacterium cell envelope lipopolysaccharide in infection site attachment. *Infect. Immun.* **13**: 1080–1083.
51. Wiese, L. 1974. Nature of sex specific glycoprotein agglutinins in *Chlamydomonas*. *Ann. N. Y. Acad. Sci.* **234**: 383–395.

Discussion of Paper by Dr. Sequeira

Tomiyama opened by observing that some conceptual difficulties seem to exist when the hypersensitive response (HR) is studied. For example, in potato-*Phytophthora* the hypersensitive reaction is a resistance phenomena, while in Sequeira's studies it appears to indicate susceptibility. Sequeira acknowledged the conceptual difficulties but pointed out that HR is associated with resistance and over the years has been assumed to be initimately involved, but has not been experimentally tested for a role. As others have pointed out, it may be a secondary response, an expression of resistance. If plants are inoculated with a avirulent bacteria, cells die very quickly in typical HR fashion. Heat-killed cells do not cause this, but still the tissue is resistant; in fact, the resistance is systemic not localized. Further, there is a threshold level of about 10^7 cells per inoculation in order to cause HR in tobacco, but if 10^2 to 10^3 cells are used there is no visible HR. Dr. Goodman would argue that the hypersensitive response is occurring in individual cells, it is not confluent and that's the reason why HR is not seen. Kuć agreed with Sequeira's summary and described his work with cucumbers showing that inoculation of the first leaf protects this leaf and all other leaves starting 4–5 days after the first inoculation, even after the inoculated leaf is removed. Daly focused on one apparently significant difference between the phenomenon described by Sequeira and Kuć, that is, the requirement in Sequeira's system for the inducing leaf to be retained, and asked if biochemicals changes had been measured in that leaf. Sequeira reported that they had looked at respiration, photosynthesis and some enzyme activity, particularly in the shikimic acid pathway, but only minor changes were found. However, the contents of the intercellular space is rich in inorganic ions and organic components but to date the significance for disease was not understood. Daly and Dunkle then asked why it was necessary to assume that a factor for resistance was exported from the inoculated leaf rather than a substance in the upper leaves becoming transported to the lower leaves. Sequeira agreed that since removing the inducing leaf shortened protection of the upper leaves the process was possible. Kuć, however, has noted no protection below the inoculated leaf as one argument for export from that leaf. Wheeler called attention to early work by T. Pirone and Wheeler in which victorin applied to a non-host bean leaf induce nearly complete resistance to local lesion formation by TMV. Recent results suggest that the effect can be induced with 1 hr of exposure to toxin followed by immediate inoculation with TMV and is fully developed by 4 hr. Sequeira acknowledged interest in the original report because they also considered and have not abandoned the idea of a repair mechanism coming into play as suggested by Wheeler. In response to his comment that the situation may be dissimilar from bacteria, Wheeler pointed to the fact that bean is considered to be hypersensitivity resistant to virus. Since treatment with victorin still permits virus multiplication, perhaps victorin is preventing necrosis *per se*. In response to Daly's question as to whether the cytological events saw localized protection in the challenged leaf were also observed in the systemically protected leaves, Sequeria reported they had not established this but noted that purified LPS causes the same systemic protection and that the response in the treated leaf is identical to heat-killed cells. Uritani asked if LPS might be recognized by a lectin and called to the possible role of lectins in virus infection such as those described by Wheeler. Although feeling that possibility existed, Sequeira observed that some viruses have only protein coats. A considerable discussion developed among Keen, Uritani, and Sequeira as a consequence of Keen's question about a potencial role for ethylene in protection. Sequeira cited work from his laboratory and others suggesting that ethylene production does occur and may be important. Further, in his work, a new peroxidase increases in tissue protected by heat-killed cells. However, it does not increase with LPS protection and thus its role, particularly for ethylene biosynthesis, remains obscure.

Recognition and Specificity in Plant Host-Parasite Interactions, pp. 253-272, 1979

RECOGNITION AND SPECIFICITY IN PLANT VIRUS INFECTION

ALBERT SIEGEL

Department of Biology, Wayne State University, Detroit, Michigan U.S.A.

There appears to be a commonality in at least some aspects of the interaction of pathogens with higher plants because it has been observed that plants sometimes respond in a similar manner to infection by viruses, bacteria and fungi. It is not unlikely, therefore, that some of the general principles governing higher plant-pathogen interaction may be deduced from a comparative view of plant response to the different kinds of pathogens. It is to help provide such an overview that a brief survey is presented here of some of the responses of higher plants to virus infection together with a review of current knowledge concerning the plant virus life cycle.*

Just as with plant pathogenic fungi, the association of a virus with its host is an intimate one, whether the host be a plant, animal, fungus, protist or bacterium. The intimacy of the association derives from the fact that viruses can only replicate inside living cells and, thus, are in all cases obligate parasites. Viruses are inert in the extracellular stage of their life cycle when they consist at a minimum of either one or a few nucleic acid molecules

* The reader is referred to textbooks (*16, 24, 33*) for more extensive coverage of much of the subject matter dealt with here. In addition, reviews of specialized topics of plant virology can be found in Advances in Virus Research and Annual Review of Phytopathology.

usually encased in a capsid composed of many protein molecules, either all identical or of only a few different types. In addition, some virus particles contain membranous material and carbohydrate moieties. Viruses can be thought of as bits of genetic material packaged in a coat which protects the genetic material from degradation and which also sometimes aids in the initiation of infection.

As far as is known the genetic material of all cellular organisms is DNA and, as Watson and Crick (*52*) have shown, it has a double-stranded structure. The genetic material of viruses, however, may be other than double-stranded DNA and Baltimore (*3*) has classified viruses on the basis of their genomic constitution as follows:

Class I	double-stranded DNA
Class II	single-stranded DNA
Class III	double-stranded RNA
Class IV	single-stranded RNA of the same polarity as viral messenger RNA (+ strand)
Class V	single-stranded RNA opposite in polarity to viral messenger RNA (− strand)
Class VI	single-stranded RNA (+ strand) which is transcribed to DNA for replication
Class VII	single-stranded RNA which does not contain structural genes and does not become encapsidated (viroid)

Most of the plant viruses so far characterized contain single plus stranded RNA genomes and, thus, belong to Class IV. Plant viruses are also known which are members of all of the other classes with the exception of Class VI which so far appears to be limited to vertebrates.

There are a number of different groups of Class IV plant viruses of which 19 have so far received official recognition by the International Committee on Taxonomy of Viruses (*11*). The groups are distinguished on the basis of a number of properties, primary among which are morphology and the number of pieces of RNA which comprise the genome. The extracellular virus particles of the different groups are either rod-shaped (rigid or flexous) or icosahedral (crudely resembling a sphere). Within each morphological class, there are groups which contain undivided genomes and groups in which the genetic material is divided among several (*2–4*) RNA strands. The Class IV split genome viruses are unique in having the parts of their genomes separately encapsidated so that several different virus particles are required for successful infection in contrast to the undivided genome groups where only one is necessary.

I. THE VIRUS LIFE CYCLE

The steps in the life cycle of plant viruses can be summarized as follows:

1) An infecting virus particle gains entry into a living cell.
2) The genome of the virus particle is released from its protein coat.
3) The viral RNA is translated.
4) The viral RNA is replicated.
5) New virus particles are assembled from preformed nucleic acid and protein molecules.
6) Virus particles spread to previously uninfected cells and hosts.

1. *Methods of Inoculation*

1) Vectors: In order for infection to occur virus particles must be transferred from an external source to at least one cell of a previously uninfected host plant. In nature, this is most frequently mediated by a living non-plant vector which obtains infectious virus particles from either an infected plant or plant debris and then introduces virus particles into cells of another plant incidentally to feeding or other type of vector-plant relationship. Among the vectors of plant viruses are a variety of insects, mites, fungi, and nematodes. Prominent among the insect vectors are aphids and leafhoppers, although certain species of white flies, thrips, mealy bugs, beetles, and grasshoppers are also known to be vectors. Most of the fungal vectors are species of *Olpidium, Spongospora,* and *Polymyxa.* A range of vector-virus relationships have been recognized, at the extremes being the non-persistant and persistant types. The non-persistant, or what is in many cases synonymous, stylet born relationship, describes the situation in which the vector acquires virus after a short feeding period on an infected host plant (*2–5* min), can immediately transmit the virus to a healthy plant, and then rapidly (minutes) loses the ability to infect. Although it might seem at first sight that in this type of transmission the virus is carried passively from one plant to another on the vector mouth parts, there are a number of compelling reasons for believing that the situation is considerably more complicated. In the persistant, or circulative, relationship the time of feeding for acquisition of virus by the vector is usually longer than in the non-persistant relationship and, following acquisition, there is a latent period of hours to days before virus can be transmitted to a new host but once the vector does become infective, it remains so for an extended period of time, days to weeks. In extreme cases of the persistant relationship, the virus multiplies in both the plant host and the vector and this situation is called propagative. Most instances of the propagative relationship are found to occur with some of the Class III and Class V plant viruses which can multiply usually both in a leafhopper vector and in the plant host. In some cases of the propagative relationship the virus is transmitted vertically through the vector by transovarian passage.

The reason for dwelling on the different modes of vector transmission is to point out that a large part of recognition and specificity in the plant host-virus interaction in nature does not depend directly on virus and host but rather is frequently mediated indirectly by recognition and specificity between virus and vector and between plant and vector. Thus, some viruses are transmitted by a number of different species all of which, however, are usually closely related. In like manner some vectors are known to transmit only one or at most a few different viruses, whereas others, such as the aphid *Myzus persicae*, become important virus disease spreading agents because they can transmit many different viruses and can feed on many different plants. The interactions which lead to successful virus transmission, those between vector and virus and between vector and plant, are in some cases highly specific and in others the specificities are somewhat, but not altogether relaxed.

2) Mechanical inoculation: Not all viruses are transmitted from plant to plant by vectors but instead are spread by rubbing of an infected plant against a previously virus-free plant or by an animal first rubbing against one plant and then another. Such viruses are said to be mechanically or sap-transmitted. Man frequently becomes an agent in the transmission of such viruses particularly in those crops where manipulation of plants is part of horticultural practice. Not only are viruses without other known or suspected vectors sap-transmissable but so are many viruses that are normally vector transmitted. There are, however, a number of viruses which so far have been resistant to attempts at mechanical inoculation primarily, it is thought, because they appear to be localized in the phloem. In the case of viruses which are normally vector transmitted but can also be sap-transmitted, the latter inoculation route bypasses the vector-plant and vector-virus interactions in providing recognition and specificity between plant and virus. In such cases it is frequently found that the host range of the virus is greater by experimental sap-inoculation than by the known vector transmission routes.

It is a common observation that plants are completely resistant to virus penetration and can be immersed in solutions containing high concentrations of virus without becoming infected. In order to become infected by mechanical inoculation, the tissue must first sustain injury. Experimentally, this is accomplished by gentle rubbing of the surface of a leaf, usually in the presence of virus and a mild abrasive. The number of infections induced by this procedure is a function of the concentration of virus in the inoculum and this procedure forms the basis of an assay for amount of infectious virus under circumstances where the individual infections can be visualized. Quantitative analysis of the mechanical inoculation process leads to the conception that abrasion of a leaf surface creates a number of infectible sites which have a distribution in the ease with which they can be converted to infective centers. The infectible sites are converted to infective centers if they came into contact with virus particles before they decay (*14, 15, 44*). Although the foregoing is a valid description of the infectious process, its initimate details are little more known except that somehow a virus particle must gain entry into a living cell, perhaps through ectodesmata (*34*) to start an infection.

3) *Protoplasts:* A third type of inoculation is that accomplished when plant protoplasts are exposed to virus under appropriate conditions, the appropriate conditions appearing to be adjustment of the surface charge of the virus particles so they will interact with and not be repelled by the plasma membrane (*40, 53*). It is most appropriate to discuss plant protoplasts especially as they apply to virus study because of the pioneering work done in this field by Japanese colleagues (*49, 50*). It is found that recognition and specificity of the plant-virus interaction is reduced below that found with mechanical inoculation when the virus-protoplast system is examined. For instance, several viruses such as cucumber mosaic, cowpea chlorotic mosaic, pea enation mosaic, brome mosaic, cowpea mosaic, and cucumber green mottle mosaic that do not visibly react with or cause apparent infection of tobacco plants can, nevertheless, infect and multiply to high titer in protoplasts derived from tobacco leaf mesophyll.

It is seen from the foregoing that the specificity of the plant-virus reaction depends on the route of inoculation, being most restrictive when mediated by a vector, less so with direct mechanical inoculation and apparently least with the protoplast system. The precise mechanism of virus entry into a host cell may be different depending on the inoculation technique, whether *via* vector, by mechanical inoculation or by exposure of protoplasts and in all cases a complete understanding of the processes remains to be obtained.

2. *Removal of the Protein Coat*

The second stage of the virus life cycle that may be concomitant with cell entry is the freeing of the viral nucleic acid from its capsid so that its genetic information may be expressed in the cell. Although a number of methods have been devised for the *in vitro* recovery of both the protein(s) and nucleic acid of many viruses, little is known of the mechanism by which this is accomplished by the cell or upon entry into the cell. It is known that upon mechanical inoculation of a leaf, the few virus particles in the inoculum that become responsible for the further events of infection are removed from the extracellular milieu almost immediately after inoculation, for at this time they can neither be washed from the leaf nor be inactivated by anti-serum although the bulk of the inoculum virus can be readily recovered from the leaf in still infectious form by washing (*13, 15, 44*). Estimates have been made of the time involved for stripping from the differences observed in the time course of infection induced by virus particles as compared with free nucleic acid. The limited number of estimates that have been made indicate a 2-hr period for release of the viral RNA from its capsid (*25, 45*).

3. *Translation of Viral RNA*

Cellular RNA is transcribed from cellular DNA and no known mechanism is present in uninfected cells for the replication of RNA from an RNA template. Thus, the replication of Class IV viral RNA requires the generation of an RNA-dependent RNA polymerase and, according to our present surmise, such an enzyme, or at least part of one, must be coded for by the viral RNA. Thus, it is reasonable to assume that translation of the infecting RNA must occur before its replication (somewhat different considerations apply to the Class V and VI single-stranded RNA viruses). The viral RNA genome must contain genes which specify several proteins as well as recognition sequences for an RNA replicating enzyme. At a minimum, nucleotide sequences must be present to code for the RNA replicase (or part of it) and the capsid protein(s) although, it would not be surprising to find others. The point is that the viral genome is by necessity multi-genic. This presents a difficulty because eucaryotic cells differ from procaryotes in an important aspect of translation mechanism. Whereas procaryote translation machinery can make starts at several different places on a polycistronic RNA and synthesize several different proteins from a single messenger RNA molecule, eucaryotes normally can initiate at only one place on an RNA and, thus, normally synthesize and translate primarily monocistronic RNAs (*22, 26*). Several strategies have evolved for the translation of the multigenic viral RNA genomes. The animal polio virus translation strategy stands at one extreme. In this case the undivided genome is translated into a polyprotein which is then split into functional virus-specific proteins by limited, specific protease action (*22, 26*). The tobacco mosaic virus strategy stands at the other extreme. Here, the undivided genome is processed during infection to form at least one monocistronic messenger RNA, that for capsid protein (*20, 48*). Whether other virus-specific monocistronic messengers are produced during infection or whether the remaining gene product(s) is translated from a viral RNA length messenger is not clear. The split-genome viruses have evolved still another strategy. In this case the genome comes in several, mostly monocistronic pieces so that problems concerned on the one hand with polyprotein synthesis and cleavage and, on the other, with RNA processing are largely, but not completely, obviated (*30*). To take an example, the brome mosaic virus genome is divided among three RNA molecules; two are monocistronic messengers for proteins whose functions have yet to be defined and the third, which is dicistronic, is processed during infection to give rise to a fourth RNA species which proves to be the monocistronic messenger for capsid protein (*42, 43*). Although the details of plant virus RNA translation are not completely known, it can be deduced that the appearance of monocistronic messengers offers an opportunity for control of the relative rates of synthesis of the different virus-specified proteins. The monocistronic capsid protein messenger RNAs prove to be extremely efficient in stimulating the synthesis of the specified protein in cell free systems (*19, 42*) and probably are also efficient *in vivo* messengers. When protoplasts are synchronously infected with tobacco mosaic virus and then pulse-labeled with a radioactive protein precursor for sequential 2 hr periods it is found that synthesis of capsid protein can first be detected between 5 and 7 hr post-inoculation and that by 24 hr fully 50% of the cellular protein synthesis is that of viral capsid protein. By 2 days after inoculation this number increases to 70% (*46*).

4. *Replication of Viral RNA*

As pointed out earlier, one of the products of translation of the viral genome is presumed to be a protein(s) involved in the replication of viral RNA. Such an enzyme has been well characterized for a Class IV bacterial virus, where it has been found that the viral RNA replicase is a tetramer composed of three host-coded proteins and one that is viral-coded (*9*). As yet, complete characterization of a plant virus induced RNA replicase is not at hand although, in the several cases examined, it has been found to be membrane bound (*7, 37, 41*). Perhaps the best characterized enzyme to date is that for turnip yellow mosaic virus which has been solubilized without appreciable loss of activity and shown to be rather specific in its acceptance of the inciting viral RNA as template (*35*). Two new species of RNA are found in extracts of infected tissue with properties that suggest that they might be intermediates in the replicative process. They are called replicative forms (RF) and replicative intermediate (RI), the former being a double stranded structure composed of one strand of viral RNA and one strand of its complement and the latter resembling RF but containing, in addition, single stranded tails. Although the details of the replicative process are still to be solved, the available evidence points particularly to RI as being an intermediate in the synthesis of new viral RNA strands (*21, 27*). The active participation of a double-stranded structure in viral RNA replication indicates that this process resembles DNA replication in the sense that viral RNA acts as a template for its complement and the complement, in turn acts as a template for new strands of viral RNA.

5. *Assembly of Virus Particles*

The replication of virus is unique in that, unlike cells, viruses do not grow in mass and then divide to form two. Rather, the viral components are synthesized separately and new virus particles are formed by the assembly of these presynthesized molecules. The *in vitro* conditions for assembly of a number of different plant viruses have been determined (*29*) and, although these are in most cases quite different from the conditions which might prevail intracellularly, the fact that *in vitro* assembly is possible at all without enzymatic aid leads to the supposition that the self-assembly process is also operative *in vivo*.

6. *Spread of Infection to New Cells*

This final step in the viral life cycle to be considered is that of spread of infection to new cells and to a new host. We have already considered vector and mechanical transmission of virus from one plant to another and also quite briefly the spread of virus to new cells within a plant. I wish at this point to consider some additional points of intraplant virus movement with the reminder that there are two aspects to consider. One is cell to cell spread, presumable *via* plasmodesmata, and the other is movement over longer distances in the vascular system. In regard to cell to cell movement the question is raised as to what is the nature of the infectious agent that moves from one cell to another. It is known that nucleoprotein virus particles are unnecessary for cell to cell spread because two cases are known in which infection spreads from cell to cell despite the fact that the infectious entity is a replicating nucleic acid without virus particle formation (*31, 47*). It has been suggested that the usual mode of cell to cell spread is *via* nucleic acid rather than virus particles (*38*) but this notion is in dispute because a number of observations of virus particles in plasmodesmata have been recorded (*8, 10, 28*). However, in those cases for which evidence is available, only nucleoprotein virus particles and not virus nucleic acid can be transported through the vascular system to reinitiate infection at a site distant from the original infection locus (*34, 35*).

II. PLANT RESPONSE TO VIRUS INOCULATION

1. The Systemic Response

In the systemic response virus replicates in the initially infected cell and the infection then spreads to neighboring cells probably *via* plasmodesmata. Virus also enters the conducting elements and is moved to sites distant from the initial infective center where secondary infection is established. In many cases very young leaves near the growing point become infected and disease symptoms then usually become apparent on these leaves when they expand. An inoculated mature leaf usually supports the multiplication of virus to a high concentration but whether or not symptoms develop depends on the virus-host combination and environmental conditions. The relationship between virus multiplication and consequent disease symptoms is poorly understood but is known to be dependent upon, among other factors, environmental conditions, the virus-host combination, and the physiological condition and age of the host tissue at the time it becomes infected.

2. The Hypersensitive Response

The hypersensitive or local lesion host response is characterized by the spread of virus from initially infected cells to neighboring cells followed by death of the patch of infected cells to form a necrotic lesion. Lesions usually became apparent from 2 to 6 days following inoculation and some reach their final size immediately upon tissue collapse whereas others spread with time (*32, 38*). In most cases virus is confined to the lesion and immediately adjacent tissue although there can be escapes of virus for systemic infection dependent on the host-virus system and environmental conditions, particularly temperature. The hypersensitive response is genetically determined both on the part of the plant and the virus. For example, the local lesion response towards tobacco mosaic virus has been shown to be determined by a dominant allele at a single gene locus. *Nicotiana tabacum* cv. Xanthi and *N. glutinosa* have this allele and respond in a hypersensitive manner to all strains of tobacco mosaic virus but also support the systemic multiplication of a large number of other viruses. A different situation applies to *N. sylvestris*. This "differential host" is hypersensitive when inoculated with some strains of tobacco mosaic virus but is invaded systemically by others. "Necrotizing" varients arise when a systemic strain is treated with a mutagenic agent indicating that whether or not a hypersensitive response occurs in *N. sylvestris* depends not only on the genetic constitution of the host but on that of the virus as well (*36*).

An interesting feature of the hypersensitive response is that it is a tissue and not a cellular response to infection. This conclusion is reached from the observation that protoplasts derived from a hypersensitive host support the multiplication of virus to high levels and do not exhibit the type of cytopathological phenomena of infected cells that are part of a leaf. As a matter of fact the course of infection in protoplasts derived, respectively, from hypersensitive and systemic hosts is indistinguishable. Apparently it is not the differentiated state that is necessary for the expression of hypersensitivity but merely the aggregation of cells into a mass for, as Beachy and Murakishi (*5*) have observed, callus derived from a hypersensitive host will necrotize.

When plants undergo hypersensitive response as a consequence of virus infection they can acquire both a localized and systemic resistance to further infection. The localized resistance is present in the immediate vicinity of local lesions, whereas systemic resistance is present throughout the plant so that inoculation of a leaf other than the one initially inoculated with virus will result in the formation of fewer and smaller lesions than would appear on a comparable leaf of a plant not previously exposed to virus. An interesting feature of this type of acquired resistance is that it is relatively nonspecific so that the number of infections by non-inciting viruses as well as by the inciting virus is reduced (*39*). Both novel proteins (*51*) and RNA-like anti-viral factors (*1*) have been detected in extracts made from the non-lesion tissue of plants undergoing hypersensitive response. The appearance of acquired resistance can be blocked by the timely treatment of actinomycin D and, thus, one proposed interpretation of the relationship between hypersensitivity and acquired resistance is that upon infection a host gene is activated whose product is responsible for virus localization. This product keeps being synthesized not only locally but throughout the plant, thus activating, before virus introduction, the localizing response. Acquired resistance, according to this hypothesis, results from a very rapid localizing response upon secondary inoculation so that many of the lesions produced are too small to be visible (*32*). However, both the nature of the hypersensitive response and the associated acquired resistance are still poorly understood and the details of these processes, when they are elucidated, may differ considerably from the above working hypothesis.

3. *The Blocking Response*

Although the systemic and necrotic responses to virus inoculation are by far the most common and obvious ones, two others will be discussed briefly for the light they may shed on possible host-pathogen reactions. One of these is what I shall call the blocking response. An example of this is seen in the reaction of pinto bean leaves to inoculation with two strains of tobacco mosaic virus, one (U1) which induces the appearance of clearly recognizable necrotic local lesions and the other (U2) which is apparently non-infectious to this host. However, although the U2 strain does not give rise to symptoms and does not multiply to a detectable level, it does block infection by the U1 strain. The phenomenon of cross-protection, by which prior (or sometimes simultaneous) infection by one strain of a virus will block multiplication and symptom expression of a closely related strain, is well known in plant virology so that the above cited interference is only remarkable in that it is accomplished by a strain which by itself is apparently incapable of infection. Two observations reveal that matters are not always as they seem for apparently the blocking virus does undergo limited infection. The first is that the U2 strain is actually capable of inducing visible necrotic lesions on pinto bean but only if the leaves are heat-shocked at a defined time period following inoculation (*54*). It appears then that infection proceeds to a point where it is prevented from progressing further by a heat sensitive block. The second observation is that the U2 strain does actually induce microscopic lesions on pinto bean leaves without heat shock but that these are so small that they are not visible to the naked eye (*18*). My purpose in dwelling on this situation is several fold. One is to indicate that sometimes the hypersensitive host response may operate in such a way as to give superficial appearance of no infection at all. Another is to point out that as Yarwood (*56*) discovered, the course of virus infection may in some situations have a heat sensitive block. Finally, the details of the blocking reaction serve as an introduction to the final type of host response to virus infection which is no apparent response at all.

4. *No Apparent Response*

Host-ranges of viruses have been determined primarily by observing the response of a number of species and cultivars to mechanical inoculation. In those cases where symptoms develop or there is easily detectable virus-multiplication the responding plant is designated a host and the type of response, whether systemic or localized, is noted. Non-responding plants are put in the non-host list. The lack of apparent response is a form of resistance to virus disease and I shall consider possible reasons for this in the next section.

III. FORMS OF RESISTANCE TO VIRUS DISEASE

There are several possible types of effective resistance to virus disease and these shall now be considered. Susceptibility and resistance are narrowly considered in this discussion in terms of whether disease is produced or, in the case of agronomic and horticultural crops, whether there is economic or aesthetic loss. Basic to our consideration will be the adoption of the hypothesis that viruses are indiscriminate in their ability to multiply in living plant cells, this hypothesis being an extension of the observation that protoplasts are capable of supporting the multiplication of viruses for which the plants from which they were derived are not ordinarily considered hosts.

1. *Hypersensitivity*

There are two types of host reaction which lead to effective resistance. The first we have already considered and consists of the hypersensitive response in which local necrotic lesions result from inoculation. The second we have delayed considering and is more complex, being the situation in which there is no apparent host response.

2. *No Apparent Response*

Below are listed a number of possible causes for lack of a visible reaction following mechanical inoculation.

1) Failure of virus to enter a living cell: Such cases are known because there are a group of viruses which appear to be restricted to specialized tissue for their multiplication usually the vascular bundles. Infectible sites are not easily created in such tissue by the type of leaf rubbing associated with mechanical inoculation and, thus, transmission of such viruses is limited to vectors and grafting. The nature of the requirement for the specialized cells is not known at present.

2) Failure of RNA release from the capsid: Ever since it was demonstrated that infection could be initiated with the nucleic acid portion of Class IV viruses (*12*), it has been postulated that one form of resistance might derive from the inability of certain hosts to free the nucleic acid from the protein capsid. However, it does not appear that such inability can be widespread and, as a consequence, be an important source of resistance because there has been no confirmed case, as yet, of a viral nucleic acid having a greater host range than the virus from which it was derived (*cf. 4, 17*). It has been demonstrated, however, that artificial encapsidation of the nucleic acid of one virus with protein from another will, in some cases, prevent infection of plants that are host for the virus from which the RNA was drived. The basis for this phenomenon is unknown (*2*).

3) Tolerance: Tolerance of virus multiplication can be considered another type of disease resistance. Plants that are tolerant to infection may exhibit some slowing of growth rate but there is otherwise no obvious disease symptom while at the same time virus multiplies to a fairly high level. Agronomic use is made of this phenomenon under appropriate circumstances by deliberately inoculating crop plants with a viral strain to which they are tolerant in order to provide protection against a disease producing strain of the same virus (*6*). The induction of disease symptoms as a consequence of virus infection is a poorly understood subject and, likewise, is the failure of disease symptoms to develop.

4) Failure of spread of virus from an initially infected cell to adjacent cells: No evidence exists at the present time for resistance based on such a phenomenon although its possibility cannot be ruled out.

5) Failure of systemic virus spread: Systemic spread of virus infection fails to take place in a number of virus-host combinations where the hypersensitive reaction is not a factor. In these cases the virus replicates and spreads from cell to cell in the inoculated leaf and remains confined to that leaf; infection does not spread to the rest of the plant. This phenomenon is known not only for the few cases where nucleoprotein particles are not formed but also for some cases where virus particles are synthesized (*23*). The biochemical or structural basis for failure of systemic spread where this occurs is not known.

6) Invisible lesions: Another possible type of disease resistance without obvious host manifestation may result from what I shall term an invisible hypersensitive response. The likelihood that such a phenomenon may account for the type of resistance exhibited by many plants that are considered non-hosts of a virus may be appreciated from the observation that the size of visible necrotic lesions formed as a consequence of the hypersensitive reaction differ over a broad range dependent on the host-virus system. In addition, some lesions expand with time after appearance and others do not. As an example, the U1 strain of tobacco mosaic virus induces fairly large spreading lesions on the host *N. glutiosa* whereas the U2 strain induces smaller lesions (*38*) and the VM strain very small lesions (*55*). With such a large size range of lesions it is not unreasonable to suppose that some virus-host combinations yield lesions that are so small as to be invisible to the naked eye. The U2 strain of tobacco mosaic virus inoculated to pinto bean leaves has already been mentioned as a system in which only microscopically visible lesions are produced. The size of lesion is determined by a number of factors and it is probable that there may be many instances in which tissue collapse and necrosis occurs before the infected tissue becomes very large.

7) Inability of virus replication: Consideration is given to the possibility that types of resistance exist in which one or another of the steps of the intracellular life cycle is blocked such as translation, RNA replication or assembly. However, although it may exist, evidence is lacking for this type of resistance. As a matter of fact, the ability to infect protoplasts derived from "non-host" plants would argue that most plant viruses may be able to replicate in almost any plant cell.

SUMMARY

This brief review has concerned itself with recognition and specificity factors determining susceptibility and resistance in the plant virus-host reaction. The plant virus life cycle involves entry of a virus particle into a living cell, release of the nucleic acid portion of the virus particle from its capsid, translation of the viral nucleic acid, replication of the virus nucleic acid, assembly of new virus particles, spread of the infection to new cells and tissue of the plant and, finally transfer of virus particles to a new host. Many, but not all, viruses depend on vectors for transmission from plant to plant and, thus, a good deal of recognition and specificity residues in plant-vector and vector-virus relationships rather than on the plant-virus interaction directly. Infection can also be initiated by mechanical inoculation of plants and by exposure of protoplasts to virus particles under appropriate conditions. Specificity is greatest when inoculation is vector mediated, less so with mechanical inoculation and least when protoplasts are exposed to virus.

Four types of host response to virus infection are systemic multiplication of virus in many parts of the plant, the hypersensitive response, the blocking response and no obvious response. Hypersensitive response depends on the genomes of both the virus and the host and frequently leads to induced acquired resistance. Plants that support systemic multiplication of virus with production of disease symptoms are considered to be susceptible to virus disease; those that respond with the hypersensitive response, the blocking response or no obvious response are considered to be resistant. Plants have no obvious response to virus inoculation for a number of reasons, the more likely of which are failure of virus particles to enter living cells, a situation that may be confined to phloem limited viruses; failure of symptom development to accompany systemic virus multiplication (tolerance); failure of virus to spread from an initially infected cell or leaf; and hypersensitive response which does not give rise to apparent symptoms.

REFERENCES

1. Antignus, Y., I. Sela, and I. Harpaz. 1977. Further studies on the biology of an antiviral factor (AVF) from virus-infected plants and its association with the N-gene of *Nicotiana* species. *J. Gen. Virol.* **35**: 107–116.
2. Atabekov, J. 1965. Host specificity of plant viruses. *Annu. Rev. Phytopathol.* **13**: 127–145.
3. Baltimore, D. 1971. Expression of animal virus genomes. *Bact. Rev.* **35**: 235–241.
4. Bawden, F. C. 1961. The susceptibility of *Rhoeo discolor* to infection by tobacco mosaic virus. *J. Biol. Chem.* **236**: 2760–2761.
5. Beachy, R. and H. Murakishi. 1971. Local lesion formation in tobacco tissue culture. *Phytopathology* **61**: 877–878.
6. Broadbent, L. 1976. Epidemiology and control of tomato mosaic virus. *Annu. Rev. Phytopathol.* **14**: 75–96.

7. Clark, G. L., K. W. Peden, and R. H. Symons. 1974. Cucumber mosaic virus induced RNA polymerase: partial purification and properties of the template-free enzyme. *Virology* **62**: 434–443.
8. De Zoeten G. and G. Gaard. 1969. Possibilities for inter- and intracellular location of some icosahedral plant viruses. *J. Cell. Biol.* **40**: 814–823.
9. Eoyang, L. and J. T. August. 1974. Reproduction of RNA bacteriophages. *In*: H. Fraenkel-Conrat and R. Wagner (eds.). *Comprehensive Virology*. vol. 2. Plenum Press, New York, pp. 1–59.
10. Esau, K., J. Cronshaw, and L. Hoefert. 1967. Relation of beet yellows virus to the phloem and to movement in the sieve tube. *J. Cell. Biol.* **32**: 71–87.
11. Fenner, F. 1976. Classification and nomenclature of viruses: Viruses of plants. *Intervirology* **7**: 65–90.
12. Fraenkel-Conrat, H. 1956. The role of nucleic acid in the reconstitution of active tobacco mosaic virus. *J. Am. Chem. Soc.* **78**: 882–883.
13. Fraenkel-Conrat, H., S. Veldee, and J. Woo. 1964. The infectivity of tobacco mosaic virus. *Virology* **22**: 432–441.
14. Furumoto, W. and R. Mickey. 1967. A mathematical model for the infectivity-dilution curve of tobacco mosaic virus. *Virology* **32**: 216–226.
15. Furumoto, W. and S. Wildman. 1963. Studies on the mode of attachment of tobacco mosaic virus. *Virology* **20**: 45–53.
16. Gibbs, A. and B. Harrison. 1976. *Plant Virology, The Principles*. John Wiley and Sons, New York, p. 292.
17. Gordon, M. and C. Smith. 1960. Multiplication of tobacco mosaic virus in a normally unsusceptible host. *J. Biol. Chem.* **235**: PC28.
18. Helms, K. and G. McIntyre. 1962. Studies on size of lesions of tobacco mosaic virus on Pinto bean. *Virology* **18**: 535–545.
19. Higgins, T., P. Goodwin, and P. Whitfeld. 1976. Occurrence of short patricles in beans infected with the cowpea strain of TMV. II. Evidence that short particles contain the cistron for coat protein. *Virology* **71**: 486–497.
20. Hunter, T., T. Hunt, J. Knowland, and D. Zimmer. 1976. Messenger RNA for the coat protein of tobacco mosaic virus. *Nature* **260**: 759–764.
21. Jackson, A., M. Zaitlin, A. Siegel, and R. I. B. Francki. 1972. Replication of tobacco mosaic virus III. Viral RNA metabolism in separated leaf cells. *Virology* **48**: 655–665.
22. Jacobson, M., J. Asso, and D. Baltimore. 1970. Further evidence on the formation of Polio virus proteins. *J. Mol. Biol.* **49**: 657–668.
23. Johnson, J. 1947. Virus attenuation and the separation of strains by specific hosts. *Phytopathology* **37**: 822–837.
24. Kado, C. and H. O. Agrawal. 1972. *Principles and Techniques in Plant Virology*. Van Nostrand Reinhold Co., New York, p. 688.

25. Kassanis, B. 1960. Comparison of the early stages of infection by intact and phenol-disrupted tobacco necrosis virus. *Virology* **10**: 353–360.
26. Kiehn, E. and J. Holland. 1960. Synthesis and clevage of enterovirus polypeptides in mammalian cells. *J. Virol.* **5**: 358–371.
27. Kielland-Brandt, M. and T. Nillson-Tilgren. 1973. Studies on the biosynthesis of TMV RNA and its complimentary RNA at different times after infection. *Mol. Gen. Genet.* **121**: 229–238.
28. Kitajima, E. and J. Laurifis. 1969. Plant virions in plasmodesmata. *Virology* **37**: 681–685.
29. Klug, A. and P. Butler. (eds.) 1976. A discussion on the assembly of regular viruses. *Philos. Trans. R. Soc. B* **276**: 1–204.
30. Lane, L. and P. Kaesberg. 1972. Multiple genetic components in bromegrass mosaic virus. *Nature New Biol.* **232**: 40–42.
31. Lister, R. 1968. Functional relationships between virus-specific products of infection by viruses of the tobacco rattle type. *J. Gen. Virol.* **2**: 43–52.
32. Loebenstein, G. 1972. Localization and induced resistence in virus infected plants. *Annu. Rev. Phytopathol.* **10**: 177–206.
33. Matthews, R. E. F. 1970. *Plant Virology*. Academic Press, New York, p. 778.
34. Merkins, W., G. de Zoeten, and G. Gaard. 1972. Observations on ectodesmata and the virus infection process. *J. Ultrastruct. Res.* **41**: 397.
35. Mouches, C., C. Bove, C. Barreau, and J. Bove. 1976. TYMV RNA replicase: formation of a complex between the purified enzyme and TYMV RNA. *Ann. Microbiol. (Inst. Pasteur)* **127A**: 75–90.
36. Mundry, K. and A. Gierer. 1958. Die Erzengung von Mutationen des tabakmosaik virus durch chemische Behandlung seiner Nucleinsaure *in vitro*. *Z. Vererbungsl.* **89**: 614–630.
37. Ralph, R., S. Bullivant, and S. Wojick. 1971. Cytoplasmic membranes as a possible site of tobacco mosaic virus RNA replication. *Virology* **44**: 473–479.
38. Rappaport, I. and S. G. Wildman. 1957. A kinetic study of local lesion growth on *Nicotiana glutinosa* resulting from tobacco mosaic virus infection. *Virology* **4**: 265–274.
39. Ross, A. 1966. Systemic effects of local lesion formation. *In*: A. Beemster and J. Dijkstra (eds.). *Viruses of Plants*. North-Holland Publ., Amsterdam, pp. 127–150.
40. Sarkar, S., M. Upadhya, and G. Melchers. 1974. A highly efficient method of inoculation of tobacco mesophyll protoplasts with ribonucleic acid of tobacco mosaic virus. *Mol. Gen. Genet.* **135**: 1–9.
41. Semal, J. and J. Kummert. 1971a. Sequential synthesis of double-stranded and single stranded RNA by cell-free extracts of barley leaves infected with brome mosaic virus. *J. Gen. Virol.* **10**: 79–89.

42. Shih, D. and P. Kaesberg. 1973. Translation of brome mosaic viral ribonucleic acid in a cell-free system derived from wheat embryo. *Proc. Natl. Acad. Sci. U.S.* **80**: 799–1805.
43. Shih, D., L. Lane, and P. Kaesberg. 1972. Origin of the small component of brome mosaic virus RNA. *J. Mol. Biol.* **64**: 353–364.
44. Siegel, A. 1966. The first stages of infection. *In*: A. Beemster and J. Dijkstra (eds.). *Viruses of Plants*. North-Holland Publ., Amsterdam, pp. 3–18.
45. Siegel, A., W. Ginoza, and S. Wildman. 1957. The early events of infection with tobacco mosaic virus nucleic acid. *Virology* **3**: 554–565.
46. Siegel, A., V. Hari, and K. Kolacz. 1978. The effect of tobacco mosaic virus infection on host and virus specific protein synthesis in protoplasts. *Virology* **85**: 494–503.
47. Siegel, A., M. Zaitlin, and O. Sehgal. 1962. The isolation of defective tobacco mosaic virus strains. *Proc. Natl. Acad. Sci. U.S.* **48**: 1845–1851.
48. Siegel, A., V. Hari, I. Montgomery, and K. Kolacz. 1976. A messenger RNA for capsid protein isolated from tobacco mosaic virus-infected tissue. *Virology* **73**: 363–371.
49. Takebe, I. 1975. The use of protoplasts in plant virology. *Annu. Rev. Phytopathol.* **13**: 105–125.
50. Takebe, I. and Y. Otsuki. 1969. Infection of tobacco mesophyll protoplasts by tobacco mosaic virus. *Proc. Natl. Acad. Sci. U.S.* **74**: 843–851.
51. Van Loon, L. and A. Van Kammen. 1970. Polyacrylamide disc electrophoresis of the soluble leaf proteins from *Nicotiana tabaccum* var. Samsun and Samsun NN. II. Changes in protein constitution after infection with tobacco mosaic virus. *Virology* **40**: 199–211.
52. Watson, J. D. and F. H. C. Crick. 1953. The structure of DNA. *Cold Spring Harbor Symp. Quant. Biol.* **18**: 123–134.
53. Watts, J., D. Cooper, and J. King. 1975. Plant protoplasts in transformation studies; some practical considerations. *In*: R. Markham, D. Davies, D. Hopwood, and R. Horne (eds.). *Modification of the Information Content of Plant Cells*. North-Holland Publ., Amsterdam, pp. 119–132.
54. Wu, J. H. 1963. Extension of the host range of tobacco mosaic virus by heat activation of latent infections. *Nature* **200**: 610–611.
55. Wu, J. H., A. Hildebrandt, and A. Riker. 1960. Virus-Host relationships in plant tissue culture. *Phytopathology* **50**: 587–594.
56. Yarwood, C. 1961. Heat activation of plant virus infections. *Virology* **14**: 312–319.

Discussion of Paper by Dr. Siegel

J. VanEtten opened the session by remarking on the intriguing breakdown in host specificity when isolated protoplasts are inoculated and asked if plant protoplasts could be infected by animal or fungal viruses. Siegel was not aware of any attempts to inoculate plant protoplasts with viruses isolated from hosts of different kingdoms. He did note one unsubstantiated report of successful culture of TMV in yeast protplasts. He suspected that discoveries such as intrigued VanEtten were the serendipitous result of the difficulty in isolating protoplasts of specific hosts and the ease with which tobacco protoplasts can be prepared. He believed a key element in such attempts would be adjusting the charge of the virus so as not to be repelled by the cell membrane. Wheeler asked if attempts had been made to regenerate whole tobacco plants from protoplasts infected with a local lesion virus to see if the basic biological interaction had been altered but Siegel knew of no such attempts. A related question by Durbin raised the possibility of different responses if the protoplasts were permitted to regenerate only cell walls before viral challenge. Uritani's question directed attention to the problem of viral coding by asking how many genes are known for viral RNA. Siegel was certain of only two, for the viral capsid and one of the two large proteins. He pointed out that there is not enough information for two large proteins and so one may represent a false start or termination. In response to Uritani's suggestion that some host proteins (such as proteases) may be viral-coded, Siegel knew of no evidence and commented that it seems unlikely because, with some rare exceptions, viral multiplication occurs with only mild disturbance of host cells. The general collapse as in the hypersensitive response is a symptom that may not require synthesis. Paxton returned to the problem of recognition in host specificity and Siegel summarized his position that vector-host rather than virus-host relationships seemed most important as evidenced by the drop in specificity when vector, mechanical and protoplast inoculations are compared. Keen asked if capsule proteins might trigger the hypersensitive response even though infection *per se* was not involved. However, SIEGEL said the available scanty evidence did not support this; for example; ultraviolet inactivated virus has no visible effect on plants even though the proteins seem unaffected. WHEELER asked two related questions: in mechanical inoculation by gentle wounding, how do the virus escape the effects of RNAse known to be released?; how long do infectible sites increase and how long are their half-lives? To the first, SIEGEL noted that the mechanisms are obscure but certainly the virus particles responsible for infection become "hidden" from external influences very rapidly. With rinsing it is possible to recover almost all applied virus without reducing the number of infection sites. As to the second, he noted that infectible centers disappear rapidly but may be viable for an hour or so on certain conditions. He suspects some sort of rapid repair is operable. A final suggestion by DAY that specificity might result from the activity of restriction endonucleases led to SIEGEL's observation that restriction endonucleases for RNA have not been discovered so far.

Recognition and Specificity in Plant Host-Parasite Interactions, pp. 273-287, 1979

RNA AND PROTEIN SYNTHESIS AND ENZYME CHANGES DURING INFECTION

TOSHIKAZU TANI AND HIROYUKI YAMAMOTO

Faculty of Agriculture, Kagawa University, Kagawa, Japan

The possible significance of RNA and proteins in the determination of specificity in plant diseases has been discussed for many years (*7, 13, 30, 31*). Especially in diseases caused by obligate biotrophic fungi, metabolic changes of these high molecular compounds have been extensively studied in association with the establishment of compatibility. Stimulation of synthesis of ribosomal RNA (rRNA) and soluble RNA (sRNA) was demonstrated as a general phenomenon for infections with rust, powdery mildew, and smut fungi (*4, 6, 7, 9, 12*). In most cases, however, increased synthesis is detectable at late stages of infections coincident with the initiation of reproductive differentiation of the pathogen and is interpreted to represent fungal RNA. Although the importance of increased levels of RNA synthesis by the host at early stage of infection has been postulated (*7, 9*), no convincing evidence has been shown so far. More than ten years ago, the exchange of messenger RNA (mRNA) or enzyme subunits was speculated to occur between the specific host and pathogen (*20, 21*), but no data are available as yet indicating that the establishment of compatible infections is mediated by gene specific RNA or proteins.

With relation to the incompatible interactions with obligate pathogens, increased synthesis of RNA and protein has been suggested by some workers (*3, 33*); while Barna *et al.* (*1*) recently challenged the idea of the participation of *de novo* synthesis of protein in the resistance of wheat to incompatible races of the stem rust fungus. On the other hand, the involvement of RNA and protein synthesis in the resistance to facultative pathogens which is mediated by phytoalexin production as well as papilla formation was suggested by several workers (*11, 14, 17, 32*), but Biggs (*5*) could not find an association of RNA synthesis with the phaseollin production. Recently, Yoshikawa *et al.* (*38, 39*) demonstrated that a remarkable stimulation of mRNA synthesis and a subsequent protein synthesis by the host are linked with resistance of soybean hypocotyls to *Phytophthora* through the production of glyceollin.

We have been working with changes of RNA and protein metabolism of oat leaves following infections with compatible and incompatible races of *Puccinia coronata avenae* (26–29). In compatible infection, the synthesis of RNA species such as rRNA, sRNA, and mRNA increased markedly, when uredial formation was initiated 4 days after inoculation. However, evidence obtained so far suggested that at least a substantial portion of the increased RNA levels originated from the fungus. On the other hand, in leaves infected by the incompatible race the increased synthesis of RNA species occurred prior to the cessation of the fungal development, *i.e.*, 28 hr after inoculation, and was considered to be of host origin. In the subsequent experiments, however, we unexpectedly failed to find any increase in template activity of mRNA and any change in protein synthesis at this stage of infection. Hence we presumed that this enhanced synthesis of RNA species is the biochemical events which accompanied, but not responsible for, the expression of the resistant response.

During these experiments, however, an increase of a few proteins probably of host origin was suggested by immunoelectrophoresis of soluble proteins (*37*). Therefore, the aim of this paper was to re-examine the occurrence of RNA synthesis which may be linked with the resistance expression leading to the production of proteins (*23, 25, 36*). This paper mainly discusses our recent studies on this subject and extending them to the causal association of some enzyme activities with resistance.

I. BLOCKAGE OF RESISTANCE BY CHEMICALS

We used oat cultivar Shokan 1 and incompatible race 226 and compatible race 203 of *P. coronata avenae* as cultivar-race combinations. The growth of intercellular hyphae of race 226 in primary leaves stops between 35 and 40 hr after inoculation, and primary haustoria produced between 28 and 35 hr remain immature and secondary haustoria are seldom produced (*24*). However, in leaves supplied prior to inoculation with either cordycepin (2.5×10^{-4} M), blasticidin S (5×10^{-6} M) or puromycin (2.5×10^{-4} M) for 4 hr from the stem cut ends of seedlings, the hyphal growth and haustoria development of race 226 became identical to those of compatible race 203. Such a remarkable stimulation was not observed by the treatment of leaves with other chemicals involving five RNA synthesis inhibitors and five protein synthesis inhibitors as well as six analogues of purine and pyrimidine

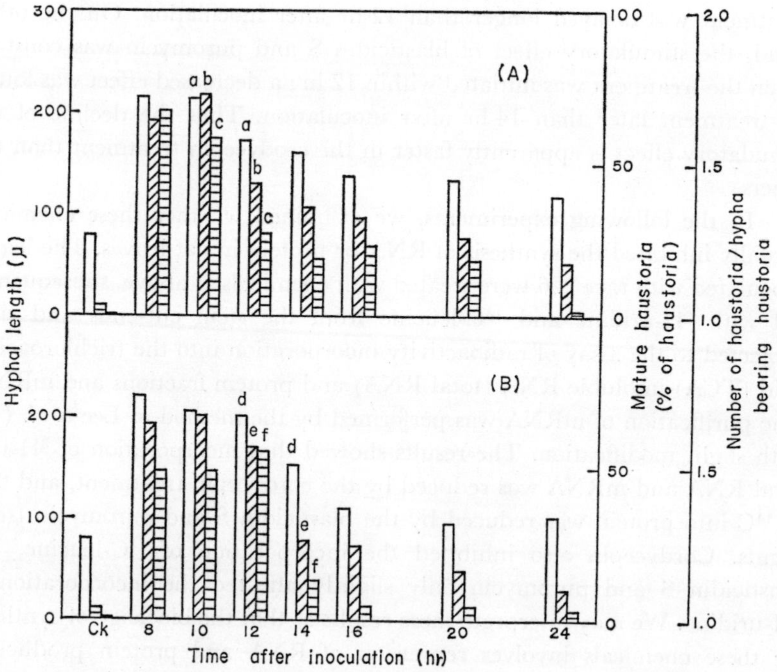

Fig. 1. Development of normally incompatible race 226 of *P. coronata avenae* in Shokan 1 oat leaves treated with cordycepin (A) and puromycin (B). Both chemicals were supplied for 4 hr from indicated hour after inoculation and the length of infection hyphae (□), number of mature haustoria (per cent of total haustoria; ▨) and number of haustoria per hypha bearing haustoria (▤) were estimated 48 hr after inoculation. The results followed by the same letter within each group are significantly different at the 1% level. Ck indicates control, for which deionized water was supplied.

bases and six amino acid analogues. Nine growth regulators involving ethylene and maleic hydrazide were also ineffective. It appeared therefore that the stimulation of fungal development by these chemicals could not be achieved by non-specific reduction of the physiological activity of host tissues, but instead by the specific blockage of a certain mechanism of resistance response.

Indeed, we could demonstrate a difference in the stimulation of fungal development between cordycepin and the other two chemicals by treating the leaves at various times before and after inoculation (Fig. 1). The effect of cordycepin was fully expressed when the treatment was initiated within 10 hr after inoculation, but gradually declined as the initiation time of the treatment was delayed longer than 12 hr after inoculation. On the other hand, the stimulatory effect of blasticidin S and puromycin was constant when the treatment was initiated within 12 hr; a decreased effect was found by treatment later than 14 hr after inoculation. Thus the decline of the stimulatory effect is apparently faster in the crodycepin treatment than the others.

In the following experiments, we examined whether these chemicals actually inhibited the synthesis of RNA or protein in oat leaves. The leaves inoculated with race 226 were treated with chemicals as above, subsequently fed with ^{3}H-uridine and ^{14}C-leucine from the stem cut-ends and then subjected to the assay of radioactivity incorporation into the trichloroacetic acid (TCA)-insoluble RNA (total RNA) and protein fractions and mRNA. The purification of mRNA was performed by the method of Lee *et al.* (*15*) with slight modification. The results showed that incorporation of ^{3}H into total RNA and mRNA was reduced by the cordycepin treatment, and that of ^{14}C into protein was reduced by the blasticidin S and puromycin treatments. Cordycepin also inhibited the incorporation of ^{14}C-leucine, but blasticidin S and puromycin only slightly affected the incorporation of ^{3}H-uridine. We may interprete these results as that the blockage of synthesis by these chemicals involves repression of RNA and protein production which determines the resistance.

II. RNA, mRNA, AND PROTEIN SYNTHESIS DURING INFECTION

Based on the results described in the above section, we re-examined the changes in RNA and protein synthesis between 10 and 24 hr after inoculation with incompatible race 226. A double-labeling technique using a mixture

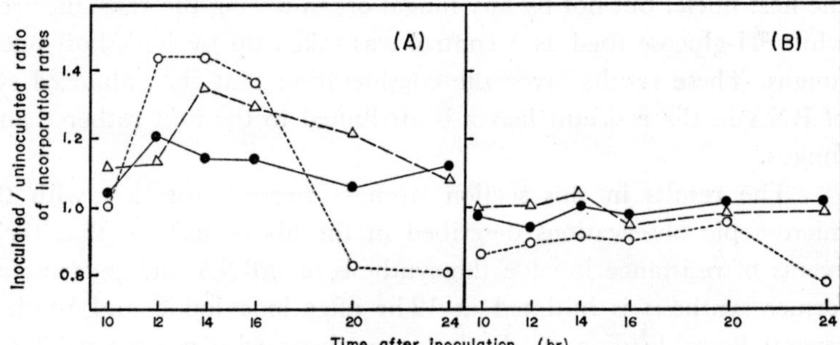

Fig. 2. Incorporation of ^{3}H-uridine (●) and ^{14}C-leucine (△) into acid insoluble fraction and of ^{3}H-uridine into mRNA (○) of Shokan 1 oat leaves inoculated with incompatible race 226 (A) and compatible race 203 (B) of *P. coronata avenae.* Labeled compounds were supplied for 1 hr from indicated hour after inoculation and subsequently assayed for radioactivity incorporation.

of ^{3}H-uridine and ^{14}C-leucine was employed in this experiment in order to compare accurately the changes in synthesis between RNA and protein (Fig. 2A). The mixture was fed for 1 hr from the indicated time after inoculation, and the inoculated/uninoculated ratio of incorporation was estimated. In leaves inoculated with race 226, the ratio of ^{3}H incorporation increased from 12 hr after inoculation, to 1.25, then the increased level declined gradually. On the other hand, an increased ratio of ^{14}C incorporation was not clearly evident at 12 hr, but became apparent at 14 hr, increasing up to 1.4, then declined gradually. Although these trends were relatively low, additional single-labeling experiments confirmed that the increased ratios were statistically significant at 12, 14, and 16 hr for the RNA synthesis and at 14, 16, and 20 hr for the protein synthesis.

Changes in the synthesis of mRNA following infection were also examined by applying ^{3}H-uridine as a precursor for 1 hr (Fig. 2A). The inoculated/uninoculated ratio of incorporation increased at 12 hr after inoculation to 1.4 in the resistant leaves. The increased level was fairly constant for the subsequent 4 hr, then declined rapidly. Comparison of the increased ratio of ^{3}H-uridine into RNA species indicated that the enhanced synthesis of mRNA is more pronounced than that of cytoplasmic and chloroplast rRNAs at this stage of infection.

Microautoradiographic determination of the distribution of ^{3}H-uridine within host and fungal cells indicated that this precursor was taken up by the host nuclei but not by any fungal organ during the resistance response, while ^{3}H-glucose used as a control was taken up by both host nuclei and fungus. These results favor the consideration that the enhanced synthesis of RNA in the resistant leaves is attributed to the host rather than to the fungus.

The results in this section strongly suggest, together with those of microscopic observations described in the above section, that the causal events of resistance involve the synthesis of mRNA and protein; and the former synthesis is initiated at 12 hr after inoculation and continues for several hours leading to the latter synthesis with a lag period of about 2 hr.

Contrary to the incompatible infection with race 226, leaves inoculated with compatible race 203 showed that the incorporation of ^{3}H-uridine into total RNA and mRNA and that of ^{14}C-leucine into protein were close to those of uninoculated controls throughout the experimental period (Fig. 2B). This may indicate that the establishment of compatibility requires no

TABLE I

Fungal Development and Incorporation of ^{14}C-Leucine into Acid Insoluble Fraction of Susceptible Oat Leaves Treated with Blasticidin S after Inoculation with *P. coronata avenae*

Inoculum race	Treatment with blasticidin S	Infection hypha (μm)	Mature haustorium (%)	Uredial differentiation (%)	Incorporation rate of ^{14}C-leucine (%)
Shokan 1 oat					
226	−	67	2	9	20.0
226	+	276	78	62	1.17
203	−	262	67	82	16.6
203	+	237	69	80	0.80
Victoria 226-S oat					
226	−	241	83	80	17.8
226	+	226	80	83	1.15
203	−	256	71	85	18.5
203	+	255	73	80	0.99

Blasticidin S was supplied for 4 hr from 12 hr after inoculation. Infection hyphae and mature haustoria were measured as in Fig. 1 at 48 hr, and uredial differentiation (in total infection sites) was recorded at day 7. ^{14}C-leucine was supplied for 4 hr from 16 hr after inoculation and subsequently harvested for the radioactivity assay.

additional synthesis of RNA and protein by the host. Indeed, vegetative development and uredial production of race 203 were not affected by the treatment of leaves with cordycepin and blasticidin S. Table I demonstrates that the compatible infection of Shokan 1 with race 203 and that of another oat cultivar Victoria 226-S with races 226 and 203 was unchanged under the condition that the protein synthesis was remarkably reduced by the blasticidin S treatment. It is thus likely that the transcription and translation of the host genes during infections are the events which mediate the expression of resistance rather than susceptibility.

III. RNA AND PROTEIN SYNTHESIS IN NON-HOST RESPONSE

To evaluate whether the synthesis of RNA and protein is responsible to the induced resistance against non-pathogenic rust fungi, as in the case of the cultivar-race resistance, we made further studies. We first observed the stomatal penetration using uredospores of twenty rust fungi; eight were pathogenic to certain gramineous plants other than oat, and the remainder were non-pathogenic to any gramineous plant. The results showed that only the former group was successful in penetrating through stomata, with one exception, and six of these showed stimulatory growth of intercellular hyphae producing haustoria abundantly by the treatment of leaves with cordycepin and blasticidin S. Several fungi belonging to the latter group produced infection structures on the leaf surface without finding stomata, resulting in failure to infection. It is therefore likely that the resistance of oat leaves to the latter group can be attributed to certain static factors on leaf surfaces.

The tracer experiments for the former group revealed that the incorporation of ^{3}H-uridine and ^{14}C-leucine was greater in all inoculated leaves at 12 or 16 hr after inoculation, compared with corresponding uninoculated controls. These results are in accord with those with the incompatible race of the pathogen, indicating that the synthesis of RNA and protein at the prehaustorial stage of infection is also responsible to the expression of induced resistance of oat leaves.

IV. CHANGES OF PROTEIN COMPOSITION AND ENZYME ACTIVITIES

Since the participation of RNA and protein synthesis in the resistance responses was indicated, the following studies were designed to elucidate changes in protein composition and enzyme activities linked with the resistance expression of the Shokan 1-race 226 system. As to the protein composition, we tried qualitative analysis by means of the two-dimensional electrophoresis of O'Farrell (*18*). Water soluble fractions from intact leaves revealed 143 protein spots on an electrophoresed gel plate. An additional minor 6 spots were detectable for leaves inoculated with incompatible race 226, as estimated 20 hr after inoculation, but none of these new spots appeared when the leaves were treated wit blastichidin S at 12 hr after inoculation. It is therefore very likely that the resistance expression requires *de novo* synthesis of certain soluble proteins.

We previously reported that the blasticidin S treatment reduced the cross protection effect to race 203 induced by the previous inoculation with race 226 and simultaneously reduced an increased level of antifungal activity during infection, suggesting that protein synthesis activated by the resistance induction involved a production of enzymes related to antifungal activity (*27*). Since it is unclear as yet what kinds of antifungal substances are produced in oat leaves responding with rust infection, we (*35*) first investigated changes in the activity of phenylalanine-ammonia lyase (PAL), because this enzyme had been implicated in the mechanism of resistance in various fungal diseases through the control of biosynthesis of phenolic compounds (*8, 30*).

The PAL activity in leaves inoculated with incompatible race 226 increased with two distinctive phases, one occurring between 8 and 16 hr and the other between 35 and 48 hr after inoculation, exhibiting activity four and six times greater than that of uninoculated controls at 12 and 35 hr, respectively. The activity was also two times greater at 20 and 28 hr. In leaves inoculated with compatible race 203, only the first phase of the increase was detected. However, possible participation of such characteristic increases in the resistant leaves was negated by the experiment using blasticidin S (Table II). When leaves were supplied with this chemical at 12 hr after inoculation with race 226, the PAL activity increased at 28 hr to 4.7-fold that of the race 226-inoculated and -untreated leaves, despite the fact that the host reaction reversed to susceptible by the treatment. The activity increase by the blasticidin S treatment was also observed in leaves inoculated with compatible race 203 without affecting susceptibility. In addition, parallel experiments showed that the contents of total phenol and flavonol and major three flavonoids in leaves were roughly constant throughout the period responding with resistance. We may conclude from

TABLE II

Phenylalanie-ammonia Lyase Activity and Peroxidase Isozymes in Shokan 1 Oat Leaves Treated with Blasticidin S after Inoculation with *P. coronata avenae*

Inoculum race	Treatment with blasticidin S	Host reaction	PAL activity at		Intensity of PO isozyme bands		
			16 hr	28 hr	10	11	12
—	—	—	8.6	10.4	1	0	0
226	—	Resistant	33.0	20.0	3	2	1
226	+	Susceptible	40.4	93.7	3	2	1
203	—	Susceptible	21.6	11.9	3	1	0
203	+	Susceptible	37.4	74.2	3	1	1

Blasticidin S was supplied for 4 hr from 12 hr after inoculation. Phenylalanine-ammonia lyase (PAL) activity was measured at indicated hour and expressed as cinnamic acid produced (nmoles/g fr. wt./hr). Intensity of peroxidase (PO) isozyme bands was estimated at 48 hr after inoculation, rating 0 (no band) to 3 (highest intensity).

these results that the PAL activation characterisitic of the resistance response is induced independently of the resistance determination.

The second aim of our investigation on enzyme changes was to elucidate the causal association of polyphenol oxidative enzymes to the resistance (*34*), since these enzymes are known to be responsible to numerous disease resistance (*10*), although several workers have negated the perticipation of peroxidase (PO) in the stem rust resistance of wheat (*2, 19*). Gel electrophoretic resolution of PO and polyphenol oxidase activities reacting with various substrates showed that the infection of Shokan 1 leaves by incompatible race 226 was accompanied by the characterisitic increase in intensity of two anionic PO isozymes including one new isozyme. This change in isozyme composition was detectable from 20 hr after inoculation and therefore appeared to be responsible to the resistance. However, it was experimentally possible to detect these isozymes under conditions of susceptible (Table II). In leaves supplied with either blasticidin S or puromycin at 12 hr after inoculation, the fungal development of race 226 was identical to that of compatible race 203. Nevertheless, the PO isozyme pattern on the gel was the same as that of resistance-responding leaves. Similar results were obtained by an experiment using heat treatment and stem detachment to reverse the host response.

It was confirmed in additional experiments that the change in total

PO activity was negligible between 8 and 35 hr after inoculation with race 226, and that no substance specifically reacting with the increased isozymes could be detected in inoculated and uninoculated leaves. No lignification of the host cell walls in tissues around the infected sites was detected by histochemical as well as electron microsconic observations. Thus the changes in PO isozymes may also be non-significant in this cultivar-race association.

Recently a contribution of preformed substances to the resistance of oat leaves was suggested (*16*). Bisdesmosidic furostanol saponins avenacosid A and B are present in intact leaves and are easily converted into the corresponding monodesmosidic derivatives 26-desglucoavenacosid A and B (26-DGA A and B), when the leaves are attacked by avirulent fungi. A β-glucosidase named as 26-desgluco-avenacosidase (26-DGase) has been considered to specifically catalize this reaction and hence to be responsible for resistance. We isolated from Shokan 1 leaves two extremely strong inhibitors to germ tube growth of various rust fungi (ED_{80}=14 μg/ml) and identified them as 26-DGA A and B. Therefore, the enzyme 26-DGase seemed to be important for the rust resistance. We established the procedure of detecting 26-DGase isozymes and found 12 isozymes in uninoculated leaves; but number and intensity of these isozyme bands were unchanged by the inoculation of leaves with both races 226 and 203. We consider, therefore, that the increased synthesis of 26-DGase is not required for rust resistance of oat leaves.

SUMMARY

We propose that the activation of RNA (mRNA) and protein synthesis by the plant is required for the resistancc expression to the pathogenic and non-pathogenic rust fungi, but probably not for the establishment of susceptibility. The time schedule of the events in Shokan 1 oat leaves in response to incompatible race 226 of *P. coronata avenae* is summarized in Fig. 3.

We previously indicated that in this cultivar-race system the cellular conditioning of host tissues towards the resistant state is irreversibly established when the fungus produced substomatal vesicles (*22, 24*). The induction of RNA synthesis is interpreted as the event which occurs subsequent to the resistance determination. This first biochemical evcnt may lead to the specific protein synthesis. At present, we have no evidence to demonstrate

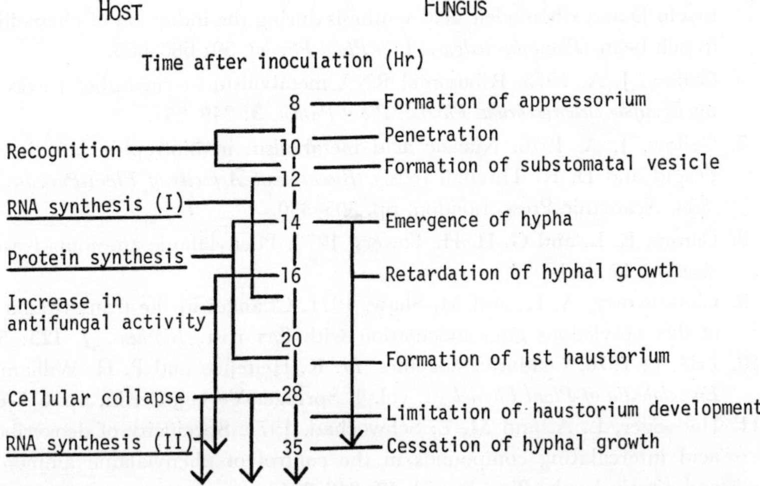

Fig. 3. Time schedule of the resistance expression of Shokan 1 oat leaves against incompatible race 226 of *P. coronata avenae*.

how these events contribute to the limitation of fungal development, but it is likely that the proteins responsible to the resistance are the enzyme(s) other than PAL, PO, PPO, and 26-DGase.

The second phase of the RNA synthesis which is activated 28 hr after inoculation seems to be non-significant for the retardation of fungal development. Perhaps this reflects a state of host cells irritated to the point of collapse as a consequence of a hypersensitive response.

REFERENCES

1. Barna, B., E. Bálazs, and Z. Király. 1975. Proteins and resistance of wheat to stem rust: non-involvement of some serologically and electrophoretically determined proteins. *Physiol. Plant. Pathol.* **6**: 137–143.
2. Barna, B., T. Érsek, and S. F. Mashaâl. 1974. Hypersensitive reaction of rust-infected wheat in compatible host-parasite relationships. *Acta Phytopathol. Acad. Sci. Hung.* **9**: 293–300.
3. Battacharya, P. K. and M. Shaw. 1968. The effect of rust infection on DNA, RNA and protein in nuclei of Khapli wheat leaves. *Can. J. Bot.* **46**: 96–99.
4. Bennet, J. and Scott, K. J. 1971. Ribosomal metabolism in mildew-infected leaves. *FEBS Lett.* **16**: 93–95.

5. Biggs, D. R. 1972. Studies on phytoalexins. The relationship between actinomycin D and ribonucleic acid synthesis during the induction of phaseollin in the french bean (*Phaseolus vulgaris* L.). *Plant Physiol.* **50**: 660–666.
6. Callow, J. A. 1973. Ribosomal RNA metabolism in cucumber leaves infected by *Erysiphe cichoracearum*. *Physiol. Plant Pathol.* **3**: 249–257.
7. Callow, J. A. 1976. Nucleic acid metabolism in biotrophic infections. *In*: J. Friend and D. R. Threlfall (eds.). *Biochemical Aspecits of Plant-Parasite Relationships.* Academic Press, London, pp. 305–330.
8. Camm, E. L. and G. H. H. Towers. 1973. Phenylalanie ammonia lyase. *Phytochemistry* **12**: 961–973.
9. Chakravorty, A. K. and M. Shaw. 1971. Changes in the transcription pattern of flax cotyledons after inoculation with flax rust. *Biochem. J.* **123**: 551–557.
10. Frić, F. 1976. Oxidative enzymes. *In*: R. Heitefuss and P. H. Williams (eds.). *Encyclopedia of Plant Physiology*. vol. 4. Springer-Verlag, Berlin, pp. 617–631.
11. Hadwiger, L. A. and M. E. Schwochau. 1971. Specificity of deoxyribonucleic acid intercalating compounds in the control of phenylalanie ammonia lyase and pisatin levels. *Plant Physiol.* **47**: 346–351.
12. Heitefuss, R. 1968. The significance of changes in nucleic acid metabolism for the relations between host and obligate parasites. *Neth. J. Plant Pathol.* **74**: 9–18.
13. Heitefuss, R. and G. Wolf. 1976. Nucleic acid in host-parasite interactions. *In*: R. Heitefuss and P. H. Williams (eds.). *Encyclopedia of Plant Physiology*. vol. 4. Spriger-Verlag, Berlin, pp. 480–508.
14. Hess, S. L. and L. A. Hadwiger. 1971. The induction of phenylalanine ammonia lyase and phaseollin by 9-aminoacridine and other deoxyribonucleic acid intercalating compounds. *Plant Physiol.* **48**: 197–202.
15. Lee, S. Y., J. Mendecki, and G. Brawerman. 1971. A polynucleotide segment rich in adenylic acid in the rapidly-labeled polysomal RNA component of mouse sarcoma 180 ascites cells. *Proc. Natl. Acad. Sci. U.S.* **68**: 1331–1335.
16. Lünning, H. U. and E. Schlösser. 1976. Role of saponins in antifungal resistance VI. Interactions *Avena sativa-Drechslera avenacea*. *Z. Pflanzenkr. Pflanzenschutz.* **83**: 317–327.
17. Ōba, K., H. Tatematsu, K. Yamashita, and I. Uritani. 1976. Induction of flavoterpene production and formation of the enzyme system from mebaronate to isopentenyl pyrophosphate in sweet potato root tissue injured by *Ceratosystis fimbriata* and by toxic chemicals. *Plant Physiol.* **58**: 51–56.
18. O'Farrell, P. H. 1975. High resolution two-dimensional electrophoresis of proteins. *J. Biol. Chem.* **250**: 4007–4021.
19. Seevers, P. M., J. M. Daly, and F. F. Catedral. 1971. The role of peroxidase isozymes in resistance to wheat stem rust diseases. *Plant Physiol.* **48**: 353–360.
20. Shaw, M. 1963. The physiology and host-parasite relations of the rusts. *Annu. Rev. Phytopathol.* **1**: 259–294.

21. Stahmann, M. A., W. Woodbury, L. Lovrekovich, and V. Macko. 1968. The role of enzymes in the regulation of disease resistance and host-pathogen specificity. *In*: T. Hirai, Z. Hidaka, and I. Uritani (eds.). *Biochemical Regulation in Diseased Plants or Injury*. The Phytopathol. Soc. Japan, Tokyo, pp. 263–274.
22. Tani, T., S. Ouchi, T. Onoe, and N. Naito. 1975. Irreversible recognition demonstrated in the hypersensitive response of oat leaves against the crown rust fungus. *Phytopathology* **65**: 1190–1193.
23. Tani, T. and H. Yamamoto. 1978. Nucleic acid and protein synthesis in association with the crown rust resistance of oat leaves. *Physiol. Plant Pathol.* **12**: 215–223.
24. Tani, T., H. Yamamoto, T. Onoe, and N. Naito. 1975. Initiation of resistance and host cell collapse in the hypersensitive reaction of oat leaves against *Puccinia coronata avenae*. *Physiol. Plant. Pathol.* **7**: 231–242.
25. Tani, T., H. Yamamoto, G. Kadota, and N. Naito. 1976. Development of rust fungi in oat leaves treated with blasticidin S, a protein synthesis inhibitor. *Tech. Bull. Fac. Agric. Kagawa Univ.* **27**: 95–103.
26. Tani, T., M. Yoshikawa, and N. Naito. 1971. Changes in ^{32}P-ribonucleic acids in oat leaves associated with susceptible and resistant reactions to *Puccinia coronata*. *Ann. Phytopathol. Soc. Japan* **37**: 43–51.
27. Tani, T., M. Yoshikawa, and N. Naito. 1973. Effect of rust infection of oat leaves on cytoplasmic and chloroplast ribosomal ribonucleic acids. *Phytopathology* **63**: 491–494.
28. Tani, T., M. Yoshikawa, and N. Naito. 1973. Template activity of ribonucleic acid extracted from oat leaves infected by *Puccinia coronata*. *Ann. Phytopathol. Soc. Japan* **39**: 7–13.
29. Tani, T., M. Yoshikawa, and N. Naito. 1975. Selective enhancement of ribosomal RNA synthesis of crown rust-infected oat leaves by stem excision. *Physiol. Plant. Pathol.* **5**: 193–199.
30. Uritani, I. 1971. Protein changes in diseased plants. *Annu. Rev. Phytopathol.* **9**: 211–234.
31. Uritani, I. 1976. Protein metabolism. *In*: R. Heitefuss and P. H. Williams (eds.). *Encyclopedia of Plant Physiology*. vol. 4. Springer-Verlag, Berlin, pp. 509–525.
32. Vance, C. P. and R. T. Sherwood. 1976. Cycloheximide treatments implicate papilla formation in resistance of reed canarygrass to fungi. *Phytopathology* **66**: 498–502.
33. von Broembsen, S. L. and Hadwiger, L. A. 1972. Characterization of disease resistance responses in certain gene-for-gene interactions between flax and *Melampsora lini*. *Physiol. Plant Pathol.* **2**: 207–215.
34. Yamamoto, H., H. Hokin, and T. Tani. 1977. Peroxidase and polyphenoloxidase in relation to the crown rust resistance of oat leaves. *Phytopathol. Z.* **91**: 193–202.
35. Yamamoto, H., H. Hokin, T. Tani, and G. Kadota. 1977. Phenylalanie-ammonia

lyase in relation to the crown rust resistance of oat leaves. *Phytopathol. Z.* **90**: 203–211.

36. Yamamoto, H., T. Tani, and H. Hokin. 1976. Protein synthesis linked with resistance of oat leaves to crown rust fungus. *Ann. Phytopathol. Soc. Japan* **42**: 583–590.
37. Yamamoto, H., T. Tani, and N. Naito. 1975. Changes in protein contents of oat leaves during the resistant reaction against *Puccinia coronata avenae*. *Phytopathol. Z.* **82**: 138–145.
38. Yoshikawa, M., H. Masago, and N. T. Keen. 1977. Activated synthesis of poly(A)-containing messenger RNA in soybean hypocotyls inoculated with *Phytophthora megasperma* var. *sojae*. *Physiol. Plant Pathol.* **10**: 125–138.
39. Yoshikawa, M., K. Yamauchi, and H. Masago. 1978. *De novo* messenger RNA and protein synthesis are required for phytoalexin-mediated disease resistance in soybean hypocotyls. *Plant Physiol.* **61**: 314–317.

Discussion of Drs. Tani and Yamamoto

In the discussion following TANI's paper, WYNN and DALY noted that the resistance of Shokan 1 oats to *P. coronata* var. *avenae* is unusually fast and accompanied by considerable necrosis; however, in response to BUSHNELL, TANI emphasized that induced resistance, as determined by reversal *via* heat treatments or metabolic inhibitors, occurs at *ca.* 10 hr, when the fungus has only begun infection of the host and well before the occurrence of fungus growth stoppage or hypersensitive necrosis. In response to DAY, TANI stated that the genetics of resistance in Shokan 1 are not known, but that the well-known variety Bond reacts similarly to his incompatible crown rust race; he also pointed that several other resistant genotypes of oats that were tested all gave slower and less pronounced resistance than Shokan 1 or Bond. In response to DALY, TANI emphasized that the metabolic inhibitors completely blocked Shokan 1 hypersensitive resistance, leading to freely sporulating pustules; they did not visibly affect expression of normally compatible interactions, although they did block the synthesis of proteins normally occurring in the compatible plants. This strongly indicates that resistance but not susceptibility, is an inducible, energy-requiring process in oats. BELL suggested that perhaps the HR is only a "wound response," but TANI noted that it involves neither activation of 26-DGase nor liberation of detectable 26-desgluco-avenocoside's in hypersensitive leaves. Since their liberation occurs in response to mechanical wounding, the HR would not appear to involve the same sort of wounding.

Recognition and Specificity in Plant Host-Parasite Interactions, pp. 289–300, 1979

MOLECULAR STUDIES ON CROWN GALL TUMORS

EUGENE W. NESTER

Department of Microbiology and Immunology, Seattle, Washington, U.S.A.

In 1907, Smith and Townsend identified the first organism inducing cancer, *Agrobacterium tumefaciens* (*21*), a gram negative, rod-shaped organism closely related to the symbiotic nitrogen fixing organisms of the genus *Rhizobium* (*11*). The crown gall tumors induced by this organism occur on at least 93 different families of dicotyledenous flowering and gymnospermous plants (*7*). Crown gall has been intensively studied over the past 70 years for several reasons. First, the disease has serious economic consequences in plant nurseries. Secondly, and perhaps more importantly, crown gall tumors behave like animal tumors in a number of respects and an understanding of how *Agrobacterium* transforms plant cells might provide insight into cancer biology in general (*3*).

I. TRANSFORMED PLANT CELLS

Transformed cells differ from normal plant cells in a number of respects (Table I). There are two significant aspects to this table. First, the pioneering studies of Dr. Braun demonstrated that the transformed phenotype is stably maintained in the absence of viable bacteria (*2*). Although the induction of the tumor requires wounding of the plant surface followed by contact

TABLE I

Differences between Normal and Transformed Tumor Callus Tissue

Normal	Tumor
Requires exogenous auxin and cytokinen for growth	Does not require addition of auxin and cytokinen for growth
Do not graft onto normal plants	Graft onto normal plants and develop into tumors
Do not synthesize octopine or nopaline	Synthesize octopine or nopaline

with viable actively metabolizing bacteria, after a few days the bacteria can be eliminated without altering the development of the tumor. Because these observations make it perfectly clear that the whole bacterial cell is not required for maintenance of the tumorous state, Braun coined the term, tumor inducing principle (TIP) to indicate that portion of the bacterial cell which is responsible for transformation of the plant cell. The identification of TIP has been the focus of research for several laboratories over the past decade. With the availability of newer techniques of nucleic acid methodology, the TIP has now been identified (*6*).

II. METHOD OF SEARCHING FOR TUMOR INDUCING PRINCIPLE

Because of the stability of the transformed phenotype, the most reasonable candidate for TIP was a molecule capable of self replication in the plant cell. Of the two types of nucleic acids, the best candidate is DNA. For much of the past 10 years several laboratories looked for bacterial DNA in tumor tissue without any definitive positive results (*4, 20*). However, in 1974, a paper appeared which provided a new clue as to the identity of TIP. Schell and his colleagues in Belgium reported that all oncogenic strains of *Agrobacterium* harbored a very large plasmid (molecular weight greater than 100×10^6 daltons) (*26*). Our group in Seattle and Schell's group in Belgium independently demonstrated that oncogenic strains cured of these large plasmids lost their ability to induce tumors (*23, 24*) and reintroduction of the plasmid into a plasmidless, non-oncogenic cell either by conjugation or DNA-mediated transformation resulted in the bacteria gaining the ability to induce tumors (*5, 12*). These data strongly implied that the large plasmid was required for tumor induction and it suggested that part or all of this plasmid was related to the tumor inducing principle.

We looked for the presence of plasmid DNA in the tumor by the technique of DNA-DNA hybridization in solution (*25*). In this analysis, plasmid DNA was isolated from an oncogenic strain and labeled *in vitro* with ^{32}P by the technique of nick translation (*16*). This DNA, termed the proble, was heat denatured and then allowed to reassociate to its double-stranded form in the presence of a large excess of unlabelled DNA isolated from either tobacco tumor callus or normal tobacco callus in the absence of plant DNA. The rate of reassociation of the plasmid was also determined. The rate of the reassociation of the radioactive probe depends on the concentration of the plasmid in the reaction mixture. The higher the concentration of these DNA sequences, the more rapid the rate of reassociation. If only a part of the plasmid is present in the tumor, then the reassociation of that part of the plasmid present in the tumor will be more rapid, but the part of the plasmid not represented will reassociate at the same rate as the plasmid in the absence of plant DNA. Thus, a break in the curve of reassociation indicates the percentage of the DNA molecule (plasmid) which is present in the plant DNA. The data from a reassociation experiment of this sort is plotted on a Pot plot (Fig. 1) in which the ordinate represents the percent double stranded DNA and the abscissa represents the concentration of the probe DNA at the beginning of the experiment (P_0) multiplied by the time (t) the mixtures are incubated. The curve marked "whole" in Fig. 1 represents a theoretical curve that would be generated if the entire fragment of probe DNA were present in the tumor DNA. The middle curve (labeled half) would be generated if only half of the probe sequences were present in the tumor DNA. The

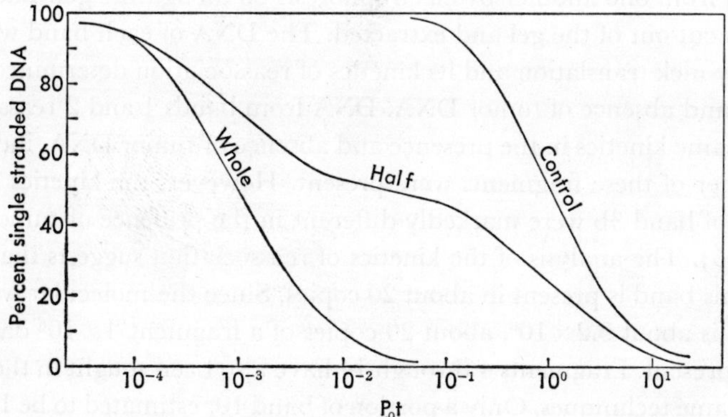

Fig. 1. Model curves of reassociation of DNA.

extent to which the curve shifts to the left is a reflection of the number of copies of the probe that are present in the tumor DNA; the more copies, the greater the shift. In our actual experiments, we always measure the reassociation of a known amount of plasmid DNA in the presence of salmon DNA in order to calibrate the experimental hybridization reactions. This allows us to calculate the concentration of plasmid DNA sequences in tumor.

III. IDENTIFICATION OF PORTION OF THE PLASMID AS THE TUMOR INDUCING PRINCIPLE

In our initial experiments, we used the entire plasmid, as the probe and studied its reassociation in the presence and absence of cloned tobacco tumor DNA (*6*). The results of these experiments indicated that the entire plasmid was certainly not present. However, the kinetics of reassociation of the plasmid in the presence of tumor DNA suggested that a small fragment of the plasmid was present in the tumor DNA. In order to amplify the signal of the probe and identify the fragment of the plasmid we suspected was present in the tumor, we decided to cleave the entire plasmid into discrete fragments and study the kinetics of reassociation of each fragment in the presence and absence of tumor DNA. If any fragment was present, its reassociation should be significantly increased in the presence of tumor DNA. Other fragments which were absent should show identical kinetics of reassociation in the presence and absence of tumor DNA. The plasmid was isolated from *Agrobacterium* and cleaved with a restriction endonuclease from *Serratia marcesens* (Sma I) into approximately 25 fragments. The fragments were separated from one another by electrophoresis on an agarose gel. Each fragment was cut out of the gel and extracted. The DNA of each band was then labeled by nick translation and its kinetics of reassociation determined in the presence and absence of tumor DNA. DNA from bands 1 and 2 reassociated with the same kinetics in the presence and absence of tumor DNA, indicating that neither of these fragments were present. However, the kinetics of reassociation of band 3b were markedly different in the presence of tumor DNA (Fig. 2) (*6*). The analysis of the kinetics of reassociation suggests that about 40% of this band is present in about 20 copies. Since the molecular weight of this band is about 9.2×10^6, about 20 copies of a fragment 4×10^6 daltons in length is present. Fragments 4 through 14 have also been sought in the tumor by these same techniques. Only a portion of band 10, estimated to be 1.6×10^6 daltons could be detected.

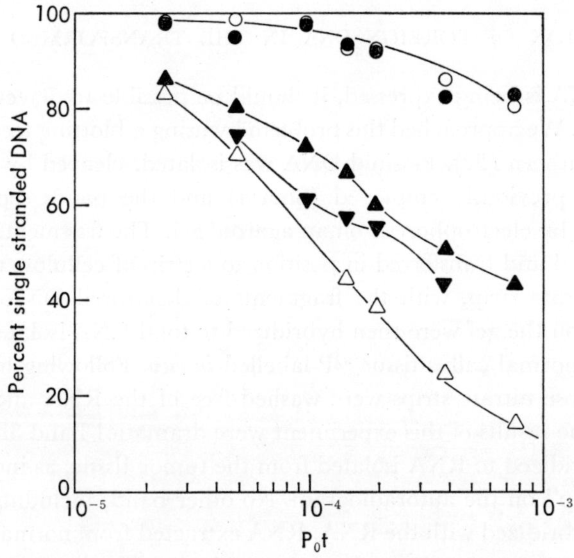

Fig. 2. Renaturation kinetics of *A. tumefaciens* fragment number 3b in the presence of tumor and control DNAs. Band 3b DNA (3.5×10^6 cpm/μg, 8.6×10^{-3} μg/ml was allowed to reassociate in the presence of DNA; ○ 2.2 mg/ml salmon DNA; ● 1.9 mg/ml normal tobacco callus DNA; ▲ 2.2 mg/ml crown gall tumor DNA; ▼ 4.4 mg/ml crown gall tumor DNA; △ 1.8 mg/ml salmon DNA + 0.035 μg/ml plasmid DNA (10 copy model).

IV. IDENTIFICATION OF TUMOR INDUCING PRINIPLE IN OTHER CROWN GALL TUMORS

All of the above studies were conducted on one cloned tobacco tumor. We next set out to determine whether other independently derived cloned tobacco tumors contained the same fragments of the plasmid (termed the T region). We analyzed a total of four tumor lines for the presence of foreign DNA previously shown to be present by the hybridization experiments we have already discussed. The results of these experiments can be summarized as follows. All three tumor lines contain a common fragment of plasmid DNA. In addition, one line contains an additional fragment. Thus, we conclude that different tumors may contain variable amounts of foreign DNA, but a specific region of the plasmid must be present in order for the tumor phenotype to be maintained (Merlo, D. *et al.* manuscript in prep.).

V. TRANSCRIPTION OF FOREIGN DNA IN THE TRANSFORMED CELLS

If the foreign DNA is being expressed, it should be possible to detect transcription products. We approached this problem by using a blotting technique developed by Southern (*22*). Plasmid DNA was isolated, cleaved by the restriction enzyme previously employed (Sma I) and the bands separated from one another by electrophoresis on an agarose gel. The fragments in the gel were denatured and transferred in position to a strip of cellulose nitrate. The cellulose nitrate strip, with the fragments of denatured DNA in the same position as on the gel were then hybridized to total RNA isolated from tumor and from normal callus tissue ^{32}P labelled *in vivo*. Following hybridization, the cellulose nitrate strips were washed free of the RNA and autoradiographed. The results of this experiment were dramatic! Band 3b of the tumor DNA hybridized to RNA isolated from the tumor tissue, as indicated by its "lighting up" on the autoradiogram. No other band, including band 10, apparently hybridized with the RNA. RNA extracted from normal callus did not hybridize to any fragment. From these data we can conclude that some, but perhaps not all of the foreign DNA is transcribed in the tumor.

VI. TRANSLATION OF RNA TRANSCRIPTS

The next question we addressed was whether we could gain any insight into any protein product that might be synthesized from these transcripts. The approach to this problem rested on observations made over 10 years ago by Morel and his colleagues (*17*). Crown gall tumors contain one or another unique amino acid, octopine [N^2-(D-1-carboxyethyl)-L-arginine] (*17*) or nopaline [N^2-(1,3-dicarboxypropyl) arginine] (*9, 10*). Neither of these compounds is present in normal tissue (*1*). Agrobacteria have a unique capacity, not shared by any other genera of bacteria, the ability to degrade either octopine or nopaline (a few strains can degrade both) (*15*). The French group first made the startling observation that those strains of *Agrobacterium* that degraded octopine induced tumors that synthesized octopine and those strains that degraded nopaline induced tumors that synthesized nopaline (*19*). From this strong correlation, Morel and his colleagues suggested that the same enzyme was carrying out the biosynthetic and degradative reactions. This idea received strong support when it was shown that the genes in the bacteria concerned with octopine and nopaline degradation map on the plasmid associated with virulence (*23, 24*). However, more recent data make this hypothesis highly unlikely. Bacterial mutants have been isolated in several laboratories which no longer can degrade octopine or nopaline. However, in all cases, the tumors induced by these mutants synthesize the normal amounts of these amino acids (*13, 18*). Therefore it seems highly likely that the gene coding for the synthesis of the degradative and biosynthetic enzymes are the same. However, it is possible and indeed quite likely that the structural genes responsible for octopine and nopaline synthesis in the tumor reside on the portion of the plasmid which is stably maintained in transformed plant cells.

VII. PARASITISM AT THE MOLECULAR LEVEL

Why has a bacterium evolved an ability to transform plant cells? The answer appears related to the ability of the bacteria to induce the synthesis of octopine and nopaline in the tumors. These compounds provide the bacteria with a utilizable source of carbon and nitrogen which only agrobacteria can utilize. Octopine and nopaline serve agrobacteria in another regard. Octopine induces the transfer of octopine plasmids to a plasmidless strain and nopaline promotes transfer of nopaline plasmids (*8, 14*). Thus, the presence of these compounds in the environment serves to increase the size of the population of bacteria capable of utilizing them. Thus, it is clear that agrobacteria have evolved very sophisticated mechanisms which provide the bacteria with an ecological niche uniquely adapted for their growth and survival.

SUMMARY

Agrobacteria induce crown gall tumors by incorporating a specific fragment of a plasmid present in all virulent strains into the plant cell. The minimum size of foreign DNA required for transformation has not been determined but it probably encompasses no more than a few genes. Part, but apparently not all, of the incorporated DNA is transcribed into RNA. It is quite likely that the incorporated DNA may code for enzymes concerned with the synthesis of octopine and nopaline, compounds only found in tumor cells. These compounds can be utilized by the agrobacteria inducing the tumor and promote the transfer of plasmids to plasmidless strains. Thus, the bacteria serve as genetic engineers and subvert the metabolism of the host plant to synthesize unique compounds which only agrobacteria can utilize.

Acknowledgments

The studies conducted in Seattle were supported by Public Health Service grant CA-13015 from the National Cancer Institute and by Grant NP 194 from the American Cancer Society. The studies in Seattle were conducted by an interdepartmental group of Biochemistry, Botany, Genetics, and Microbiology. The members include (in alphabetical order): A. J. Bendich, R. Bowman, M.-D. Chilton, T. C. Currier, M. H. Drummond, F. Eden, D. J. Garfinkel, S. K. Farrand, M. P. Gordon, R. Jensen, R. Johnson, D. J. Merlo, A. L. Montoya, R. C. Nutter, D. Sciaky, R. Saiki, B. Watson, F. White, and F. M. Yang.

REFERENCES

1. Bomhoff, G. H. 1974. Studies on crown gall—a plant tumor. Investigations on protein composition and on the use of guanidine compounds as a marker for transformed cells. Ph. D. Thesis, University of Leiden, The Netherlands.
2. Braun, A. C. and P. R. White. 1943. Bacteriological sterility of tissues derived from secondary crown gall tumors. *Phytopathology* **33**: 85–100.
3. Braun, A. C. 1977. *The Story of Cancer.* Addison-Wesley Publ., Reading, Massachusetts.
4. Chilton, M.-D., S. K. Farrand, F. Eden, T. C. Currier, A. J. Bendich, M. P. Gordon, and E. W. Nester. 1975. Is there foreign DNA in crown gall tumor DNA. *In*: R. Markham, D. R. Davies, D. A. Hopwood, and R. W. Horne (eds.). *Modification of the Information Content of Plant Cells.* North-Holland Publ., Amsterdam, pp. 247–311.
5. Chilton, M.-D., S. K. Farrand, R. L. Levin, and E. W. Nester. 1976. RP4 promotion of transfer of a large *Agrobacterium* plasmid which confers virulence. *Genetics* **83**: 609–618.
6. Chilton, M.-D., M. H. Drummond, D. J. Merlo, D. Sciaky, A. L. Montoya, M. P. Gordon, and E. W. Nester. 1977. Stable Incorporation of plasmid DNA into higher plant cells: the molecular basis of crown gall tumorigenesis. *Cell* **11**: 263–271.
7. DeCleene, M. and J. De Ley. 1976. The host range of crown gall. *Bot. Rev.* **42**: 389–466.
8. Gentello, C., N. Van Larabeke, M. Holsters, M. Van Montagu, and J. Schell. 1977. Ti plasmids of *Agrobacterium* as conjugative plasmids. *Nature* **265**: 561–563.

9. Goldman, A., J. Tempe, and G. Morel. 1968. Quelques particularites de diverses souches d'*Agrobacterium tumefaciens*. *Comp. Rend. Seances Soc. Biol. (Paris)* **162**: 630–631.
10. Goldman, A., D. W. Thomas, and G. Morel. 1969. Sur la structure de la nopaline metabolite anormal de certaines tumerus de crown gall. *Comp. Rend. Acad. Sci. (Paris)* **268**: 852–854.
11. Heberlein, G. T., J. De Ley, and R. Tijtgat. 1967. Deoxyribonucleic acid homology and taxonomy of *Agrobacterium, Rhizobium* and *Chromobacterium*. *J. Bacteriol.* **94**: 116–124.
12. Holsters, M., D. Dewaele, A. Depicker, E. Messens, M. Van Montagu, and J. Schell. 1978. Transfection and transformation of *Agrobacterium tumefaciens*. *Mol. Gen. Gen.* **163**: 181–189.
13. Klapwick, P. M., P. J. J. Hookyaas, H. C. M. Kerster, R. A. Schilperoort, and A. Rorsch. 1976. Isolation and characterization of *Agrobacterium tumefaciens* mutants affected in the utilization of octopine, octopinic acid and lysopine. *J. Gen. Microbiol.* **96**: 155–163.
14. Kerr, A., P. Manigault, and J. Tempe. 1977. Transfer of virulence *in vivo* and *in vitro* in *Agrobacterium*. *Nature* **265**: 560–561.
15. Lippincott, J. A., R. Biederbeck, and B. B. Lippincott. 1973. Utilization of octopine and nopaline by *Agrobacterium*. *J. Bacteriol.* **116**: 368–383.
16. Maniatis, T., A. Jeffrey, and D. G. Kleid. 1975. Nucleotide sequence of the rightwards operator phage λ. *Proc. Natl. Acad. Sci. U.S.* **72**: 1184–1188.
17. Menage, A. and G. Morel. 1964. Sur la presence d'octopine dans les tissue de crown gall. *Comp. Rend. Acad. Sci. (Paris)* **259**: 4795–4796.
18. Montoya, A. L., M.-D. Chilton, M. P. Gordon, D. Sciaky, and E. W. Nester. 1977. Octopine and nopaline metabolism in *Agrobacterium tumefaciens* and crown gall tumor cells: Role of plasmid genes. *J. Bacteriol.* **129**: 101–107.
19. Petit, A., S. Delhaye, J. Tempe, and G. Morel. 1970. Recherches sur les guanidines des tissues de crown gall. Mise en evidence d'une relation biochimique specifique entre les souches d'*Agrobacterium tumefaciens* et les tumeurs qu'elles induisent. *Physiol. Veg.* **8**: 205–213.
20. Schilperoort, R. A., J. J. M. Dons, and H. Ras. 1975. Characterization of the Complex formed between PS8 cRNA and DNA isolated from A6-induced sterile crown gall tissue. *In*: R. Markham, D. R. Davies, D. A. Hopwood, and R. W. Horne (eds.). *Modification of the Information Content of Plant Cells*. North-Holland Publ., Amsterdam, pp. 253–286.
21. Smith, E. F. and C. O. Townsend. 1907. A plant tumor of bacterial origin. *Science* **25**: 671–673.
22. Southern, E. M. 1975. Detection of specific sequences among DNA fragments separated by gel electrophoresis. *J. Mol. Biol.* **98**: 503–517.
23. Van Larebeke, N., C. Genetello, J. Schell, R. A. Schilperoort, A. K. Hermans,

J. P. Hernalsteens, and M. Van Montagu. 1975. Aquisition of tumor-inducing ability by non-oncogenic agrobacteria as a result of plasmid transfer. *Nature* **255**: 742–743.

24. Watson, B., T. G. Currier, M. P. Gordon, M. D. Chilton, and E. W. Nester. 1975. Plasmid required for virulence of *Agrobacterium tumefaciens*. *J. Bacteriol.* **123**: 255–264.
25. Wetmur, J. G. 1976. Hybridization and renaturation kinetics of nucleic acids. *Annu. Rev. Biophys. Bioengng.* **5**: 337–361.
26. Zaenen, I., N. Van Larebeke, H. Teuchy, M. Van Montagu, and J. Schell. 1974. Supercoiled circular DNA in crown gall inducing *Agrobacterium* strains. *J. Mol. Biol.* **86**: 109–127.

Discussion of Paper by Dr. Nester

NESTER responded to questions from HANCHEY and URITANI by emphasizing that there are at least 4 distinct tumor types and that in two of them (nopaline-less and octopine-less tumors) there seems to be less plasmid DNA in the tumor cells; therefore the portion of the Ti plasmid conferring octopine and nopaline synthesis may be superfluous for tumorgenesis. He acknowledged the hypothesis recently proposed by EINSET and SKOOG that at least one of the essential cistons on restriction fragment 3 might code for a cytokinin synthetase, but that this has not been experimentally tested. As pointed out by SCHEFFER, we are not yet sure that any of the plasmid tumor-inducing DNA is transcribed and translated but may merely affect normal regulation of endogenous plant hormone biosynthesis. In response to VANETTEN, NESTER stated that no one has initiated tumors with isolated plasmid DNA or a restriction fragment and noted the interesting possibility that the active plasmid fragment might code for a polycistronic message, despite the fact that plants are thought to only process monocistronic messenger RNAs. How this might occur is not known. SCHEFFER said that Armin Braun could obtain plants from some tobacco crown gall cultures and that these regenerated plants still synthesized nopaline, although appearing normal. NESTER agreed and further noted that the nopaline synthesizing ability was lost in the seed progeny of such plants. This might indicate that the nopaline-synthesizing determinant was cytoplasmically carried. In this line, NESTER reported that experiments are in progress to determine where plasmid DNA is located in tumor cells. For instance, by using highly labelled RNA that is complementary to plasmid fragment 3 DNA, one could attempt to see where it hybridizes in the crown gall cell (nucleus, mitochondria, chloroplasts?). In response to DAY, NESTER said that the Ti plasmids from about 40 *Agrobacterium* strains varied from 98 to 168 Mdaltons. This indicates that a minimum size of 98 million is probably required for an active Ti plasmid. Since only a small portion of this appears to be present in tumors, the function of the remaining DNA is obscure but could be involved in plasmid transfer to the plant. Nester emphasized that many smaller plasmids are found in *Agrobacterium* as well as other bacteria, but they seem to have no role in tumorgenesis. In response to BRAKKE, NESTER indicated that we don't know if the plasmid DNA occurs as a circular DNA fragment in the host although recent data suggest that plasmid DNA is integrated into plant DNA.

In response to SEQUEIRA, NESTER said that his laboratory is attempting to clone all the crown gall plasmid restriction fragments, but that this has not yet succeeded with restriction fragment 3. Wheeler raised the crucial question of whether live *Agrobacterium* cells could have been present in the gall tissue used for preparation of nucleic acid in the hybridization experiments. NESTER said that all callus gall tissue used was routinely tested for bacteria by plating and that since only restriction fragment 3 hybridized with tumor DNA, it was not likely that the tumors contained bacteria; if they did, one would have expected hybridization of the entire plasmid to the tumor DNA.

Recognition and Specificity in Plant Host-Parasite Interactions, pp. 301-316, 1979

RELATIONSHIP BETWEEN TOLERANCE TO ISOFLAVONOID PHYTOALEXINS AND PATHOGENICITY

HANS D. VANETTEN

Department of Plant Pathology, Cornell University, Ithaca, New York, U.S.A.

The phytoalexin concept was developed and has continued to be used in an attempt to give a mechanistic explanation for the phenomena of induced and active resistance in higher plants. Studies involving phytoalexins consequently have emphasized those interactions which result in a resistant response. In this paper I would like to discuss isoflavonoid phytoalexins in the context of certain susceptible interactions. If phytoalexin production by higher plants is the basis of a resistance mechanism, then a pathogen in a susceptible interaction must somehow circumvent this response. Two main hypotheses relative to the phytoalexin concept have been proposed to explain susceptibility. It has been proposed that either the successful pathogen is tolerant of the phytoalexin produced, or that the successful pathogen does not elicit phytoalexin accumulation to toxic levels. I shall be dealing primarily with the proposal that phytoalexin tolerance is associated with susceptibility in certain host-parasite interactions.

In this paper I shall concentrate on pisatin, one of the phytoalexins produced by garden pea, *Pisum sativum* L., and phaseollin, one of the phytoalexins produced by kidney bean, *Phaseolus vulgaris* L. I will be describing the accumulation of these phytoalexins in susceptible interactions, their phytotoxicity, the differential sensitivity of fungi to these compounds, the relationship between tolerance and phytoalexin catabolism, the evidence for *in situ* interactions between these phytoalexins and pathogens, and the possible requirement of phytoalexin tolerance for pathogenicity. I shall use examples primarily from our own studies on these compounds and the three *formae speciales* of *Fusarium solani* (Mart.) Sacc. identified as *pisi, phaseoli,* and *cucurbitae. Fusarium solani* f. sp. *pisi* and *F. solani phaseoli* cause a cortical rot on the lower stem and upper root area of pea and bean, respectively. *F. solani* f. sp. *cucurbitae*, a pathogen of cucurbits, is included as a representative non-pathogen of bean and pea.

I. PRODUCTION OF ISOFLAVONOID PHYTOALEXINS IN HOST-PARASITIC INTERACTIONS

Müller and Börger (*16*) initially proposed that the discriminating event that determines resistance or susceptibility is the rate of phytoalexin synthesis. Other authors (*11, 13*) have also endorsed the basic concept that there is a faster rate and/or larger amount of phytoalexin synthesis in a resistant than in a susceptible interaction. Generally these discussions pertain to race-specific interactions which may involve gene-for-gene systems. Only a few race specific interactions involving isoflavonoid phytoalexins have been investigated and in those interactions phytoalexins accumulate at a faster rate and/or to higher concentration in the resistant than in the susceptible interactions (*2, 9, 12*). However, if non-race specific interactions are examined, one finds examples in which resistance can occur with very little phytoalexin accumulation and susceptibility can occur even in the presence of high concentrations of phytoalexin. The recent report by Duczek and Higgins (*8*) on the interaction of *Stemphylium botryosum* Wallr. and red clover is an example of a resistant reaction occurring in a phytoalexin-producing plant with only a slight accumulation of the plant's phytoalexins. In contrast, our work provides examples of susceptible interactions in which high concentrations of phytoalexins occur in the infected tissue. Very high amounts of pisatin that can accumulate in *P. sativum*-infected tissue during the susceptible interaction with *F. solani* f. sp. *pisi* (*17*) (Fig. 1A and B). In three separate experiments the lesion volume steadily increased after inoculation (Fig. 1B). Very high concentrations of pisatin accumulated in this same tissue sometime during the course of lesion development, reaching a maximum in one case of over 5 mg per cm^3 (Fig. 1A). A similar situation has been observed during the infection of bean hypocotyl tissue by *F. solani* f. sp. *phaseoli* (*25*). This

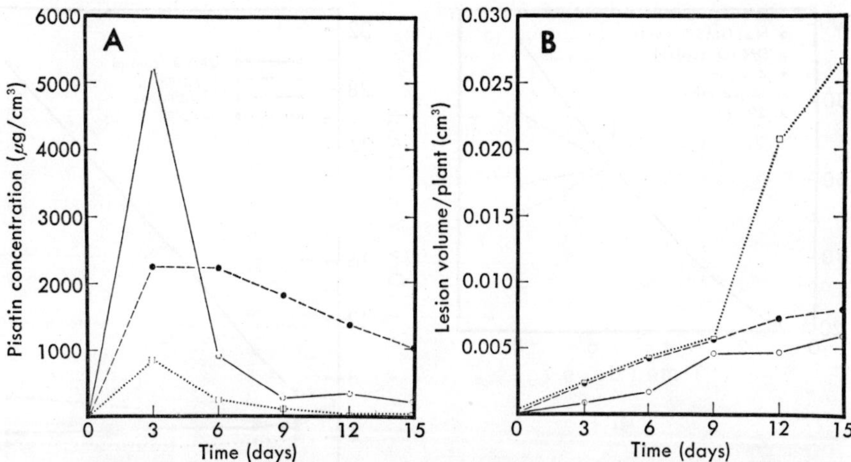

Fig. 1. A, Pisatin concentration in the lesion, and B, lesion volume per plant in pea epicotyls inoculated with *F. solani* f. sp. *pisi*. The results of three separate experiments are plotted as dashed, dotted, or solid lines (*17*).

pathogen causes a spreading lesion in bean tissue even though the infected tissue can contain phytoalexin concentrations as high as 5% of the dry weight. The prevention of phytoalexin accumulation would, therefore, not appear to account for the susceptibility of pea and bean to *F. solani* f. sp. *pisi* and *F. solani* f. sp. *phaseoli*, respectively.

II. THE PHYTOTOXICITY OF PISATIN AND PHASEOLLIN

The antifungal properties of pisatin and phaseollin have been demonstrated repeatedly (*24*), but in only a few cases has the toxicity of these phytoalexins to their source plants been examined. Although Cruickshank and Perrin (*6*) failed to observe any toxicity of pisatin to endocarp cells of pea pods, Bailey (*1*) demonstrated that concentration of <10 μg of pisatin/ml inhibited the growth of pea callus tissue and recently Shiraishi *et al.* (*19*) showed that concentrations of ≥ 300 μg of pisatin/ml are toxic to stemepiderm is cells of pea and to protoplasts prepared from leaf epidermis tissue. Exogenously added phaseollin can cause permeability changes in *P. vulgaris* hypocotyl and leaf tissue (*9, 23*) and is toxic to cells in cell suspension cultures of *P. vulgaris* (*10*). When such cultures were treated with phaseollin, the cells failed to accumulate and retain the vital stain neutral red and the growth rate of the phaseollin-treated cultures was altered (*10*) (Fig. 2).

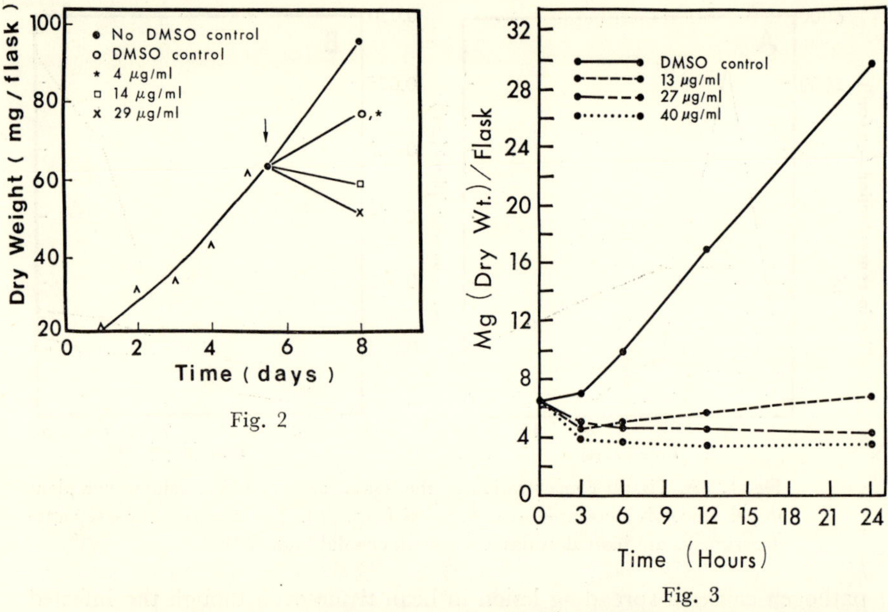

Fig. 2. Effect of phaseollin on the growth of kidney bean cell suspension cultures. Growth (as mg dry wt./flask) was recorded for 5.5 days (∧), and then cultures (50 ml in 125 ml flasks) were treated. Phaseollin in dimethylsulfoxide (DMSO) at a final concentration of 4, 14, and 29 μg of phaseollin/ml of medium was added to the cultures at the time indicated by the arrow, and the cultures were harvested after an additional incubation period of 60 hr. Controls consisted of cultures receiving no DMSO or cultures receiving the same amount of DMSO as used for phaseollin treatment (final DMSO conc.=0.3%) (*10*).

Fig. 3. Effect of phaseollin on the growth of *F. solani* f. sp. *cucurbitae* in liquid shake culture (4.0 ml/25 ml flasks). Phaseollin in DMSO at a final concentration of 13, 27, and 40 μg of phaseollin/ml of medium was added to the cultures at time 0 and growth was recorded as mg dry wt./flasks. Final DMSO concentration in the phaseollin treatments and the DMSO control was 0.5% (*26*).

When one compares the effects of phaseollin on the growth of bean cell suspension cultures with the effect of phaseollin on the growth of phaseollin-sensitive fungi in shake cultures (*23, 26*), one realizes that phaseollin is as inhibitory to *P. vulgaris* as it is to a sensitive fungus such as *F. solani* f. sp. *cucurbitae* (Fig. 2 *vs.* Fig. 3). The concentration of phaseollin per ml of media, the ratio of phaseollin per mg dry weight of the test organisms, and the environmental culturing conditions were similar (*10, 23, 26*). At 4 μg of phaseollin per ml (data for *F. solani* f. sp. *cucurbitae* not shown) the phytoalexin had little effect, but at concentrations above 13–14 μg/ml growth of both types of organisms is prevented and an actual loss in dry weight occurs. Phaseollin and pisatin appear to be broad spectrum toxins and which are as toxic *in vitro* to their source plant tissues as to most fungi.

The phytotoxicity of pisatin and phaseollin to pea and bean, respectively, is consistent with the obvious necrosis of the plant tissue routinely observed in both susceptible and resistant interactions in which these compounds accumulate to high concentrations. Whether the observed necrosis is the result or the cause of phytoalexin accumulation is unresolved.

III. DIFFERENTIAL SENSITIVITY OF FUNGI TO PISATIN AND PHASEOLLIN

The presence of high phytoalexin concentration in resistant interactions is consistent with cessation of growth of a potential parasite in such interactions. However, when a high concentration of phytoalexin accumulates in a susceptible interaction, it might appear paradoxical that the pathogen continues to ramify through the infected tissue in what is a potentially toxic environment. One explanation of this apparent paradox is that a successful pathogen, unlike the host itself or non-pathogens, is tolerant of the phytoalexin (*5*). The classic studies of Cruickshank and colleagues (*4, 7*) on pisatin and phaseollin demonstrated that in general pathogens were more tolerant of their host's phytoalexin than non-pathogens of those plant species. Numerous exceptions to this pattern exist and the type of bioassay conditions employed can markedly influence the apparent antifungal activity of phytoalexins (*3, 24*). Nevertheless, if one selects a biased sample, a dramatic difference in sensitivity to these phytoalexins can be demonstrated. The response of the three *formae speciales pisi, phaseoli,* and *cucurbitae* of *F. solani* to pisatin or phaseollin is a case in point. When these three *formae speciales* are tested in radial growth bioassays on phytoalexin-amended semi-solid media, the nonpathogen of bean or pea, *F. solani* f. sp. *cucurbitae,* is strongly inhibited by both pisatin and phaseollin while the pea pathogen, *F. solani* f. sp. *pisi* is tolerant of pisatin and the bean pathogen, *F. solani* f. sp. *phaseoli,* is tolerant of phaseollin (Fig. 4A and B).

The relatively high degree of sensitivity of *F. solani* f. sp. *cucurbitae* to pisatin and phaseollin and the relative high degree of tolerance of *F. solani* f. sp. *pisi* to pisatin remained constant when these isolates were tested under

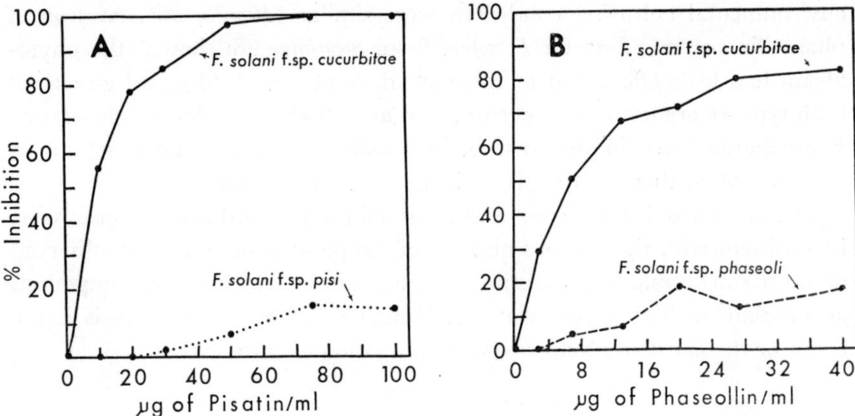

Fig. 4. A, Effect of pisatin on the radial growth of *F. solani* f. sp. *cucurbitae* and *F. solani* f. sp. *pisi* and B, effect of phaseollin on the radial growth of *F. solani* f. sp. *cucurbitae* and *F. solani* f. sp. *phaseoli*. A 40 mm (diam.) mycelial plug was placed on the surface of a semi-solid medium amended with phytoalexin dissolved in DMSO or DMSO alone (final DMSO conc.=0.5%). The percent inhibition was determined when the DMSO controls had a net growth of 27±4 mm (4 days for *F. solani* f. sp. *pisi* and *F. solani* f. sp. *cucurbitae* and 8 days for *F. solani* f. sp. *phaseoli*) (*26*).

a variety of bioassay conditions (*26*). The response of *F. solani* f. sp. *phaseoli* to phaseollin, however, varied considerably and depended on what type of bioassay conditions were employed. The response also sometimes varied between experiments employing the same type of bioassay. Examples of this latter type of variation are illustrated in Fig. 5A and B, which show the results of two duplicate experiments designed to measure the effect of phaseollin on dry weight increases of *F. solani* f. sp. *phaseoli* in shake culture. In a given experiment (Fig. 5A) this organism may appear relatively sensitive to phaseollin while in a repeated experiment it may appear quite tolerant of the compound (Fig. 5B). The reasons for the variability of response are not known, but we speculate that some of the variation may be related to the rapid fungicidal potential of phaseollin (*20, 26*) and to the possible presence of an adaptive tolerance mechanism as *F. solani* f. sp. *phaseoli* to phaseollin.

Two types of observations suggest an adaptive tolerance mechanism to phaseollin in *F. solani* f. sp. *phaseoli*. Its growth rate in phaseollin-supplemented liquid shake cultures occasionally was comparable to that in the controls after an initial lag period (Fig. 5A and B). Secondly, a short exposure

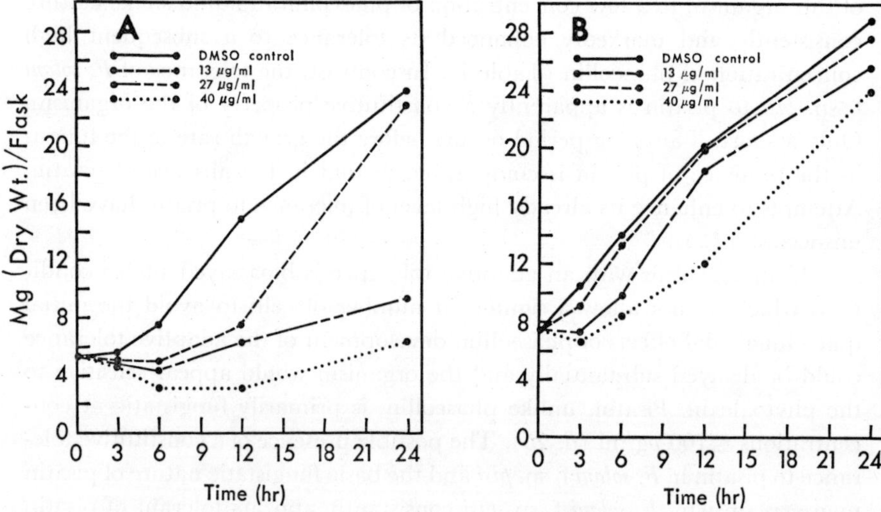

Fig. 5. A and B, Effect of phaseollin on the growth of *F. solani* f. sp. *phaseoli* in liquid shake culture in two separate experiments. The fungus was bioassayed as described in Fig. 3 (*26*).

TABLE I

Effect in Shake Culture of a Pretreatment with a Low Concentration of Phaseollin on the Response of *F. solani* f. sp. *phaseoli* to a Subsequent Treatment with a Higher Concentration of Phaseollin (*26*)[a]

Treatment	Dry wt. (mg/flask) at		
	0 hr	1.5 hr	13.5 hr
None	5.9		
DMSO at 0 hr		6.6	
3 µg phaseollin/ml at 0 hr		6.7	
DMSO at 0 hr and DMSO at 1.5 hr			26.4
3 µg phaseollin/ml at 0 hr and DMSO at 1.5 hr			25.8
DMSO at 0 hr and 27 µg phaseollin/ml at 1.5 hr			12.4
3 µg phaseollin at 0 hr and 27 g phaseollin/ml at 1.5 hr			22.7

[a] Approximately 6 mg (dry wt.) of the fungi were suspended in 4.0 ml of medium contained in 25 ml flasks. Samples were treated with phaseollin (3 µg/ml of medium) in DMSO or a comparable volume of DMSO and incubated at 24±2°C on a reciprocal shaker (125 strokes/min) for 1.5 hr. Some samples then were treated with additional phaseollin (27 µg/ml medium) or DMSO. The final DMSO concentration for each treatment was 0.5%.

of this organism to a low concentration of phaseollin in liquid shake culture consistently and markedly enhanced its tolerance to a subsequent high concentration of phaseollin (Table I). In contrast, the tolerance of *F. solani* f. sp. *pisi* to pisatin is apparently a constitutive property of the organism. Only a short, if any, lag period occurs before the growth rate of the fungus in the presence of pisatin is comparable to that in the absence of pisatin. Attempts to enhance its already high level of tolerance to pisatin have been unsuccessful (*26*).

If an organism with an adaptive tolerance is bioassayed under conditions which do not allow a significant number of cells to avoid the initial quick fungicidal effects of phaseollin, development of the adaptive tolerance could be delayed substantially and the organism would appear sensitive to the phytoalexin. Pisatin, unlike phaseollin, is primarily fungistatic at concentrations $\leq$100 μg/ml (*6, 26*). The possible presence of a constitutive tolerance to pisatin in *F. solani* f. sp. *pisi* and the basic fungistatic nature of pisatin may explain why *F. solani* f. sp. *pisi* consistantly appears tolerant of pisatin regardless of the bioassay conditions.

IV. RELATIONSHIP BETWEEN TOLERANCE AND ABILITY TO CATABOLIZE PHYTOALEXINS

F. solani f. sp. *pisi* demethylates pisatin to the less inhibitory compound 3,6a-dihydorxy-8,9-methylenedioxypterocarpan (DMDP) (*24, 27*). *F. solani* f. sp. *phaseoli* oxidizes phaseollin to the less inhibitory compound 1a-hydroxyphaseollone (*21, 22, 25*). *Fusarium solani* f. sp. *cucurbitae* is not able to metabolize either phaseollin or pisatin (*26*) and is sensitive to both phytoalexins. Although this might suggest that the mechanism of phytoalexin tolerance in *F. solani* is due to metabolic detoxification of the compounds, other data indicate that fungal metabolism of isoflavonoid phytoalexins may not always be a detoxification mechanism and that other tolerance mechanisms are likely (*24, 26*). For example, *F. solani* f. sp. *pisi* grows substantially in shake cultures supplemented with pisatin prior to significant catabolism of the compound (Table II). Thus, mechanisms in addition to or instead of metabolic detoxification of pisatin must account for the tolerance of *F. solani* f. sp. *pisi* to pisatin *in vitro*.

Both tolerance to phaseollin and metabolism of phaseollin are enhanced in *F. solani* f. sp. *phaseoli* by a prior exposure to phaseollin (*21, 26*). We have been unable to demonstrate growth of *F. solani* f. sp. *phaseoli* in

TABLE II

Metabolism of Pisatin by *F. solani* f. sp. *pisi* in Relation to Growth (*26*)[a]

Treatment	Dry wt. (mg/flask) at		% Pisatin recovered at	μg/ml of DMDP[b] at
	0 hr	6 hr	6 hr	6 hr
98 μg of pisatin/ml at 0 hr	6.4	9.0	95	1 μg/ml

[a] Cultures prepared and treated with phytoalexin as described in Table I. [b] DMDP, 3, 6a-dihydroxy-8, 9-methylenedioxypterocarpan.

shake culture before all the phaseollin is metabolized, whether or not it has been pretreated with that compound (*26*). Our data thus do not clarify whether the adaptation to phaseollin by *F. solani* f. sp. *phaseoli* depends on enhanced catabolism.

V. DOES PISATIN OR PHASEOLLIN INTERACT *IN SITU* WITH CERTAIN PATHOGENIC *F. SOLANI* ISOLATES?

Of paramount importance to the possible involvement of phytoalexins in disease resistance is the location of these compounds in infected plant tissue. Little biological activity by them would be expected if they are physically (or chemically) sequestered from the invading parasite. The site of occurrence of pisatin or phaseollin in plant tissue is not known. Failure to isolate intact protoplasts containing pisatin from pisatin-producing leaf tissue suggests but does not prove that the phytoalexin may be released into the cell wall or intercellular spaces in leaves (*18*).

Even though there is no direct evidence for where pisatin or phaseollin are located in plant tissue, circumstantial evidence suggests that phaseollin interacts with the bean pathogen *F. solani* f. sp. *phaseoli in situ*. The product of *in vitro* phaseollin catabolism by *F. solani* f. sp. *phaseoli*, 1a-hydroxyphaseollone, can be isolated from bean tissue infected with that fungus (*25*). To date we have not been able to induce the formation of this compound in *P. vulgaris* tissue abiotically (VanEtten, unpublished results). Cell suspension cultures of *P. vulgaris* metabolically alter exogenously-added phaseollin, but 1a-hydroxyphaseollone was not detected as one of the products produced (*10*). The most straightforward explanation of the origin of the 1a-hydroxyphaseollone in *F. solani* f. sp. *phaseoli*-infected bean tissue is that this pathogen came into contact with the host's phytoalexin. Since substantial amounts of phaseollin remain in infected tissue, some of the phytoalexin must be inaccessible to the metabolic system of the pathogen.

Although *F. solani* f. sp. *pisi* can metabolize pisatin to DMDP, no DMDP was detected in pea epicotyl or root tissue infected with this pathogen (Steve Pueppke, personal communication). Whether the failure to detect DMDP is because this pathogen and pisatin do not come into contact or for some other reason is not known at this time.

VI. IS PATHOGENICITY OR VIRULENCE RELATED TO PHYTOALEXIN TOLERANCE AND/OR PHYTOALEXIN CATABOLISM?

The initial studies by Cruickshank (*4*) on the differential sensitivity of fungi to pisatin revealed an almost absolute correlation between tolerance and sensitivity to pisatin and pathogenicity and nonpathogenicity to pea, respectively. The numerous subsequent studies on the relationship between phytoalexin tolerance or phytoalexin catabolism and virulence have had contradictory results. Although the observations that the type of bioassay conditions can markedly influence the apparent sensitivity of certain fungi complicates the interpretation of *in vitro* responses, it still seems clear that the correlation is not absolute. Nor would it seem logical that such an absolute correlation would be expected. Pathogenicity surely requires a multitude of physiological attributes of which tolerance of phytoalexins may be only one. It would seem highly probable that non-pathogenic isolates can be obtained which are tolerant of a phytoalexin but lack some other attribute needed for pathogenicity. Looking at the question of phytoalexin tolerance and pathogenicity in a slightly different manner, it can be asked is this tolerance required for pathogenicity? If the phytoalexin sensitivity of fungi which initially appeared tolerant of their host's phytoalexin is increased, does their virulence decrease?

To study this possibility we are using *F. solani* f. sp. *pisi* for two primary reasons. We have tested one isolate of this pea pathogen and it consistently appears tolerant of pisatin under a variety of bioassay conditions. Thus, unlike some other fungi, any bioassay seems to give a true indication of the *in vitro* sensitivity of the organism to this phytoalexin. Secondly, this organism has a perfect stage, *Nectria haematococca* (Syn. *Hypomyces solani*) Berk. & Br., that is amenable to genetic studies. If there appears to be a correlation between increased sensitivity to pisatin and lowered virulence, genetic analysis would be required to critically evaluate such an apparent correlation.

A straightforward evaluation of the relationship between tolerance to pisatin and virulence on pea is a genetic analysis. The approach is to cross *F. solani* f. sp. *pisi* with fungi sensitivie to pisatin and to analyze the segregation of virulence to pea and pisatin sensitivity. Although *F. solani* f. sp. *cucurbitae* is sensitive and has the same perfect stage as *F. solani* f. sp. *pisi*, the two *formae speciales* are not interfertile because they belong to different mating populations (MP) (*15*). We are, therefore, forced to look elsewhere for a sensitive isolate which can be crossed by normal sexual means with isolates of *F. solani* f. sp. *pisi*. *Fusarium solani* f. sp. *pisi* belongs to MP VI and members of this MP can also be found in habitats other than infected pea tissue (*14*). If tolerance to pisatin is not linked to some other survival character, the chance of finding an isolate sensitive to pisatin may be greater in isolates of MP VI originating from habitats other than infected peas. We have identified 39 members of MP VI and these have all been tested for the virulence on pea and for their sensitivity to pisatin. None of these isolates of *N. haematococca* MP VI exhibited the extreme sensitivity observed in *F. solani* f. sp. *cucurbitae*. However, the isolates did vary in their sensitivity to pisatin and the six most sensitive isolates of the 39 were non-pathogenic or only weakly virulent on pea. In addition, the most highly virulent isolates were all very tolerant of pisatin. As expected non-pathogenic or weakly virulent isolates that were very tolerant of pisatin were found. Much further work is needed to determine if increased sensitivity to pisatin always decreases virulence on pea in *N. haematococca* MP VI, but these preliminary results are suggestive of such a relationship.

VII. CONCLUDING COMMENTS

An examination of the susceptible interactions produced by *F. solani* f. sp. *pisi* on pea and *F. solani* f. sp. *phaseoli* on bean, and of the *in vitro* responses of these pathogens to their host's phytoalexin does not reveal any obvious conflicts with the possibility that phytoalexin production may be the basis for a resistance response in some plants. In both of these susceptible interactions, high levels of phytoalexin accumulate in the infected tissue but each organism expresses a tolerance of its host's phytoalexin *in vitro*. The regulatory mechanism and the physiological basis for tolerance may be different in each organism but each organism seems capable of growth in the presence of very high concentrations of the compound. Phytoalexin tolerance by pathogens in some interactions may be a necessary requirement for pathogenicity.

This paper has dealt entirely with susceptibility and susceptible interactions. However, it is conceivable that the lack of an appropriate tolerance mechanism in an organism or an interference with the ability of a phytoalexin-tolerant organism to express its tolerance could be involved in resistance in some non-race specific or even some race specific interactions. In other words, the sitmulation of phytoalexin synthesis may be a non-specific event, but the manner in which the potential parasite responds to the phytoalexin produced or the way in which a plant might influence the potential parasite's response could be the discriminating event that determines the final outcome of the interaction.

Such a simple interpretation of the phytoalexin concept in regards to susceptibility and resistance fails to explain the cases in which a pathogen is highly sensitive to the phytoalexins from its host. In these interactions prevention of phytoalexin synthesis or accumulation may account for susceptibility. However, common root rot of pea caused by *Aphanomyces euteiches*, is an apparent exception (*17, 18*). This organism aggressively invades pea tissue even though it is very sensitive to pisatin *in vitro* and even though pisatin accumulates to concentrations substantially higher than those theoretically needed to completely prevent growth in the infected tissue. Attempts to experimentally explain this paradox within the framework of the phytoalexin concept have been unsuccessful (*18*). Results such as these point out the need for more research before it can be claimed that phytoalexin production in higher plants is the basis of a resistance response.

SUMMARY

High concentrations of pisatin occur during the susceptible interaction between *F. solani* f. sp. *pisi* and pea and likewise high concentrations of phaseollin occur during the susceptible interaction between *F. solani* f. sp. *phaseoli* and bean. These concentrations are toxic to both the host tissue and to most fungi in *in vitro* bioassays. However, both pathogens are tolerant of their host's phytoalexins. The biochemical basis of this tolerance is not clearly understood but in some cases mechanisms in addition to the metabolisms of the phytoalexin to non-toxic compounds appear to be involved.

There is circumstantial evidence that the detoxification of phaseollin by *F. solani* f. sp. *phaseoli* occurs *in situ*. Also there are preliminary indications that tolerance of pisatin by *F. solani* f. sp. *pisi* is required for a high level of virulence on pea. For some pathogens, tolerance of their host's phytoalexins may be a necessary atribute for pathogenicity.

REFERENCES

1. Bailey, J.A. 1970. Pisatin production by tissue cultures of *Pisum sativum* L. *J. Gen. Microbiol.* **61**: 409–415.
2. Bailey, J. A. and B. J. Deverall. 1971. Formation and activity of phaseollin in the interaction between bean hypocotyls (*Phaseolus vulgaris*) and physiological races of *Colletotrichum lindemuthianum. Physiol. Plant Pathol.* **1**: 435–449.
3. Bailey, J. A., G. A. Carter, and R. A. Skipp. 1976. The use and interpretation of bioassays for fungitoxicity of phytoalexins in agar media. *Physiol. Plant Pathol.* **8**: 189–194.
4. Cruickshank, I. A. M. 1962. Studies on phytoalexins. IV. The antimicrobial spectrum of pisatin. *Aust. J. Biol. Sci.* **15**: 147–159.
5. Cruickshank, I. A. M. 1965. Phytoalexins in the leguminosae with special reference to their selective toxicity. *Tagungsber. Dtsch. Akad. Landwirtschaftowiss. (Berlin)* **74**: 313–332.
6. Cruickshank, I. A. M. and D. R. Perrin. 1961. Studies on phytoalexins. III. The isolation, assay and general properties of a phytoalexin from *Pisum sativum* L. *Aust. J. Biol. Sci.* **14**: 336–348.
7. Cruickshank, I. A. M. and D. R. Perrin. 1971. Studies on phytoalexins. XI. The induction, antimicrobial spectrum and chemical assay of phaseollin. *Phytopathol. Z.* **70**: 209–229.
8. Duczek, L. J. and V. J. Higgins. 1976. The role of medicarpin and maackiain in the response of red clover leaves to *Helminthosporium carbonum, Stemphylium botryosum,* and *S. sarcinaeformae. Can. J. Bot.* **54**: 2609–2619.
9. Elnaghy, M. A. and R. Heitefuss. 1976. Permeability changes and production of antifungal compounds in *Phaseolus vulgaris* infected with *Uromyces phaseoli*. II. Role of phytoalexins. *Physiol. Plant Pathol.* **8**: 269–277.
10. Glazener, J. A. and H. D. VanEtten. 1978. Phytotoxicity to and alteration of phaseollin by cell suspension cultures of *Phaseolus vulgaris. Phytopathology* **68**: 111-117.
11. Hadwiger, L. A. and M. E. Schwochau. 1969. Host resistance responses—an induction hypothesis. *Phytopathology* **59**: 223–227.
12. Keen, N. T. 1971. Hydroxyphaseollin production by soybeans resistant and susceptible to *Phytophthora megasperma* var. *sojae. Physiol. Plant Pathol.* **1**: 265–275.

13. Keen, N. T. 1976. Specific elicitors of phytoalexin: Determinants of race specificity? *In*: K. Tomiyama, J. M. Daly, I. Uritani, K. Oku, and S. Ouchi (eds.). *Biochemistry and Cytology of Plant Parasite Interactions*. Kodansha Ltd., Tokyo, and Elsevier, Amsterdam, pp. 84–93.
14. Matuo, T. and W. C. Snyder. 1972. Host virulence and the hypomyces stage of *Fusarium solani* f. sp. *pisi*. *Phytopathology* **62**: 731–735.
15. Matuo, T. and W. C. Snyder. 1973. Use of morphology and mating populations in the identification of formae speciales in *Fusarium solani*. *Phytopathology* **63**: 562–565.
16. Müller, K. O. and H. Börger. 1940. Experimentelle Untersuchungeh über die Phytophthora-Resistenz der Kartoffel. *Arb. Biol. Reichsanst. Landu. Forstwirtsch. (Berlin)* **23**: 189–231.
17. Pueppke, S. G. and H. D. VanEtten. 1974. Pisatin accumulation and lesion development in peas infected with *Aphanomyces euteiches, Fusarium solani* f. sp. *pisi*, or *Rhizoctonia solani*. *Phytopathology* **64**: 1433–1440.
18. Pueppke, S. G. and H. D. VanEtten. 1976. The relation between pisatin and the development of *Aphanomyces euteiches* in diseased *Pisum sativum*. *Phytopathology* **66**: 1174–1185.
19. Shiraishi, T., H. Oku, M. Isono, and S. Ouchi. 1975. The injurious effect of pisatin on the plasma membrane of pea. *Plant Cell Physiol.* **16**: 939–942.
20. Skipp, R. A. and J. A. Bailey. 1976. The effect of phaseollin on the growth of *Colletotrichum lindemuthianum* in bioassays designed to measure fungitoxicity. *Physiol. Plant Pathol.* **9**: 253–263.
21. Van den Heuvel, J. and H. D. VanEtten. 1973. Detoxification of phaseollin by *Fusarium solani* f. sp. *phaseoli*. *Physiol. Plant Pathol.* **3**: 327–339.
22. Van den Heuvel, J., H. D. VanEtten, J. W. Serum, D. L. Coffen, and T. H. Williams. 1974. Identification of 1a-hydroxyphaseollone, a phaseollin metabolite produced by *Fusarium solani*. *Phytochemistry* **13**: 1129–1131.
23. VanEtten, H. D. and D. F. Bateman. 1971. Studies on the mode of action of the phytoalexin phaseollin. *Phytopathology* **61**: 1363–1372.
24. VanEtten, H. D. and S. G. Pueppke. 1976. Isoflavonoid phytoalexins. *Annu. Proc. Phytochem. Soc.* **13**: 239–289.
25. VanEtten, H. D. and D. A. Smith. 1975. Accumulation of antifungal isoflavonoids and 1a-hydroxyphaseollone, a phaseollin metabolite, in bean tissue infected with *Fusarium solani* f. sp. *phaseoli*. *Physiol. Plant Pathol. 5*: 225–237.
26. VanEtten, H. D. and J. I. Stein. 1978. Differential response of *Fusarium solani* isolates to pisatin and phaseollin. *Phytopathology* **68**: 1276–1283.
27. VanEtten, H. D., S. G. Pueppke, and T. C. Kelsey. 1975. 3,6a-Dihydroxy-8,9-methylenedioxypterocarpan as a metabolite of pisatin produced by *Fusarium solani* f. sp. *pisi*. *Phytochemistry* **14**: 1103–1105.

Discussion of Paper by Dr. VanEtten

In the discussion of H. VanEtten's paper, Paxton noted that many plants make multiple phytoalexins and in view of this asked how resistance or sensitivity of a pathogen to only one phytoalexin from a plant could reliably indicate whether the microorganism would parasitize the plant? Van Etten recognized the importance of the problem but pointed out that at least one fungus (*F. solani* f. sp. *phaseoli*) has been shown to degrade the isoflavenone kievitone as well as the pterocarpan phaseollin. Oku pointed out that the sensitivity of a pathogen to a phytoalexin may be different depending on the environment, and that different morphologic forms of the pathogen may also be differentially sensitive. Van Etten acknowledged that it is difficult to emulate the plant environment in *in vitro* experiments but said that plant extract media had been used in the Aphanomyces work and acted like other artificial media. In response to a question by Siegel, VanEtten said that the adaptive degradation of phaseollin by *F. solani* f. sp. *phaseoli* likely did not involve selection of resistant mutants because the adaptation time was short and recovery of the fungus by growing on phaseollin-less medium overcame the induced resistance.

Kuć suggested that a differential phytoalexin tolerance hypothesis might work to explain differential pathogenicity with non gene-for-gene host-parasite systems, but was not likely with gene-for-gene systems that more likely involve specific elicitors and/or specific phytoalexin suppressors. Van Etten responded that this was likely but one could propose that gene-for-gene systems involved specific invocation of phytoalexin degrading enzyme systems in pathogens, and that these are simply not activated in incompatible host-parasite interactions. In response to Bell, VanEtten reiterated that *F. solani* f. sp. *phaseoli* will not degrade pisatin and *F. solani* f. sp. *pisi* will not degrade phaseollin, but develops an adaptive tolerance to it. Bell then pointed out that *Verticillium dahliae* vegetative cells do not degrade the cotton terpene phytoalexins, but that chlamydospores and resting microsclerotia of the same fungus have an enzyme, thought to be laccase, that does degrade them. It would be of interest to know if other examples of phytoalexin degrading enzymes specific only to certain morphologic (or physiologic) forms of plant pathogens exist. In discussion with ELLINGBOE, VAN ETTEN said that heterocaryons have not been formed and sexual crosses have not been performed between the *F. solani* forms such as *pisi* and *cucurbitae*, although it would be very lucrative if this were possible. He also said that mutants had been searched for but not found that lacked the enzyme(s) involved in degradation of pisatin. In response to TANI and DALY, VAN ETTEN emphasized that in the bean-*F. solani* f. sp. *phaseoli* system, the immediate degradation product of phaseollin, 1a-hydroxy phaseollone, can be readily isolated from infected tissues in concentrations as high as phaseollin. This establishes that the fungus contacts phaseollin during infection and that the degradation readily occurs in the host.

Recognition and Specificity in Plant Host-Parasite Interactions, pp. 317–333, 1979

THE ROLE OF PHYTOALEXINS IN HOST-PARASITE SPECIFICITY

HACHIRO OKU, TOMONORI SHIRAISHI, AND SEIJI OUCHI

College of Agriculture, Okayama University, Okayama, Japan

Since the phytoalexin theory was proposed by Müller and Börger (*13, 14*), a number of papers have appeared on the isolation, chemical characterization and role of phytoalexins in disease resistance in many host-parasite combinations, and these have been the subject of several review papers (*5, 6, 10, 36*). However, the exact role of phytoalexins in resistance or in determining host-parasite specificity remains obscure, although it seems to be rather diverse and dependent on the host-parasite combination.

Most research on phytoalexins has been done with saprophytic or facultative parasitic disease and little information is available in regard to phytoalexins accumulated in disease caused by obligate parasites. Recently we presented evidence that phytoalexins are produced also in obligate parasitic diseases, powdery mildews of barley and pea (*17, 19*). A systematic research (*17–19, 21, 22, 31*) on phytoalexins produced in these powdery mildews indicated that they seem to play a very important role in the host-parasite specificity.

I. BIPHASIC PRODUCTION OF PHYTOALEXINS IN THE PATHOGENESIS OF POWDERY MILDEW DISEASE

During the pathogenesis in powdery mildews of barley and pea plants, there were two phases of phytoalexin production. The first phase coincided with the stage of hyphal penetration by incompatible fungi.

In powdery mildew of barley, activity was detected at 8 hr after inoculation and was proportional to the degree of incompatibility in the race-cultivar interaction (Fig. 1). In pea stem tissues the first phase phytoalexin (pisatin) was detected in the epidermis by 12 hr of inoculation with

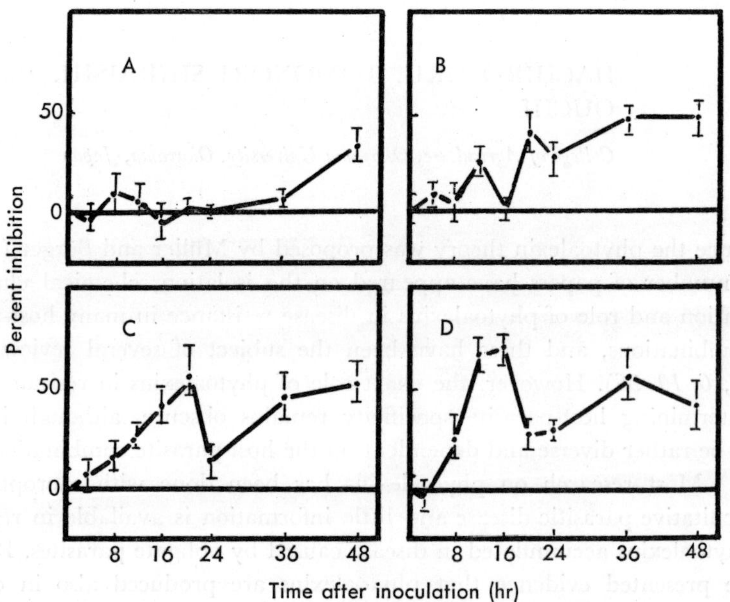

Fig. 1. Comparison of phytoalexin induction in some cultivar-race interaction of barley powdery mildew disease. A, Kobinkatagi-race 1 (reaction type 4); B, No. 21-race 1 (reaction type 3); C, No. 241-race 1 (reaction type 2); D, H.E.S.4-race 1 (reaction type 0). Percent inhibition was calculated as follows:

$$100-\left(\frac{\text{\% germination of race 1 on agarose block impregnated with exudate from inoculated leaves}}{\text{\% germination of race 1 on agarose block impregnated with exudate from noninoculated leaves}}\times 100\right)$$

nonpathogenic powdery mildew fungus, *Erysiphe graminis hordei*, at a concentration of 10 ppm. The concentration reached to 30 ppm by 15 hr post-inoculation.

In contrast to the incompatible fungus, compatible powdery mildew fungus induced phytoalexins after the infection was established.

In pea stem epidermis, pisatin was first detectable 24 hr after inoculation, then the concentration increased and reached 0.25% on a fresh weight basis in the epidermis on 6th day. The phytoalexin also accumulated in barley leaves inoculated with a compatible race of powdery mildew fungi in the tissues surrounding the colony that ceased growth.

The phytoalexin thus produced after the establishment of infection by powdery mildew fungus was called the second phase phytoalexin.

II. SUPPRESSION OF THE FIRST PHASE PHYTOALEXIN PRODUCTION BY HEAT TREATMENT, AND PRELIMINARY INOCULATION WITH COMPATIBLE RACE

The parallel activity of the first phase phytoalexin with the degree of incompatibility in barley-*E. graminis* combinations and the coincidence of the time of penetration with the appearance of the first phase phytoalexin suggested that the one in the first phase might possibly be concerned with resistance to infection.

The resistance of barley leaves against powdery mildew fungus was broken by heat treatment (*25*), and the scalded leaves which lost the resistance did not produce the first phase phytoalexin activity even when inoculated with an incompatible race (*18*).

Tsuchiya and Hirata (*33*), Ouchi *et al.* (*23, 24*) reported that the preliminary inoculation with a compatible race of *E. graminis* rendered barley leaves accessible to originally incompatible race, and also to a nonpathogenic powdery mildew fungi. The inoculation of an incompatible race induced, on the other hand, a resistance to originally compatible races.

The production of the first phase phytoalexin in the incompatible interaction was suppressed when barley leaves were inoculated with a compatible race before the incompatible race was applied. Conversely, the preliminary inoculation with an incompatible race conditioned the leaves to produce the same level of phytoalexin on subsequent inoculation regardless of the compatibility of the challenger race (Fig. 2).

The facts described above suggest the importance of the first phase

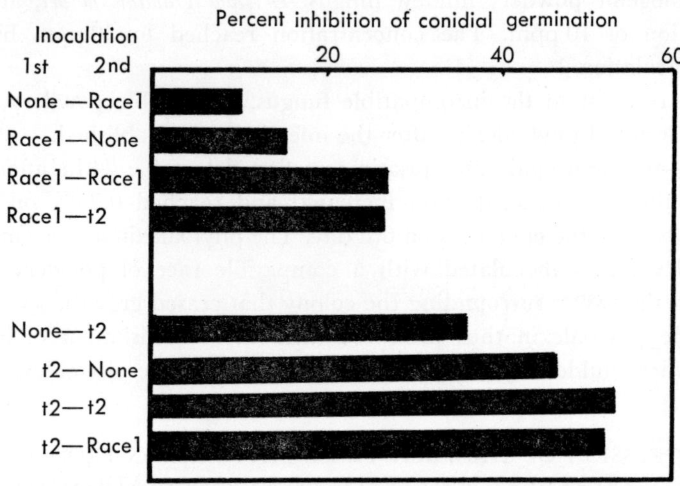

Fig. 2. Effect of accessibility and resistance induction on phytoalexin production in barley leaves. Accessibility (or resistance) was induced in barley leaves (cv. Kobinkatagi) by inoculation with race 1 (or t2) and phytoalexin production was estimated 12 hr after the second inoculation. The interval of the first and second inoculation was 48 hr.

phytoalexin in determining the host-parasite specificity, and the possibility that the pathogenic fungus can suppress the initiation of the general defense reaction to infection, leading to the induction of phytoalexin.

III. LOCALIZATION OF PHYTOALEXIN ACCUMULATION

To evaluate the real role of phytoalexin in host-parasite specificity, it is necessary to know the exact concentration of phytoalexins which accumulate at the infection sites. Sato and Tomiyama (*28*) reported that rishitin accumulated in the infected cells and the adjacent cells of potato tuber tissue inoculated with *Phytophthora infestans*.

When pea stem was inoculated with the pathogenic fungus, *E. pisi*, pisatin was found to accumulate only in the epidermal tissue, which is the actual infection site, but not in the underlying tissue. By inoculation with a nonpathogenic powdery mildew fungus, *E. graminis hordei*, pisatin was detected 12 hr after inoculation in the epidermis (Table I). The concentration at the infected site was more than 10 ppm at that time and this was enough

TABLE I

Local Accumulation of Pisatin in Pea Stem by Inoculation with Nonpathogenic (*E. graminis hordei*) and Pathogenic (*E. pisi*) Powdery Mildew Fungi

Time after inoculation (hr)	Concentration of pisatin accumulated (μg/g fresh weight)[a]			
	E. graminis hordei		*E. pisi*	
	Epidermis	Stem without epidermis	Epidermis	Stem without epidermis
10	0	0	0	0
11.5	0	0	0	0
12	10.1	0	0	0
13	15.2	0	0	0
15	33.0	0	0	0
20	34.0	0	0	0
24	20.0	0	46.2	0
48	Not tested	Not tested	232	0
96	Not tested	Not tested	697	7.7

[a] Data are the average of 4 replications.

to inhibit the infection even by the pathogenic fungus, *E. pisi*, as described later. Pisatin and barleyp hytoalexin accumulated just beneath and in the adjacent tissues of the fungal colonies, but not in tissues more than 5 mm from the colonies.

Puppke and VanEtten (*27*) also reported that pisatin accumulated at epidermal and subepidermal tissues by ultra violet (UV) irradiation or by inoculation with *Aphanomyces euteiches*.

IV. SENSITIVITY OF POWDERY MILDEW FUNGI TO PHYTOALEXINS AND THE ROLE IN HOST-PARASITE SPECIFICITY

Several races and formae speciales of *E. graminis* showed the same grade of sensitivity to the phytoalexin of barley. On the other hand, pea pathogen, *E. pisi*, was tolerant to phytoalexin, pisatin, of its own host showing an ED_{50} for conidial germination of 530 ppm, in contrast to an ED_{50} of 40 ppm with a nonpathogen, *E. graminis hordei*. That is, the pathogenic fungus was 13 times more tolerant to pisatin than the nonpathogenic one.

Müller and Börger (*14*), and Cruickshank (*5*) presented an working hypothesis in regard to the role of phytoalexins in resistance or host-parasite specificity. They postulated that the specificity between host species or variety and parasite species or strain within species are determined by both the rate of phytoalexin synthesis and differential sensitivity of parasite to the phytoalexin.

However, in cases where specificity is determined at the level of variety-strain or cultivar-race interaction theoretically no difference of sensitivity to phytoalexin should be present among races or strains, because phytoalexins are chemically host specific. The only difference among races that should determine host-parasite specificity is their ability to induce phytoalexin in the host tissue. In these diseases, therefore, the determination of specificity depends solely upon the rate of phytoalexin induction.

If there is any race insensitive to phytoalexin, it should invade all variety or cultivars, hence theoretically no variety or cultivar should be incompatible to that race. No such race of barley powdery mildew fungus has been found in Japan so far, and the races of *E. graminis* were almost equally sensitive to barley phytoalexin as described above. The races of *P. infestans* were reported to be similarly sensitive to the potato phytoalexin, rishitin (*32*), and β-, γ-, and δ-races of *Colletotrichum lindemuthianum* also showed the same degree of sensitivity to phaseollin (*2*).

On the contrary, in cases where the specificity of host and parasiste is determined in species-species interaction or species-formae speciales interaction, the specificity should be determined not only by the rate of phytoalexin induction but also by the sensitivity of pathogens to phytoalexins as the Müller's hypothesis. The pea pathogen, *E. pisi* was characterized by delayed induction of and high tolerance to pisatin, while the nonpathogen, *E. graminis*, elicited pisatin induction at an earlier stage and was sensitive to it.

V. INHIBITORY ACTIVITY OF PISATIN ON THE ESTABLISHMENT OF INFECTION BY PEA PATHOGEN AND ITS ROLE IN HOST-PARASITE SPECIFICITY

As the pea pathogen is tolerant to pisatin, there may be no necessity for the fungus to suppress pisatin induction for establishing infection. However, as mentioned before, the pea pathogen apparently suppressed the induction of pisatin at the first phase.

This suggest that the parasitism of pea pathogen is not solely determined by the antibiotic activity of pisatin. Therefore, the effect of artificial administration of pisatin in early stage of infection on the infection process of *E. pisi* on pea leaves was examined.

In practice, the epidermis of lower surface of half leaves of pea seedlings was removed and the conidia of *E. pisi* were inoculated on the upper surface. The inoculated leaves were incubated in a moist chamber at 20°C after bringing the mesophyll cells into direct contract with an aqueous solution on a glass slide. After appropriate time intervals, the leaves were transferred

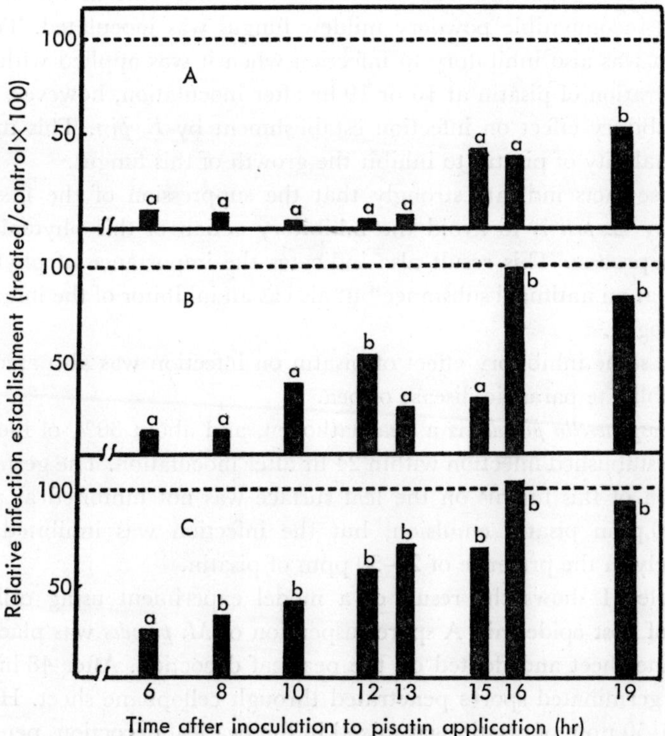

Fig. 3. Effect of pisatin on infection establishment of *E. pisi* on pea leaves. After the lower epidermis of half leaves was removed, the opposite surface was inoculated with *E. pisi*, and the stripped mesophyll tissue was brought into direct contact with (A) 100 ppm, (B) 30 ppm, or (C) 10 ppm pisatin solution at the above time intervals. Infection frequency was estimated 48 hr after inoculation. (a) represents a significant difference and (b) a non-significant difference from control respectively at $p=0.05$.

to glass slides on which 0, 10, 30, or 100 ppm pisatin solution had been applied. The leaves were then incubated under the same condition, fixed and stained with cotton blue at 48 hr after inoculation. The infectivity of the pathogen was assessed by calculating the frequency of spores producing secondary hyphae from conidia with appressoria. The uptake of pisatin into the pea leaf through the stripped mesophyll tissue was ascertained by quantitative analysis for pisatin in treated leaves.

As shown in Fig. 3, 30–100 ppm pisatin prevented infection of pea leaves by *E. pisi* when administered within 15 hr after inoculation. These are the actual concentrations accumulated at that time in the epidermis when an incompatible powdery mildew fungus was inoculated. Ten ppm of pisatin was also inhibitory to infection when it was applied within 6 hr. Administration of pisatin at 16 or 19 hr after inoculation, however, did not give inhibitory effect on infection establishment by *E. pisi*. This might be due to inability of pisatin to inhibit the growth of this fungus.

These facts indicate strongly that the suppression of the first phase pisatin by *E. pisi* is to avoid the inhibitory action of this phytoalexin on infection process. This result also indicates the importance of phytoalexin not only as an antifugal substance but also as an inhibitor of the infection by the pathogen.

The same inhibitory effect of pisatin on infection was also ascertained in non-obligate parasitic disease of pea.

Mycosphaerella pinodes is a pea pathogen, and about 30% of inoculated conidia established infection within 24 hr after inoculation. The germination of conidia of this fungus on the leaf surface was not inhibited at all even in a 500 ppm pisatin emulsion, but the infection was inhibited almost completely in the presence of 25–50 ppm of pisatin.

Table II shows the result of a model experiment using cellophane instead of host epidermis. A spore suspension of *M. pinodes* was placed on a cellophane sheet and floated on the pea leaf decoction. After 48 hr, about 24% of germinated spores penetrated through cellophane sheet. However, when 15–50 ppm of pisatin was mixed in the pea leaf decoction, penetration through the cellophane sheet was inhibited significantly, though the germination of conidia was not affected at all even in 500 ppm pisatin emulsion.

Thus, pisatin at non-inhibitory concentrations inhibits the penetrating ability of *M. pinodes*, a non-obligate parasite.

This fact that the phytoalexin-tolerant fungi could not infect their host indicates the possibility that some substances which are synthesized

TABLE II
Inhibitory Effect of Pisatin on Penetration of *M. pinodes* through Cellophane Sheet

Concentration of pisatin (μg/ml)	Percentage of germinated spores	Percentage of penetrated spores
0	100	23.6
15	100	4.9
25	100	5.8
50	100	6.6
150	92.9	0
500	96.1	0

during the infection process, but have no antibiotic activity, may play a role in determining host-parasite specificity. In this connection, Berard *et al.* (*3*) reported that a diffusate from the incompatible interaction of bean anthracnose protected the bean plant from the compatible pathogen, though the diffusate did not inhibit spore germination or fungal development on the host.

VI. MECHANISM OF INDUCTION AND SUPPRESSION OF PHYTOALEXIN SYNTHESIS

It seems the most important event in determining host-parasite specificity is whether the first phase phytoalexin is induced or not by the attacked fungus. Thus, it is important to know how the defense reaction and the subsequent phytoalexin synthesis at the first phase initiated by incompatible fungi, but not by compatible fungi.

Although Cruickshank (*7*) and Keen (*8*) reported specific elicitors for phytoalexin induction in some host-parasite combinations, the defense reaction in higher plant cells may generally be initiated by some common metabolite or metabolites produced by many microorganisms. This is supported by the evidence that phytoalexin, especially of the first phase, is produced by many incompatible and nonpathogenic fungi. Since a fungus compatible to a given cultivar or variety also initiates a defense reaction and subsequent phytoalexin induction in resistant varieties of the same species or in non-host plants, the fungus should have an ability to produce the initiating substances. Therefore, the following two molecular mechanisms may be conceivable for the compatible host-parasite relationship: (1) compatible fungi do not produce the initiating substance on their host. (2) Pathogen has some mechanism to suppress the initiation of the defense reaction.

The latter mechanism is more likely from the following experimental results. We demonstrated the presence of both elicitor and suppressor of pisatin production in the germination fluid of pycniospores of a pathogenic fungus of pea, *M. pinodes*. The elicitor was found to be a high molecular weight compound and the supressor a low molecular one. The preliminary application of the suppressor fraction on pea leaf surface reduced significantly the induction of pisatin by *E. graminis hordei* (Table III). This suppressor also inactivate the pisatin producing ability of the high molecular weight elicitor of *M. pinodes*. The suppressor seems to be a peptide from its color reaction with ninhydrin and Lowry reagents.

Thus, a pathogen produces a metabolite which suppress the initiation of phytoalexin induction, possibly through the suppression of defense reaction of its own host. Therefore, the word, "pathogenicity" could be replaced, in a certain sense, by the phrase, "the ability to suppress the defense reaction of the host plant." The fact that compatible fungi produced the second phase phytoalexin indicate the possibility that the mechanism by which compatible fungi suppress the defense reaction of their own host may operate only during the early stage of infection.

TABLE III

Effect of Low Molecular Weight Fraction from Spore Germination Fluid of *M. pinodes* on Pisatin Induction in Pea Leaves by Inoculation with *E. graminis hordei*[a]

Dilution of low molecular weight fraction	Conc. of pisatin accumulated (μg/g fresh weight leaves)
Control	57.9
1	0
2	13.7
10	16.3
20	26.4

[a] Sample of low molecular weight fraction was prepared as follows; 50 ml of pycnispore germination fluid (2 millon spores/ml) was concentrated to 2 ml, dialized, the outer dialyzate was again concentrated to dryness, and dissolved in 2 ml of deionized water. The surface of pea leaves was wetted with 60 μl of each diluent of the sample, dried for 30 min, inoculated with *E. graminis*, and the pisatin concentration was determined 24 hr later.

VII. ROLE OF THE SECOND PHASE PHYTOALEXIN IN THE PATHOGENESIS

The role of the second phase phytoalexins which accumulates at the later stage of pathogenesis in the compatible combination of powdery mildew differ from one host-parasiste combination to the other.

In barley powdery mildew, it seems apparently involved with the resistance against colony development. Colonies of barley powdery mildew fungus usually grow very rapidly in the early stage of pathogenesis, then gradually level off, finally stopping at the later stage. This might be due to the sensitivity of the barley fungus to barley phytoalexin which accumulates at a high level in colony margins.

On the other hand, the colony of pea powdery mildew grows linearly until the diseased leaves wilt. This might be due to the high tolerance of pea fungus to accumulated pisatin. The wilting of pea leaves by powdery mildew infection seemed to be due to the deleterious effect of accumulated pisatin on the plasma membrane of the host itelf (*30*).

When epidermal tissues separated from the pea stem were stained with neutral red, plasmolyzed with a hypertonic KCl solution and then treated with 300 ppm of pisatin (in hypertonic KCl solution), the plasmolyzed cells shrank within a few minutes. The membrane disappeared gradually with time after pisatin treatment, whereas cell membranes treated with KCl (control) remained unchanged. The red color of cytoplasm stained with neutral red also disappeared within 10 min after treatment.

Isolated protoplasts in a isotonic mannit solution swell immediately and the cell burst within 10 min after treatment with 300 ppm pisatin.

These results suggest that pisatin accumulated as the result of a defense mechanism of host is an important factor in symptom development of this disease (wilting) because such a powerful toxin with a wilting effect can not be produced by the mildew fungus which is a typical obligate parasite.

The injurious effect of phaseollin, a phytoalexin produced by bean, on bean hypocotyl was reported by VanEtten and Bateman (*35*). The increased respiration in powdery mildew infected pea leaves seemed also due to the effect of accumulated pisatin, though Allen (*1*) reported that the respiratory increase in powdery mildewed wheat might be due to the uncoupling effect of mildew toxin.

The pattern of respiratory increase in inoculated pea leaves was parallel to the pattern of increase in pisatin content in leaves, and rubbing of the leaf surface with a cotton ball which was wetted by 300 ppm pisatin solution stimulated oxygen uptake.

The oxidative phosphorylation by the mitochondrial fraction prepared from soaked pea seeds was found to be uncoupled by 80 ppm of pisatin. Uncoupling has also been reported for ipomeamarone, a phytoalexin from sweet potato (*Ipomoea batatas* Lam.). It prevented oxidative phosphorylation by mitochondria from mung bean and sweet potato (*34*).

Thus, some of the physiological changes and injuries in pea plant infected by powdery mildew fungus seemed to be due to the effect of accumulated pisatin resulted from the defense mechanism of host itself. In other words, some of the injury in powdery mildewed pea should be considered as "self-injury."

VIII. CONCLUDING REMARKS

Many plant pathogenic fungi are highly selective and parasitize only certain species of plant, cultivars or varieties within species, but the chemical bases of such specificity in parasitism are almost unknown. In this paper, the authors emphasize the importance of the first phase induction of phytoalexins in determining the host-parasite specificity at the infection site of powdery mildew diseases, in which two phases of phytoalexin production have been found.

The first phase phytoalexin does not appear in infection with compatible fungi. Some experimental evidence suggested that the compatible fungi have some mechanism to suppress the defense reaction of their own host, hence phytoalexin production. The same mechanism may operate in some non-obligate parasites since a suppressor of pisatin production was demonstrated in the germination fluid of *M. pinodes*, a pathogen of pea.

Thus, the most important task for a plant pathogenic fungus in order to establish infection on its own host may be overcoming the defense reaction of plants. Host-specific toxins are found to be essential for colonization and induction of disease for some host-parasite combinations, and are called primary determinants of pathogenicity (*29*). These toxins are synthesized during spore germination (*15, 16*) and break down the defense reaction by exerting deleterious effect only on the compatible host. Host-specific toxins were, however, found in limited numbers of host-parasite combinations in which parasitism is perthophytic, and such a drastic toxin may not be observed in the obligate parastitic or facultative saprophytic fungi. Therefore, the fungal metabolite which suppresses the defense reaction of its own host without injurious effect should be said to be the primary determinant in these plant pathogenic fungi.

As to the evaluation of the role of phytoalexin in resistance or host-parasite specificity, discussion centers on whether the accumulated phytoalexins in plant tissue are sufficient to inhibit the growth of the parasite or not. However, we demonstrated clearly that the administration of pisatin at non-inhibitory concentration (10–100 ppm) in early stage of infection reduced significantly the infection rate of pisatin-tolerant fungi, *E. pisi* (ED_{50} for conidial germination was 530 ppm) and *M. pinodes* ($ED_{50} > 500$ ppm).

Thus, if we direct our attention to the inhibitory effect of phytoalexins on the infection establishment of pathogens, their role in determining host-parasite specificity may be much more important than have been considered (*4, 9, 11, 26*).

Further, the endocarp of pea pod or been pod may not be a suitable material to study the role of phytoalexins. We found that the endocarp of pea pod showed incompatible, hypersensitive reaction to *E. pisi*, while leaves, stems, and exocarp are compatible (Oku *et al.* unpublished data). Therefore, to discuss the role of phytoalexin, we should use organs and tissues which are the actual infection site. Artificial injury should also be avoided for inoculation because we could not estimate the effect on penetration.

Finally, we would like to emphasize the necessity to study the toxicity of phytoalexins to mammalian cells, as Puppke and VanEtten (*26*) and Kuć (*12*) pointed out. We (*20*) also reported that pisatin destroyes human erythrocytes at 100 ppm or more, and we found it to be an uncoupler not only of the oxidative phosphorylation by pea seed mitochondria but also by rat liver mitochondria.

SUMMARY

Biphasic production of phytoalexins was found in the pathogenesis of powdery mildew disease of barley and pea. The first phase was observed by inoculation with incompatible fungi at the time just germinated-conida began to penetrate into host cellmembrane. The production of phytoalexins in this phase was not detectable by inoculation with compatible fungi. The second phase phytoalexin accumulated by inoculation with compatible fungi after the infection was established.

Artificial administration of non-inhibitory concentration of pisatin to pea leaf at an early stage of infection (correspond to the first phase) inhibited the infection of *E. pisi* and *M. pinodes* on pea leaves, notwithstanding these fungi were highly tolerant to pisatin.

Pycniospores of *M. pinodes* secretes low molecular weight peptides which suppress the pisatin production by subsequent inoculation with incompatible fungi on pea leaves.

These results suggest strongly that the compatible fungi suppress the elicitation of the first phase phytoalexin in order to avoid the inhibitory effect on infection process. Thus, whether the first phase phytoalexin was produced or not by invading fungi may play a key role in host-parasite specificity.

The role of the second phase phytoalexin is diverse depending upon host-parasite combinations. When the invading fungus is sensitive to host phytoalexin, the phytoalexin may play a role in restricting the lesion enlargement, but when the fungus is tolerant, phytoalexin may nothing to do in the symptom development. The host rather suffers "self-injuly" by the deleterious effect of phytoalexin.

Acknowledgment
This work was supported by Grant Nos. 946004, 076132, 136006, 156033, and 176028 from the Ministry of Education, Science and Culture of Japan. Financial support from Sankyo Co., Ltd. is acknowledged.

REFERENCES

1. Allen, P. J. 1953. Toxins and tissue respiration. *Phytopathology* **43**: 221–229.
2. Bailey, J. A. and B. J. Deverall. 1971. Formation and activity of phaseollin in the interaction between bean hypocotyls (*Phaseolus vulgaris*) and physiological races of *Colletotrichum lindemuthianum*. *Physiol. Plant Pathol.* **1**: 435–446.
3. Berard, D. F., J. Kuć, and E. B. Williams. 1972. A cultivar-specific protection factor from incompatible interactions of green bean with *Colletotrichum lindemuthianum*. *Physiol. Plant Pathol.* **2**: 123–127.
4. Christenson, J. A. and L. A. Hadwigger. 1973. Induction of pisatin formation in pea foot region by pathogenic and nonpathogenic clones of *Fusarium solani*. *Phytopathology* **63**: 784–790.
5. Cruickshank, I. A. M. 1963. Phytoalexins. *Annu. Rev. Phytopathol.* **1**: 351–374.
6. Cruickshank, I. A. M., D. Biggs, and D. R. Perrin. 1971. Phytoalexin as determinants of disease reaction in plants. *J. Indian Bot. Soc. Golden Jubilee* **50A**: 1–11.
7. Cruickshank, I. A. M. and D. R. Perrin. 1968. The isolation and partial charac-

terization of monilicolin A, a peptide with phaseollin-inducing activity from *Monilinia fructicola. Life Sci.* **7**: 449–458.

8. Keen, N. T. 1976. Specific elicitors of phytoalexin production: determinants of race specificity? *In*: K. Tomiyama, J. M. Daly, I. Uritani, H. Oku, and S. Ouchi (eds.). *Biochemistry and Cytology of Plant-Parasite Interaction.* Kodansha Ltd., Tokyo and Elsevier, New York, pp. 84–93.
9. Király, Z., N. Berna, and T. Érsek. 1972. Hypersensitivity as a consequence, not the cause, of plant resistance to infection. *Nature* **239**: 456–458.
10. Kuć, J. 1972. Phytoalexins. *Annu. Rev. Phytopathol.* **10**: 207–232.
11. Kuć, J. 1976. Phytoalexins and the specificity of plant-parasite interaction. *In*: R. K. S. Wood and A. Graniti (eds.). *Specificity in Plant Diseases.* Plenum Press, New York, pp. 253–271.
12. Kuć, J. and W. Currier. 1976. Phytoalexins, plants, and human health. *Adv. Chem. Ser.* **149**: 356–368.
13. Müller, K. O. and H. Börger. 1939. Studien über den "Mechanismus" der *Phytophthora*-Resistenz der Kartoffel. *Landwirtsch. Jahrb. (Berlin)* **87**: 609.
14. Müller, K. O. and H. Börger. 1940. Experimentelle Untersuchungen über die *Phytophthora*-Resistenz der Kartoffel. *Arb. Biol. Reichsanst. Land. Fortwirtsch. (Berlin)* **23**: 189–231.
15. Nishimura, S., K. Kohmoto, H. Otani, H. Fukami, and T. Ueno. 1966. The involvement of host-specific toxins in the early step of infection by *Alternaria kikuchiana and A. mali. In*: K. Tomiyama, J. M. Daly, I. Uritani, H. Oku, and S. Ouchi (eds.). *Biochemistry and Cytology of Plant-Parasite Interaction.* Kodansha Ltd., Tokyo and Elsevier, New York, pp. 94–101.
16. Nishimura, S. and R. P. Scheffer. 1965. Interactions between *Helminthosporium victoriae* spores and oat tissue. *Phytopathology* **55**: 629–634.
17. Oku, H., S. Ouchi, T. Shiraishi, and T. Baba. 1975. Pisatin production in powdery mildewed pea seedlings. *Phytopathology* **65**: 1263–1267.
18. Oku, H., S. Ouchi, T. Shiraishi, T. Baba, and H. Miyagawa. 1975. Phytoalexin production in barley powdery mildew as affected by thermal and biological predispositions. *Proc. Japan Acad.* **51**: 198–201.
19. Oku, H., S. Ouchi, T. Shiraishi, K. Komoto, and K. Oki. 1975. Phytoalexin activity in barley powdery mildew. *Ann. Phytopathol. Soc. Japan* **41**: 185–191.
20. Oku, H., S. Ouchi, T. Shiraishi, K. Utsumi, and S. Seno 1976. Toxicity of a phytoalexin, pisatin, to mammalian cells. *Proc. Japan Acad.* **52**: 33–36.
21. Oku, H., T. Shiraishi, and S. Ouchi, 1975. The role of phytoalexin as the inhibitor of infection establishment in plant disease. *Naturwissenschaften* **62**: 486–487.
22. Oku, H., T. Shiraishi, and S. Ouchi. 1976. Effect of preliminary administration of pisatin to pea leaf tissues on the subsequent infection by *Erysiphe pisi* DC. *Ann. Phytopathol. Soc. Japan* **42**: 597–600.

23. Ouchi, S., H. Oku, C. Hibino, and I. Akiyama. 1974. Induction of accessibility and resistance in leaves of barley by some races of *Erysiphe graminis*. *Phytopathol. Z.* **79**: 24–34.
24. Ouchi, S., H. Oku, C. Hibino, and I. Akiyama. 1974. Induction of accessibility to a non-pathogen by preliminary inoculation with a pathogen. *Phytopathol. Z.* **79**: 142–154.
25. Ouchi, S., H. Oku, H. Nakabayashi, and K. Oka. 1976. Biphasic heat-induced susceptibility demonstrated in powdery mildew of barley. *Ann. Phytopathol. Soc. Japan* **42**: 131–137.
26. Puppke, S. G. and H. D. VanEtten. 1974. Pisatin accumulation and lesion development in peas infected with *Aphanomyces euteiches*, *Fusarium solani* f. sp. *pisi*, or *Rhizoctonia solani*. *Phytopathology* **64**: 1433–1440.
27. Puppke, S. G. and H. D. VanEtten. 1976. The relation between pisatin and the development of *Aphanomyces euteiches* in diseased *Pisum sativum*. *Phytopathology* **66**: 1174–1185.
28. Sato, N. and K. Tomiyama. 1969. Localized accumulation of rishitin in the potato-tuber tissue infected by an incompatible race of *Phytophthora infestans*. *Ann. Phytopathol. Soc. Japan* **35**: 202–207.
29. Scheffer, R. P. and K. R. Samaddar. 1970. Host-specific toxins as determinants of pathogenicity. *Recent Adv. Phytochem.* **3**: 124–142.
30. Shiraishi, T., H. Oku, M. Isono, and S. Ouchi. 1975. The injurious effect of pisatin on the plasma membrane of pea. *Plant Cell Physiol.* **16**: 939–942.
31. Shiraishi, T., H. Oku, S. Ouchi, and Y. Tsuji. 1977. Local accumulation of pisatin in tissues of pea seedlings infected by powdery mildew fungi. *Phytopathol. Z.* **88**: 131–135.
32. Tomiyama, K., N. Ishizaka, N. Sato, T. Masamune, and N. Katsui, 1968. "Rishitin" a phytoalexin-like substance. Its role in the defence reaction of potato tubers to infection. *In*: T. Hirai, Z. Hidaka, and I. Uritani (eds.). *Biochemical Regulation in Diseased Plants or Injury*. The Phytopathol. Soc. Japan, Tokyo, pp. 287–292.
33. Tsuchiya, K. and K. Hirata. 1973. Growth of various powdery mildew fungi on the barley leaves infected preliminarily with the barley powdery mildew fungus. *Ann. Phytopathol. Soc. Japan* **39**: 396–403.
34. Uritani, I., T. Akazawa, and M. Uritani. 1954. Increase of respiratory-rate in sweet potato tissue infected with black-rot. *Nature* **174**: 1060.
35. VanEtten, H. D. and D. F. Bateman. 1971. Studies on the mode of action of the phytoalexin, phaseollin. *Phytopathology* **61**: 1363–1372.
36. VanEtten, H. D. and S. G. Puppke. 1976. Isoflavanoid phytoalexins. *Annu. Proc. Phytochem. Soc.* **13**: 239–289.

Discussion of Paper by Drs. Oku et al.

In response to AIST's question, OKU stated they had not found a method to induce phytoalexins by physical wounding. In view of H. VANETTEN's finding that phytoalexins are self-toxic to hosts, SEQUEIRA asked if the hypersensitive response might be due to difference in host sensitivity. KEEN pointed out that would be unlikely for a gene-for-gene system. ELLINGBOE noted that the 2-step accumulation of phytoalexin was found only with a cultivar that produced infection type 2 and asked if they knew the genetics of resistance for that combination. OUCHI acknowledged that only infection type 2 showed this behavior and it was observed for several different phenotypes. Genetic information is lacking now. He noted they were assuming only one compound was involved but had no genetic information. OKU stated they are currently trying to identify the phytoalexins of which there appear to be four. H. VANETTEN asked if the effect of added pisatin in suppressing *E. pisi* infections had been affirmed by experiments in which increases in endogenous pisatin were induced. OKU stated he had tried once, but induction required 20 hr and that infection occurred much earlier than this. TANI asked if another interpretation of suppressor experiments might be blockage of the accessibility response by pisatin, but OKU has experiments showing that pisatin suppresses penetration of artificial membranes by *Mycosphaerella*. NISHIMURA asked OKU to comment on the notin that the suppressor was equivalent to a host-specific toxin in disease caused by facultative parasites but OKU and OUCHI reported they found no microscopic evidence of action of their compound when applied to host tissue. KUĆ asked for clarification of the two step accumulation of pisatins and asked if there was any biological significance to second phase accumulation which reached 800–900 ppm. OKU noted that concentrations of 300 ppm of pisatin caused wilting which would prevent any further fungal development.

Recognition and Specificity in Plant Host-Parasite Interactions, pp. 335-349, 1979

DIFFERENTIAL GROWTH RESPONSE OF VARIOUS FUNGAL STRAINS TO DIVALENT CATIONS AND PHYTOALEXINS

MINEO KOJIMA, AKIRA TAKEUCHI, AND IKUZO URITANI

Faculty of Agriculture, Nagoya University, Nagoya, Japan

It is not only a logical necessity but also a well established fact that host-parasite specificity is not determined by one-way action of either host or parasite but by mutual interactions between host and parasite. In other words, both host and parasite must contribute equally to the determination of host-parasite specificity. However, it seems that many studies on host-parasite specificity, especially involving a biochemical approach, have focused on the response of host plant to the infection rather than that of parasite to plant host. We consider that more attension should be paid to the response of the parasite to host on the studies of host-parasite specificity.

In incompatible combinations, the interactions between host and parasite cause the growth of parasite to cease, whereas interactions with the compatible combinations allow the growth of parasite. Thus, the growth response of the parasite in host-parasite interactions must be directly related to host-parasite specificity.

In most plant diseases by fungi, host-parasite interactions are initiated by spore germination of the fungus on the host, being followed by a series of mutual interactions. Spore germination is also the initial step in fungal propagation. In general, spore germination of fungi is regulated by ingenious mechanisms, possibly because of the particular importance of the initial step of propagation. Spores of some fungi do not germinate in unfavorable circumstances and do germinate only in the favorable circumstances providing the opportunity for the continuing growth and development (*1*): the spores can perceive factors affecting their subsequent growth. Thus, the spore germination of plant pathogenic fungi is a crucial event in both host-parasite interactions and fungal growth. Therefore, many workers have studied spore germination of fungi and found many factors which regulate germination; self-inhibitors (*15, 22*), inhibitors (*25*), and stimulants (*16*). In the first part of this Chapter, we deal with response of various strains of *Ceratocystis fimbriata* to germination inductive factors in sweet potato in terms of host-parasite specificity.

In many host-parasite complexes, phytoalexin production is induced in host tissue as the result of host-parasite interactions (*4–6, 9, 11, 13, 19*). Some workers have studied phytoalexin productions in relation to host-parasite specificity. Cruickshank (*5*), Cruickshank and Perrin (*6*), and Van Etten (*24*) have investigated the antimicrobial spectra of pisatin and phaseollin and have shown that they are more toxic to non-pathogenic fungi than to pathogenic ones, although there are some notable exceptions. Ishizaka and Tomiyama (*11*) reported that rishitin is produced only in potatoes infected by an incompatible race of *Phytophthora infestans* and not in potatoes infected by a compatible race. Oku *et al.* (*19*) observed two phases of phytoalexin production in powdery mildews of barley and found that the intensity of the first phase was proportional to the degree of incompatibility in the race-cultivar interactions. In the sweet potato-*C. fimbriata* system also, the host tissue produces phytoalexins composed of analogous furanoterpenoids (*9, 12, 13, 18*). In the second part of this Chapter, we deal with the fungal response to furanoterpenoid phytoalexins and discuss their role in establishing host-parasite specificity of this system.

Various strains of *C. fimbriata* were isolated from black rot lesions on sweet potato, coffee, prune, cacao, oak, taro, and almond. The strains are different in their pathogenicity to different hosts. On sweet potato only the sweet potato strain is pathogenic, while all other strains are non-pathogenic. Our studies in this Chapter are concerned with the specificity in the interactions between sweet potato and these strains of *C. fimbriata*.

I. DIFFERENTIAL RESPONSE OF VARIOUS STRAINS OF *C. FIMBRIATA* TO THE GERMINATION INDUCTIVE FACTOR IN SWEET POTATO

Good germination of the oak strain occurred neither in the synthetic medium (*3*) reported for *C. fimbriata* which contained glucose, casein hydrolyzate, fumaric acid, vitamin B_1, and inorganic compounds such as KH_2PO_4 and $MgSO_4$, nor in the synthetic medium (*23*) reported for *Picricularia oryzae* which contained sucrose, glucose, vitamin B_1, biotin, and various metallic ions such as Mg^{2+}, Ca^{2+}, Fe^{2+}, Cu^{2+}, and Na^{+}. Furthermore, all of the following compounds were inactive in inducing germination of the oak strain when tested in various concentrations and in various combinations: various amino acids, malic acid, citric acid, oxalacetic acid, vitamin C, vitamin B_2, vitamin B_6, vitamin B_{12}, pantothenic acid, inositol, nicotinic acid, nicotinic acid amide, xanthine, adenosine, cytosine, cytosine monophosphate, guanosine, guanosine diphosphate, guanosine triphosphate, coenzyme A, glutathione (reduced), indole acetic acid, gibberellic acid, kinetin, and benzyl adenine. Spore germination did not occurred even in the media containing yeast extract and/or polypeptone.

On the other hand, the oak strain as well as the other six strains germinated well in tissue extract prepared from sweet potato root tissue. The results suggested that sweet potato root extract contained some germination inductive factor(s) other than the nutrients described above. Therefore, we tried to isolate the germination inductive factor(s) in sweet potato root tissue using the oak strain for bioassay.

Tissue extract was applied to an anion exchange resin (AG-1-X8, B10-RAD Lab.) column to separate the anionic substance from the non-anionic substance fraction. Good germination (100%) was observed in the non-anionic substance fraction of the tissue extract, indicating that the germination inductive factor(s) was not anionic.

Next, spore germination was examined in the unabsorbed and the absorbed fractions which had been prepared by applying tissue extract to a cation exchange resin (AG-50W-X8, B10-RAD, Lab.) column. Spore germination occurred neither in the unabsorbed fraction nor in the absorbed fraction. However, spores germinated well in the mixture of the unabsorbed and absorbed fractions. The results indicated that the oak strain required both some cationic factor(s) in the absorbed fraction and some non-cationic factor(s) in the unabsorbed fraction for its germination.

Some observations made during isolation suggested that metallic ion(s) might be involved. Atomic absorption analysis indicated that the absorbed fraction contained metallic (cationic) ions such as Ca^{2+}, Mg^{2+}, Fe^{2+}, and K^{+}. Therefore, we examined the germination inductive activities of various cations in the presence of the unabsorbed fraction. Ca^{2+} showed the highest activity in the induction of germination. Mg^{2+}, Mn^{2+}, and Zn^{2+} also induced germination. Other cations such as Fe^{2+}, Co^{2+}, Ni^{2+}, Cu^{2+}, Al^{3+}, Mo^{6+}, Ba^{2+}, Li^{+}, Na^{+}, K^{+}, and NH_4^{+} had no inductive effects on germination. They did not show any inductive activity even when tested in various combinations. It was also observed that Ca^{2+} stimulated mycelial growth very remarkably when it was added to the medium containing divalent cations such as Mg^{2+}, Mn^{2+}, and Zn^{2+}. The unabsorbed fraction could not be replaced with any nutrients examined, such as di- and monosaccharides, amino acids, organic acids, vitamins, nucleotides, plant hormones, and yeast extract.

The effect of Ca^{2+} concentration on germination of the oak strain was studied using calcium chloride. The maximum effect for germination was observed in a concentration of 1×10^{-3} M.

Determination of the contents of Ca^{2+}, Mg^{2+}, Mn^{2+}, and Zn^{2+} was carried out with sweet potato root tissue, tissue extract and the unabsorbed fraction. The concentrations of these cations in sweet potato root tissue and tissue extract were high enough to induce the germination of the oak strain. On the other hand, these cations could not be detected in the unabsorbed fraction.

The effect of Ca^{2+} on germination of seven strains was studied (Table I). Spores of the sweet potato, coffee, and cacao strains germinated well in the

TABLE I

Effect of $CaCl_2$ on Spore Germination of Various Strains of *C. fimbriata*

Medium	Germination of various strains (% of control)[a]						
	Sweet potato strain	Coffee strain	Prune strain	Cacao strain	Oak strain	Taro strain	Almond strain
Unabsorbed fraction	100	100	38	100	19	2	55
Unabsorbed fraction with addition of $CaCl_2$[b]	100	100	92	100	52	50	100

[a] Germination in sweet potato root tissue extract was regarded as 100%. [b] Maximum germination assayed in a final concentration of 1×10^{-4} to 1×10^{-2} M.

unabsorbed fraction. On the other hand, the germination of the prune, oak, taro, and almond strains in the unabsorbed fraction were poor and enhanced by the addition of Ca^{2+}. Thus the strains of *C. fimbriata* are divided into two groups in terms of Ca^{2+} requirement for germination; one group of the fungal strains such as the sweet potato, coffee, and cacao stains do not require exogeneous Ca^{2+} for, while the other group of fungal strains such as the prune, oak, taro, and almond stains require it.

The contents of Ca^{2+} and Mg^{2+} in the spores were compared for the sweet potato and oak strains which were different in the requirement of Ca^{2+} for germination. Spores of the oak strain had higher contents of both Ca^{2+} and Mg^{2+} than those of the sweet potato strain. The results indicated no relationship between the spore content of Ca^{2+} and whether or not the spores required exogeneous Ca^{2+} ion for germination.

Time course of germination was followed after administrating Ca^{2+} to spores of the oak strain which had been incubated in the unabsorbed fraction for varied periods (Fig. 1). The germ tubes emerged 1.5 hr after administration of Ca^{2+}, regardless of the time of pre-incubation in the unabsorbed fraction.

The results described above suggest that Ca^{2+} functions as a trigger of germination, not as a nutrient. In fact, it has been shown with animal cells that metallic ions, in particular Ca^{2+}, are involved in many aspects of cellular events and serve as 'second messenger' (*21*). For instance, Ca^{2+} and Mg^{2+} have key roles in intercellular communication (*14*). It was also shown that Ca^{2+} acted as a direct activator of DNA synthesis in lymphocytes treated by concanavalin A (*7*).

Participation of Ca^{2+} in fungal physiology and in host-parasite interactions has been reported by some workers. Allen and Dunkle (*2*) reported that Ca^{2+} effectively counteracted the inhibition of germ tube growth caused by monovalent cations such as K^+. Page and Stock (*20*) have presented the evidence with *Microsporum gypserum* macroconidia that Ca^{2+} induced germination by enhancing the protease facilitating germination. Hirata (*8*) found that Ca^{2+} increased the susceptibility of primary barley leaves to powdery mildew caused by *Erysiphe graminis* f. sp. *hordei*. He explained this phenomenon as an effect of Ca^{2+} on sac formation.

During infection of sweet potato root tissue by various strains of *C. fimbriata*, divalent cations such as Ca^{2+} and Mg^{2+} in the host might be involved in host-parasite interaction as one of the mediators. In addition, these divalent cations might contribute to the establishment of host-parasite

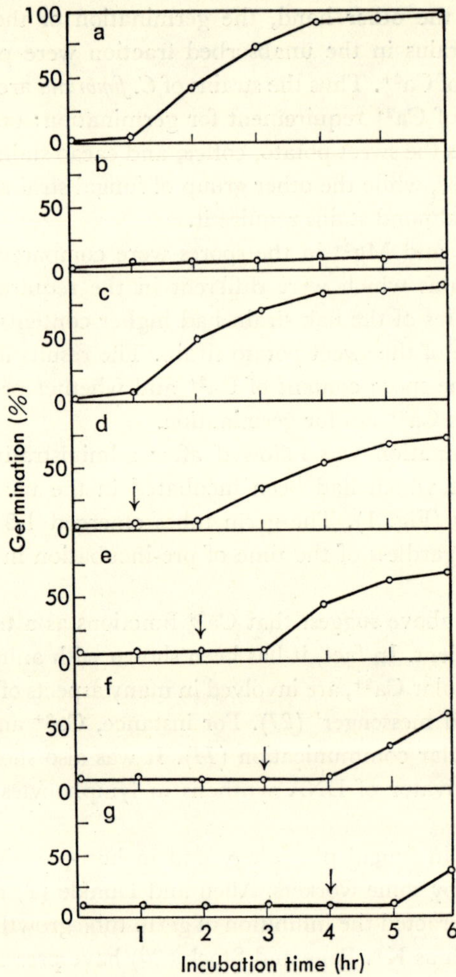

Fig. 1. Time course of germination of the oak strain of *C. fimbriata* administrated $CaCl_2$ after pre-incubation for varied periods in the cation exchange resin-unabsorbed fraction of sweet potato root tissue extract. a, germination in the sweet potato root tissue extract without addition of $CaCl_2$; b, germination in the unabsorbed fraction without addition of $CaCl_2$. $CaCl_2$ (1×10^{-3} M) was added at various times shown by arrows; c, 0 hr; d, 1 hr; e, 2 hr; f, 3 hr; g, 4 hr.

specificity through their different effects on the spore germination and growth of various strains and through their possible different availabilities in host cells among various combinations of strains and host.

II. DIFFERENTIAL RESPONSE OF VARIOUS STRAINS OF *C. FIMBRIATA* TO FURANO-TERPENOID PHYTOALEXINS IN SWEET POTATO

Spore germination of seven strains of *C. fimbriata* was examined in the water extracts of the fresh sweet potato root tissue, aged tissue and tissue infected by the sweet potato strain, which were prepared by homogenizing with an equal volume of water. In the fresh and the aged tissue extracts, spores germinated without appreciable inhibition, and no significant differences were observed in the germination patterns of the different strains. On the other hand, clear differences in spore germination of the strains were exhibited when spores were incubated in the infected tissue extract. Germination of spores of the sweet potato strain was slightly inhibited in the extract and with the exception of the cacao strain, the germination of spores of the other strains was severely inhibited. Difference was also observed in the germ tube growth of pre-germinated spores of various strains in the three-fold diluted extract from the infected tissue. All non-pathogenic strains, namely the coffee, prune, cacao, oak, taro, and almond strains, were almost completely prevented from growing after 9 hr of incubation, while the sweet potato strain showed delayed but steady mycelial growth.

Since both the infected and fresh tissue extracts had the same pH value of 6.35, a pH shift was not thought to be the cause of the inhibitory activity of the infected tissue extract. Furthermore, the inhibitory activity of the infected tissue extract was not lost by heating at 100°C for 5 min, suggesting the presence of a heat stable, inhibitory compound(s). The occurrence of such an inhibitory compound(s) was substantiated by the experiments with the sweet potato and coffee strains shown in Fig. 2. Spore germination of the coffee strain was strongly inhibited in the infected tissue extract while that of the sweet potato strain was only slightly inhibited. However, after removal of chloroform-soluble substances spores of both strains germinated in the same manner as in the fresh tissue extract (Fig. 2a and c). Furthermore, it was shown that the differential inhibitory activity was restored by re-addition of the chloroform-soluble substances to the extract that had been chloroform extracted (Fig. 2d). These results indicate that chloroform-soluble substances were responsible for the inhibitory activity of the

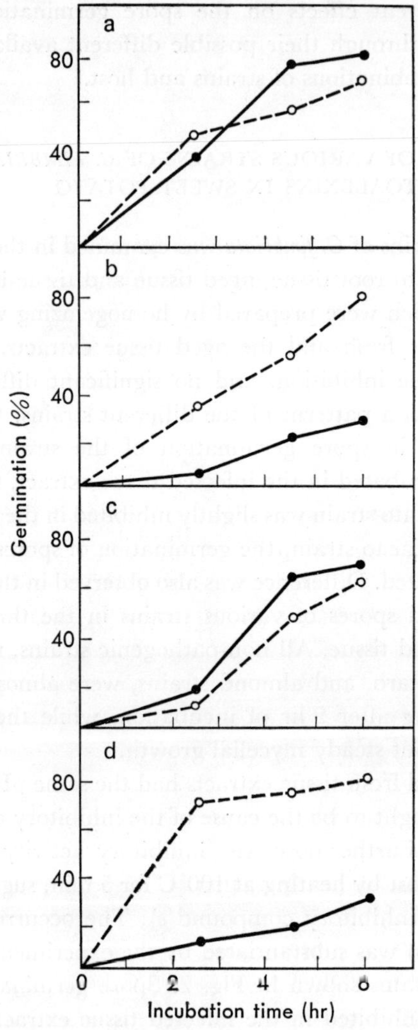

Fig. 2. Spore germination of sweet potato (○) and coffee (●) strains of *C. fimbriata* in extract of fresh sweet potato tissue and in chloroform-treated extract of sweet potato tissue infected with the sweet potato strain. a, fresh tissue extract; b, infected tissue extract; c, infected tissue extract without chloroform soluble substances; d, extract e, to which the chloroform-soluble substances from two volumes of infected extract were re-added.

infected tissue extract. The chloroform-soluble fraction from the infected tissue extract was chromatographed on silica gel thin-layer plates with *n*-hexane-ethyl acetate (3:2, v/v), a procedure which clearly separates furanoterpenoids from phenolics and coumarins in infected sweet potato roots. After chromatography, the distribution of inhibitory activity on the plates was studied using the spore germination test, with the oak strain as the test organism since it is the most sensitive of all the strains to the inhibitory activity of the infected tissue extract. Most of the inhibitory activity was distributed in the furanoterpenoid region and only small amounts of activity occurred in the regions of phenolics and coumarins.

The furanoterpenoid fraction from the infected tissue extract was chromatographed on silica gel phates using a mixture of *n*-hexane- and ethyl acetate (8:2). After chromatography, the silica gel in 2 cm wide bands scraped off, eluted, and assayed for spore germination inhibitory activity. Inhibitory activity was broadly distributed over many bands, containing such compounds as ipomeamarone (R_f 0.72), and ipomeamaronol (R_f 0.14). This result suggests that the inhibitory activity of the infected tissue extract can not be ascribed to the action of any single furanoterpenoid but to the combined action of many kinds of furanoterpenoids in the extract.

The differential inhibitory activity of furanoterpenoids was examined under conditions which were closer to those of the natural host-parasite interaction. Under natural conditions, the spores of the fungus germinate in the absence of furanoterpenoids and furanoterpenoid production occurred in later stage. Therefore, the inhibitory activity of furanoterpenoids to the various strains was studied by measuring the growth of pre-germinated spores on solid media containing varied amounts of furanoterpenoids. The sweet potato strain was rather insensitive to furanoterpenoids and could grow even on a medium containing furanoterpenoids at 12 mg/ml. On the other hand, the prune, oak, and taro strains were highly sensitive to furanoterpenoids, and their growth was completely prevented by a concentration of 6 mg furanoterpenoids/ml. The remaining strains, that is the coffee, cacao, and almond strains, were intermediate in their sensitivity to furanoterpenoids.

Differential toxicity of furanoterpenoids to fungi was also observed by Nonaka and Yasui (*17*). They examined the toxicity of ipomeamarone, the main furanoterpenoid in infected sweet-potato, to six fungi; *C. fimbriata*, three strains of *Fusarium solani, Gibberella zeae,* and *Piricularis oryzae* and found that ipemeamarone was more toxic to non-pathogenic fungi than to the pathogenic ones.

Furanoterpenoid fractions from the tissue infected by various strains were analyzed by silica gel thin-layer chromatography. The result showed that essentially the same kinds of furanoterpenoid were produced in the tissue infected by seven strains.

The site of furanoterpenoid accumulation in infected tissue was studied by histochemical techniques using Ehrlich's reagent. Two day infected tissues were used in this and the following experiments on furanoterpenoid production, because previous work in our laboratory (*10*) has shown that host-parasite specificity in this system is established within 2 days of inoculation. Clear differences were observed among tissue disks infected by the sweet potato strain and other strains in the number of cell layers containing the accumulated furanoterpenoids. In the case of tissue inoculated with the sweet potato strain, the furanoterpenoids accumulated in eight layers of cells from the inoculated surface, while they were accumulated in only three to four cell layers in tissues inoculated with the other strains. In all cases, regardless of the strain used, the outer cell layers (two or three cell layers from the surface) of the inoculated tissue were more lightly stained.

The furanoterpenoid concentration in infected tissue was determined colorimetrically after extraction with a mixture of chloroform and methanol. The furanoterpenoid concentrations in the tissue inoculated by various strains were compared on two bases, that is, the total amount of accumulated furanoterpenoids per disk and concentration in the cell layer that accumulated furanoterpenoid. The furanoterpenoid accumulation per disk infected by the sweet potato strain was higher than those of disks infected by other strains. However, when furanoterpenoid accumulation in response to the sweet potato strain was compared with accumulation in response to other strains on the base of the concentration in the cell layers that accumulated furanoterpenoids, the difference became smaller. All of the *in vivo* concentrations of furanoterpenoids in tissues inoculated by seven strains appeared to be greatly in excess of those required to prevent fungal growth *in vitro*. For example, because the sweet potato strain could not grow on solid medium containing 14 mg/ml of terpenoids, its growth *in vivo* would be completely prevented by 67 mg of terpenoid/ml which was shown to be the *in vivo* concentration in the tissue infected by the sweet potato strain. It should also be noted that the sweet potato strain has been shown to be incapable of degrading ipomeamarone (Fig. 3), yet the sweet potato strain

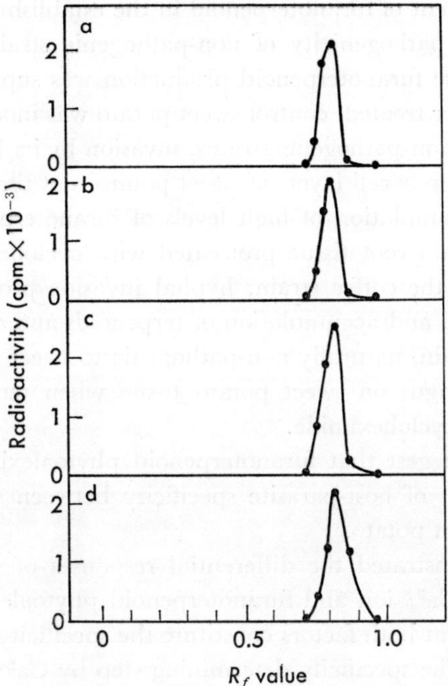

Fig. 3. Chromatogram of lipid fraction which was extracted from mixture of culture medium and mycelia of the sweet potato strain of *C. fimbriata* fed with ^{14}C-labelled ipomeamarone. Lipid fraction was prepared from the mixture of the medium and mycelia of the sweet potato strain cultured for 50 hr in the presence of ^{14}C-labelled ipomeamarone. The lipid fraction was subjected to a chromatography on a silica gel impregnated glass fiber paper (Gelman, ITLC-SA type) using *n*-hexane-ethyl acetate (8:2, v/v) as developing solvent; a, inoculated-50 hr culture; b, no inoculation; c, inoculated- no culture; d, authentic ^{14}C-labelled ipomeamarone.

continued to invade the inner cells of sweet potato under natural conditions. This apparent contradiction may be explained by a consideration of the dynamic aspect of furanoterpenoid accumulation in the cells of the infected tissue: furanoterpenoid production would continue until the cell were damaged enough to lose its furanoterpenoid producing activity. Therefore, the furanoterpenoid concentration in a cell would be low at the time that hyphae begin to penetrate, and might not reach very high concentrations until after the hypha has invaded the cell. Thus, it is inferred that the invading hyphae are in contact with lower concentrations of terpenoid than the values determined in the present study.

To confirm the involvement of furanoterpenoid in the establishment of host-parasite specificity, the pathogenicity of non-pathogenic strains was studied on sweet potato whose furanoterpenoid production was suppressed by cycloheximide. When water treated, control sweet potato was inoculated by coffee strain, one of the non-pathogenic strains, invasion by its hyphae was confined to only three to four cell layers of sweet potato root tissue and was accompanied by an accumulation of high levels of furanoterpenoids. In contrast, when sweet potato root tissue pretreated with cycloheximide was inoculated with spores of the coffee strain, hyphal invasion proceeded into seven to eight cell layers, and accumulation of terpenoids and necrosis were low. Thus the coffee strain, naturally non-pathogenic to sweet potato, behaved as a pathogenic fungus on sweet potato tissue when terpenoid production was inhibited by cycloheximide.

These results strongly suggest that furanoterpenoid phytoalexins also are involved in establishment of host-parasite specificity between various strains of *C. fimbriata* and sweet potato.

In conclusion, we demonstrated the differential responses of various strains of *C. fimbriata* to the Ca^{2+} ion and furanoterpenoid phytoalexins in sweet potato and suggested that both factors constitute the specificity determining steps of this system. The specificity determining step by Ca^{2+} seems to be in the earlier stage of infection, since Ca^{2+} exists in sweet potato as its normal constituent and can interact with the fungus from the initial stage of infection. On the other hand, the specificity-determining step by furanoterpenoid phytoalexins seems to be in the later stage of interaction, since furanoterpenoid production occurs at this time.

SUMMARY

We studied the growth response of various strains of *C. fimbriata* to constituents of sweet potato root in terms of host-parasite specificity. The strains responded differentially to germination inductive factors in sweet potato water extract. The sweet potato, coffee, and cacao strains germinated well in the cation-free fraction (the unabsorbed fraction) of sweet potato extract which had been passed through a column of cation exchange resin. On the other hand, the prune, oak, taro, and almond strains required for germination such cations as Ca^{2+} and Mg^{2+} in addition to the unabsorbed fraction. These cations likely constitute one of the steps which determine the host-parasite specificity of this system.

The strains also showed a differential response to the furanoterpenoid phytoalexins in sweet potato. The sweet potato strain, pathogenic to sweet potato, was rather insensitive to furanoterpenoid toxicity, while other non-pathogenic strains were sensitive to it. The data on the production of furanoterpenoid in the infected tissues supported that the differential toxicity of furanoterpenoid are involved in the establishment of host-parasite specificity of this system.

REFERENCES

1. Allen, P. J. 1976. Spore germination and its regulation. *In*: R. Heitefuss and P. H. Williams (eds.). *Encyclopedia of Plant Physiology*. vol. 4. Springer-Verlag, Berlin, p. 51.
2. Allen, P. J. and L. D. Dunkle. 1971. Natural activators and inhibitors of spore germination. *In*: S. Akai and S. Ouchi (eds.). *Morphological and Biochemical Events in Plant-Parasite Interaction*. The Phytopathol. Soc. Japan, Tokyo, p. 23.
3. Barnett, H. L. and V. C. Lilly. 1947. The relation of thiamin to the production of perithecia by *Ceratostomella fimbriata*. *Mycologia* **39**: 699–708.
4. Condon, P. and J. Kuć. 1960. Isolation of a fungitoxic compound from carrot root tissue inoculated with *Ceratocystis fimbriata*. *Phytopathology* **50**: 267–270.
5. Cruickshank, I. A. M. 1962. Studies on phytoalexins. IV. The antimicrobial spectrum of pisatin. *Aust. J. Biol. Sci.* **15**: 147–159.
6. Cruickshank, I. A. M. and D. R. Perrin. 1971. Studies on phytoalexins. XI. The induction, antimicrobial spectrum and chemical assay of Phaseollin. *Phytopathol. Z.* **70**: 209–229.
7. Freedman, M. H., M. C. Raff, and B. D. Gomperts. 1975. Induction of increased calcium uptake in mouse T lymphocytes by concanavalin A and its modulation by cyclic nucleotides. *Nature* **255**: 378–382.
8. Hirata, K. 1971. Calcium in relation to the susceptibility of primary barley leaves to powdery mildew. *In*: S. Akai and S. Ouchi (eds.). *Morphological and Biochemical Events in Plant-Parasite Interaction*. The Phytopathol. Soc. Japan, Tokyo, p. 207.
9. Hiura, M. 1943. Studies in storage and rot of sweet potato (2). *Rep. Gifu Agric. Coll.* **50**: 1–5.
10. Hyodo, H., I. Uritani, and S. Akai. 1969. Production of furanoterpenoids and other compounds in sweet potato root tissue in response to infection by various isolates of *Ceratocystis fimbriata*. *Phytopathol. Z.* **65**: 332–340.
11. Ishizaka, N. and K. Tomiyama. 1972. Effect of wounding or infection by *Phytophthora infestans* on the contents of terpenoids in potato tubers. *Plant Cell Physiol.* **13**: 1053–1063.

12. Kato, N., H. Imaseki, N. Nakashima, and I. Uritani. 1971. Structure of a new sesquiterpenoid, ipomeamaronol, in deseased sweet potato root tissue. *Tetrahedron Lett.* **13**: 843–846.
13. Kubota, N. and T. Matsuura. 1953. Chemical studies on black rot desease of sweet potato (6). Structure of ipomeamarone. *J. Chem. Soc. Japan* **74**: 248–251.
14. Loewenstein, W. R. 1975. Cellular communication by permeable membrane junctions. *In*: G. Weissmann and R. Claiborne. (eds.). *Cell Membranes*. HP Publ. Co., Inc., New York, p. 105.
15. Macko, V., R. C. Staples, P. J. Allen, and J. A. A. Renwick. 1971. Identification of the germination self-inhibitor from wheat stem rust uredospores. *Science* **173**: 835–836.
16. McTeague, D. M., S. A. Hutchinson, and R. J. Reed. 1959. Spore germination in Agaricus campestris. *Nature* **183**: 1736.
17. Nonaka, F. and K. Yasui. 1966. On selective toxicity of ipomeamarone towards the phytopathogens. *Agric. Bull. Saga Univ.* **22**: 39–49.
18. Oguni, I. and I. Uritani. 1974. Dehydro-ipomeamarone from infected *Ipomoea batatas* root tissue. *Phytochemistry* **13**: 521–522.
19. Oku, H., S. Ouchi, T. Shiraishi, Y. Komoto, and K. Oti. 1975. Phytoalexin activity in barley powdery mildew. *Ann. Phytopathol. Soc. Japan* **41**: 185–191.
20. Page, W. J. and J. J. Stock. 1971. Regulation and self-inhibition of *Microsporum gypseum* macroconidia germination. *J. Bacteriol.* **108**: 276–281.
21. Rasmussen, H. 1975. Ions as 'second messenger.' *In*: G. Weissman and R. Claiborne. (eds.). *Cell Membranes*. HP Publ. Co., Inc., New York, p. 203.
22. Tanaka, Y., K. Yanagisawa, Y. Hashimoto, and M. Yamaguchi. 1974. True spore germination inhibitor of a cellular slime mold *Dictyostelium discoideum*. *Agric. Biol. Chem.* **38**: 689–690.
23. Tochinai, Y. and T. Nakano. 1940. Studies on the synthetic nutrient solution being suitable for the mycelial growth of *Piricularia oryzae* CAV. *Ann. Phytopathol. Soc. Japan* **10**: 110–118.
24. Van Etten, H. D. 1973. Differential sensitivity of fungi to pisatin and to phaseollin. *Phytopathology* **63**: 1477–1482.
25. Weaver, R. F., K. V. Rajagopalan, P. Handler, P. Jeffs, W. L. Hyrne, and D. Rosenthal. 1970. Isolation of v-L-glutamynyl-4-hydroxybenzene and γ-L-glutaminyl 3,4-benzoquinone: a natural sulfhydryl reagent, from sporulating gill tissue of the mushroom *Agaricus bisporus*. *Proc. Natl. Acad. Sci. U.S.* **67**: 1050–1056.

Discussion of Paper by Drs. Kojima et al.

In view of the variability in sensitivity of the incompatible strains of *C. fimbriata* to furanoterpenoid phytoalexins, YODER asked if compatible strains also varied in sensitivity. KOJIMA pointed out that their laboratory had a number of strains isolated from sweet potato but all were compatible and appear to have the same sensitivity. For this reason they tested their hypothesis with strains isolated from other hosts. TOMIYAMA mentioned how accumulation of furanoterpenoids in the inoculated surface was observed with *Phytophthora infestans* infections of white potato, where accumulation occurs at a distance from the surface. TOMIYAMA's concept of the white potato system is that synthesis of phytoalexins takes place at a distance and is transported to the surface. DALY asked if there was direct measurement of the transport since the concentrations at any location of phytoalexin may be steady state concentrations independent of movement. TOMIYAMA replied that some evidence with isotopes was available. KUĆ noted that even such data were open to question if only healthy tissue around lesion could degrade phytoalexin, because cells in the lesions were dead or dying. KUĆ also remembered an early published experiment by URITANI's group which showed that an incompatible isolate apparently protected sweet potato from compatible strains, but that very little furanoterpenoids were elicited. After removing the infected area the underlying tissue was still protected. URITANI responded that they had some evidence that in this situation the tissue apparently contained polyphenols and amino acids which acted together to inhibit the penetration, forming a physical barrier.

SUBJECT INDEX

Accessibility (susceptibility) 50
Actinomycin D, effect on infection establishment 57
ADP, effect on hypersensitivity reaction 74
Agglutinin (lectin)
  role in resistance 39
  sweet potato root 181
AK-toxin (toxin of *Alternaria kikuchiana*) 134
Allelic genes, incompatible relationship 7
Alternariol, monomethyl ether of 137
Alternariolide 137
AM-toxin (toxin of *Alternaria mali*) 134
Apple 131
ATP, effect on hypersensitivity reaction 74
ATPase, membrane-bound 175
Avirulence 7

Barley 319
Blasticidin S 275
  effect on development of hypersensitivity potential 72
  effect on infection establishment 57
Brassica oleracea L. *gongyloides* (Kohlrabi) 88

Calcium ion
  binding to victorin 201
  contents in spores 339
  effect on spore germination 338
  role in fungal physiology 339
  stimulation of K efflux by 141
Cell permeability, the relation with disease 193
Cell wall
  elasticity of 171
  extensibility of 171
  plasticity of 171
Cerato-ulmin
  effect on elms 149
  semi-pathotoxin of *Ceratocystis ulmi* 147
Chloroplasts, ultrastructural change in infected barley 56
Compatibility
  host parasite 211
  origin 219
  pistil-pollen 211
Coniferyl alcohol 101
Cordycepin 275
Coronatine (toxin produced by *Pseudomonas coronafaciens* var. *atropurpurea*) 167
  derivatives of 168
  effect on plasmolysis of Italian ryegrass 174
  effect on potato tuber 170
  effect on protoplasmic streaming 174
Coupling factor 1, a target of tentoxin 122
Cross-protection, virus disease 231
Crown gall tumor 289
Cutin, role in disease resistance 34
Cycloheximide, effect on infection establishment 57

Datura stramonium 241
Defense, coordinated 38
26-Desglucoavenacosid 282
Differential sensitivity

fungi to pisatin and phaseollin 305
parasite to phytoalexin 322
3,6a-Dihydroxy-8,9-methylenedioxy-pterocarpan 308
2,4-Dinitrophenol, effect on hypersensitivity reaction 74
Divalent cations, contents in sweet potato 338
Dominance, evaluation of 8

Elicitor
definition 153
phytoalexin 37
Phytophtora megasperma 155
pisatin production 326
Erwinia amylovora 199
Evolution, host-parasite relationships 11

Gladiolus gandavensis 219
Gene-for-gene hypothesis 20
Gene-for-gene theory 3, 212
postulates of 13
Genetics, host-parasite interaction 3
Germ-tube growth, inhibitor in sweet potato 181
Growth
fungus in the extract of diseased tissue 341
parasite 335
Guaiacylpropane unit, lignin 100

Heat treatment, barley leaf 57
Hordeum vulgare (barley) 88
Host response 91
Host-selective toxin, *Helminthosporium sacchari* 200
Host-specific toxin 133
role in determination of host-parasite specificity 320
Hybridization, DNA 291
p-Hydroxycinnamyl alcohol 101
la-Hydroxy phaseollone 308
Hypersensitivity reaction 69
cell death by 71
potential of 72
relation with electrolyte leakage 197
Hypertrophy 166

Incompatibility, interspecific in angiosperms 217
Incongruity, pistil-pollen interaction 220
Induced resistance 33
localized 237
systemic 237
Inducer
disease resistance 240
synonym of elicitor 154
Inductive factor, spore germination in sweet potato 337
Infection, spread of viral 260
Infectivity of pathogen 324
Interferon-like substance, *Datura stramonium* 241
Ipomeamarone
concentration in infected sweet potato 344
differential toxicity 343
site of accumulation 344
Isogenic line, barley 56
Italian ryegrass (*Lolium multiflorum* Lam.) 165

Japanese pear 134

Lectin, involvement in induced resistance 243
Lignin
diseased radish 101
induction of formation of 105
lignification-inducing factor 100
role in disease resistance 35

Localization, induced resistance and succeptibility 54

Magnesium ion, stimulation of K efflux by 141
Microautoradiography 277
Monilicolin A 155
Mutant
  auxotrophic 21
  resistance to fungicides 23
  temperature senistive 22
Mutation, pathogen 20

Nectria haematococca Berk. & Br. 310
Nicotiana 122, 262

Oat, infected by *Puccinia coronata avenae* 274
Octopine 290
Outgrowth, potato tuber 166
Oxidative phosphorylation, inhibition by pisatin 328

Papillae 85, 215
Pathogenicity 301
  definition 326
Pea 317
Penetration 85
Pepper 199
Peroxidase
  infected oat 281
  infected radish root 100
  resistance response 243
Phaseollin 301
Phenylalanine ammonia lyase
  infected oat 280
  radish root 102
Phytoalexin 153
  degradation of 38
  isoflavonoid 301
  potato 36
  production 336
  production in early phase of disease 318
  production in later phase of disease 319
  role in symptom development 199
  sweet potato 36
Phytotoxicity, pisatin and phaseollin 303
Pinto bean 244
Pisatin 301
  concentration in infected pea stem 321
Plasma membrane, perforation by haustorium 107
Plasmid, *Agrobacterium* 290
Populus alba 219
Populus deltoides 219
Potato (*Solanum tuberosum* L.) 71, 170
Primary defense action 181
Protein
  change in composition of infected oat 279
  synthesis in infected oat 276
Protoplast
  effect of pisatin on 327
  infection by virus 257
  potato 77
Puromycin 275

Quadratic check, host-parasite specificity 212

Raphanus sativus 99
Reaction body, pistils 215
Reassociation, DNA 291
Recognition
  genes for 59
  self- 214
Resistance 7, 153
  induced 20

induced and active in higher plants 301
mechanism 85
non-specific mechanism for 36
virus disease 264
Response, plant to virus infection 261
Rishitin, accumulation 71
RNA
synthesis in infected oat 276
translation of viral 258
m-RNA, synthesis in infected oat 277

S-alleles 212
Self-incompatibility
gametophytic 215
sporophytic 211
Self-recognition, pistil-pollen 214
Sodium azide (NaN_3), effect on hypersensitivity reaction 74
Specificity 153
determing factors in sweet potato-*Ceratocystis fimbriata* system 346
plant host-virus interaction 256
Specific recognition, an incompatible relationship 7
Spore germination, *Ceratocystis fimbriata* 336
Steroid glycoalkaloid 36
Sterol, diseased maize 198
Suberin, role in disease resistance 34
Suppression
gene for resistance 53
pisatin production 326
Suppressor gene 22
Susceptibility
induced 50
induced by heat 50
relation to phytoalexin theory 301
Sweet potato 337
Ipomoea batatas Lam. 182
Symptom
hypersensitive or local by virus 261
systemic by virus 261
Syringylpropane unit, lignin 100

Temperature sensitivity, genes controlling host-parasite interaction 9
Tentoxin
mode of action 122, 203
structure 137
Tenuazonic acid 137
Tolerance, fungi to phytoalexins 301
Tobacco mosaic virus 236, 259
Toxin
biochemical specificity of 117
biological specificity of 117
mathematical model for specificity of 118
specificity 115
Transmembrane potential
depolarization by victorin 194
infected potato 75
Trigger
incompatibility 217
self-recognition 217

Variability, naturally-occurring host-parasite interactions 7
Vector 255
Victorin, effect on cell permeability 194
Virulence 20
Virus
assembly of 260
inoculation of 255
replication of 259
uncoating of 258

Wall apposition 85
Wound healing 85
Wound plug 85
Wound response 35

LIST OF MICROORGANISMS

Agrobacterium tumefaciens 12, 23, 231, 289
Alternaria alternata 118
Alternaria alternata f. sp. *lycopersici* 134
Alternaria citri 135
Alternaria kikuchiana 134
Alternaria mali 134
Aphanomyces euteiches 38, 312

Ceratocystis fimbriata 36, 336
Ceratocystis fimbriata Ell. and Halst 182
Ceratocystis ulmi (Buism.) C. Moreau 147
Chlamydomonas 244
Colletotrichum lagenarium 40
Colletotrichum lindemuthianum 12, 156, 238
Corynebacterium insidiosum 235
Curvularia lunata 196

Erwinia amylovora 39, 157
Erwinia chrysanthemi 241
Erysiphe cichoracearum 218
Erysiphe graminis hordei 50, 88, 319, 326
Erysiphe graminis f. sp. *hordei* 339
Erysiphe graminis tritici 50

Fusarium solani 157
Fusarium solani (Mart.) Sacc. 302

Hansenula 244
Helminthosporium carbonum 139, 196
Helminthosporium maydis 195
Helminthosporium sacchari 200
Helminthosporium victoriae 139
Hypomyces solani f. sp. *cucurbitae* 197

Linum usitatissimum 8

Melanospora lini 8, 23
Microsporum gypserum 339
Monilina fructicola 155
Mycosphaerella pinodes 324

Olpidium brassicae 88
Olpidium viceae 86

Peronospora parasitica 99
Peronospora tabacina 236
Phaseolus vulgaris 195
Phytophthora infestans 36, 71, 232, 320, 336
Phytophthora megasperma var. *sojae* 155
Piricularia oryzae 27
Pseudomonas 23, 39, 197
Pseudomonas coronafaciens var. *atropurpurea* 165
Pseudomonas lachrymans 40
Pseudomonas solanacearum E.F. Sm 233
Pseudomonas tabaci 197
Puccinia coronata avenae 274
Puccinia graminis f. sp. *tritici* 9, 157
Puccinia hordei 25

Rhizopus stolonifer 157
Rhynchosporium secalis 196

Sclerotinia sclerotium 196
Sphaerotheca fuliginea 50
Stemphylium botryosum Wallr. 302

Thielaviopsis basicola 236
Triticum aestivum 9

Uromyces phaseoli var. *vignae* 86

Xanthomonas malvacearum 198
Xanthomonas vesicatoria 199